Tools of the Trade

Tools of the Trade
Medical Devices and Practice in Sweden and Denmark, 1855–1897

Kristin Halverson

Södertörns högskola

History of Ideas
Historical Studies
School of Historical and Contemporary Studies
Baltic and East European Graduate School

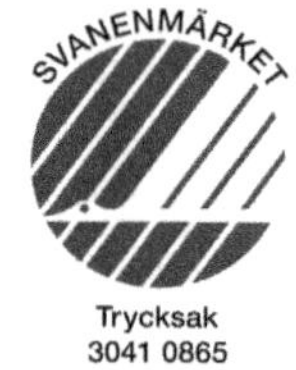

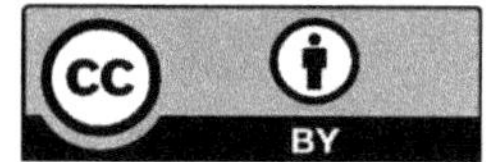

Södertörns högskola
(Södertörn University)
Library
SE-141 89 Huddinge

www.sh.se/publications

Cover image: from a photograph by Frederik Riise (1863–1933) of Danish surgeon
Oscar Wanscher (1846–1906). Dated 1888–1913. The photograph is available in the
Royal Library of Denmark's portrait collection. Det Kgl. Biblioteks bildesamling. Danske
portrætter. Wanscher, Oscar (1846–1906).
Graphic form: Per Lindblom & Jonathan Robson

Stockholm 2022

Södertörn Doctoral Dissertations 203
ISSN 1652–7399

ISBN 978-91-89504-03-5 (print)
ISBN 978-91-89504-04-2 (digital)

Abstract

Nineteenth-century medicine is characterised by rapid technological change, new methods of diagnostics and treatments of disease, far-reaching developments in medical science, and professionalisation. This has led to great interest in the period and a large body of scholarly and popular research. However, much of this scholarship studies British, German and French contexts. There is a pressing need to study how knowledge and practice were transferred between regions and how medical technologies were adapted locally.

In this study, I examine changes in medical practice in Sweden and Denmark by centring medical devices, as they were described and discussed in Swedish and Danish medical journals between 1855 and 1897. This is done by exploring the relationships between device, practice, and knowledge in four technological areas and how their use was explained in these journals. The four technological areas are lensed and mirrored instruments for examining the nose, throat, and eyes; orthopaedic treatment; antisepsis according to Joseph Lister; and asepsis. All four areas are well-researched internationally but entail a number of local particularities. These are significant in understanding local circumstances involved in their practical adoption.

The analysis of these areas illustrates that, despite the international exchange of medical knowledge, knowledge was not always translated into practice seamlessly, in particular when involving the use of devices. Because of this, many of the articles exploring these technologies were instructional and attuned to local conditions. Practice unfolded in different ways, accounting for local circumstances. This thesis highlights the importance of examining the proliferation of nineteenth-century medical technologies on the local level and in practice, in order to better understand the practical predicaments involved in their use.

Keywords: history of medicine, medical devices, nineteenth century medicine, medical technologies, Swedish history of medicine, Danish history of medicine.

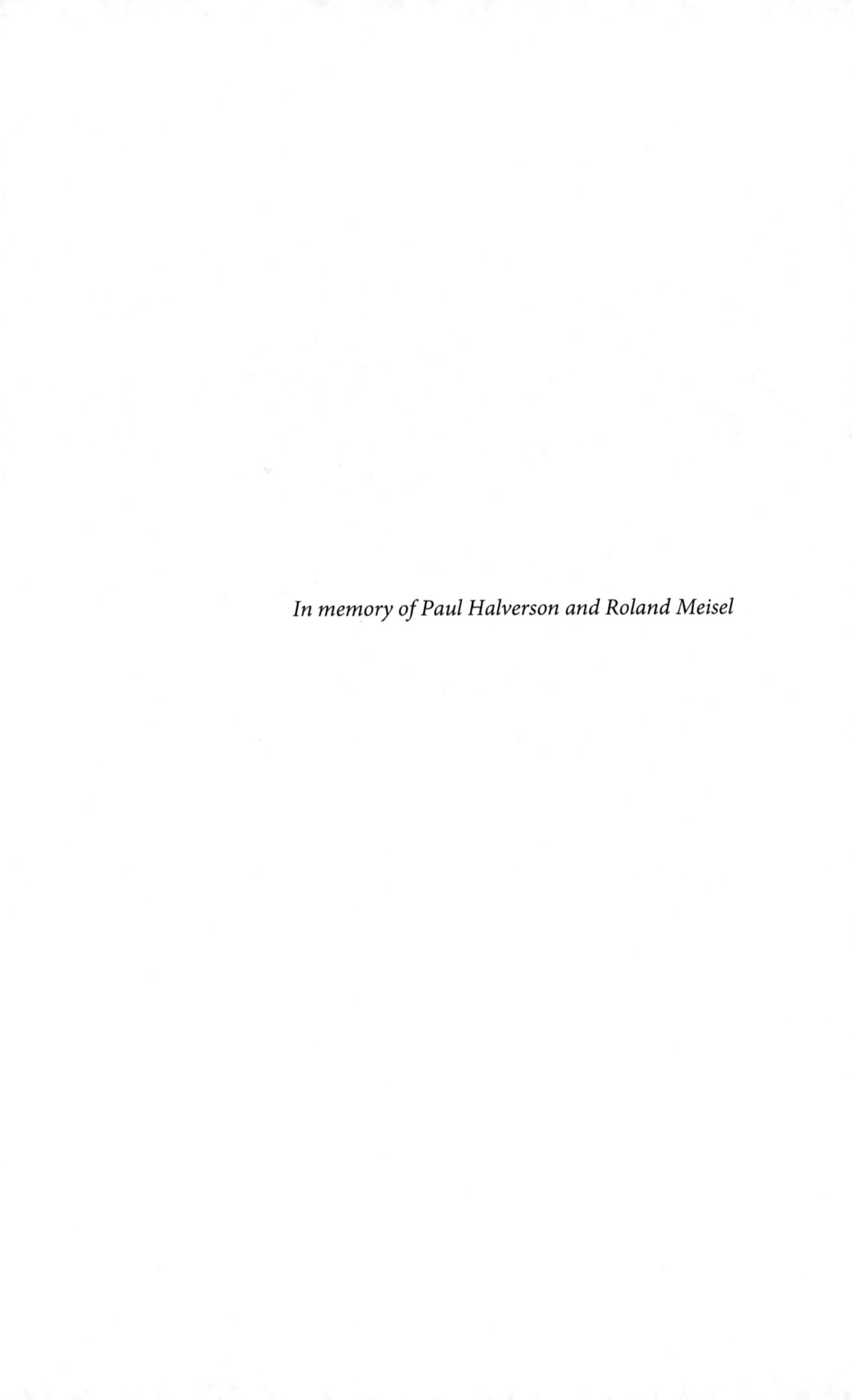

In memory of Paul Halverson and Roland Meisel

Contents

1. Introduction

There has been a long-standing research interest in the nineteenth century in the history of medicine: in scholarly studies, in popular histories, and by healthcare professionals interested in the history of their profession. The century's medical practice is characterised by rapid technological change, changes in disease diagnostics and treatment, developments in medical science, and professionalisation. Much of the interest lies in the relationships nineteenth-century medicine has with medicine we recognise today. William Bynum states for instance that the profession changed so significantly between 1850 and 1900 that medicine in 1900 is more recognisable to us today than medicine in 1790 was to practitioners in 1900.[1] However, the significant change over the course of the latter half of the nineteenth century has informed a somewhat linear portrait of the era. Furthermore, the prevailing attraction of nineteenth-century medicine has led to the establishment of grand narratives around these developments and their proliferation, in particular the influence of scientific developments on medical practice. None of these developments, whether technical, professional or scientific, occurred in a linear fashion. On the local level, some of the grand narratives might not be applicable at all. Changes may have taken shape differently and technologies may have been contested. There is a need to problematise these narratives by attending to and highlighting the importance of local practices, something that many researchers have already done.[2]

Another persisting problem in the history of medicine is the prevalence of research examining British, German and French phenomena. Extrapolating from British, German, and French circumstances might lead to drawing conclusions that in fact go against local developments. Even if many of the scientific and diagnostic changes were initiated in Britain, France, and German-speaking territories, there is still an urgency in examining how knowledge and practice were transferred between regions and how techniques and technologies in medicine were adapted locally and in practice. There are many studies that already tackle these issues and attempt to problematise these narratives. More recent scholarship points to local nuance, translation between different sites, and highlights the specific circumstances involved in the implementation of techniques and technologies

---

[1] William F. Bynum. *Science and the Practice of Medicine in the Nineteenth Century.* Cambridge: Cambridge University Press, 1994, xi–xiii; 222–226.

[2] Some of these studies will be discussed in my overview of previous research, see pg. 14ff.

in nineteenth-century medicine. These studies have underlined the significance of local practice and call the relevance of grand narratives into question. This is also my ambition with this thesis, and in the following chapters I will examine four technological developments in Sweden and Denmark more closely by examining their use in practice and by attending to their local circumstances.

In doing so, the initial point of reference in this study is medical devices and their relationships with practice and knowledge. Devices appear frequently in nineteenth-century Swedish and Danish medical journals. Sometimes they were presented as tools to solve practical problems. In other cases, they were noted as being modified or reconstructed to suit the needs of the practitioner. Sometimes practitioners had to work around them rather than with them, and be mindful of their sensitivity, weight, construction, or materials. And still, sometimes a new technology or practical method required devices to be modified, perhaps turning them into new or different devices. Swedish and Danish medical journals that cover the latter half of the nineteenth century are teeming with articles about treatment methods, diseases or case studies, and are rich sources of practical matters. Physicians were deeply concerned about modifying, correcting and instructing their techniques, especially those involving the use of instruments and other medical devices. And, although there was plenty of information, discussion, and explanation of new, scientific understandings of the body, its functions and illnesses, practical matters and clinical results were significant factors in the adoption and adaptation of techniques and technologies. This thesis is concerned with the interrelationships between device, practice, and knowledge and will study some of these stories more closely, in particular, the everyday technologies involved in examinations of the throat, nose, and eyes, wound management, and orthopaedics.

Contemporaries did not use the term "device", or any similar, general categorisation that is common now, like the World Health Organisation's, or more geographically specific, those from the Swedish Medical Products Agency [*medicintekniska produkter*] and the Danish Medicines Agency [*medicinsk udstyr*].[3] I define device as a mechanical product of labour applied

---

[3] See World Health Organization. *Medical devices: Medical Device–Full Definition.* 2019. http://www.who.int/medical_devices/full_deffinition/en/ (Accessed 18 November 2019); Swedish Medical Products Agency. *Medical Devices.* 9 July 2009. https://lakemedelsverket.se/english/product/Medical-devices/ (Accessed 14 January 2020); Danish Medicines Agency. *Medical devices.* 13 February 2019. https://laegemiddelstyrelsen.dk/en/devices (Accessed 14 January 2020). These are broad definitions that include things from bandages and disposable gloves to complicated, implantable devices.

professionally in medicine that was used to solve practical and/or technical problems or otherwise assist practice. I apply this term to a category of things that serve nineteenth-century medical practice, and this definition works from how devices manifest in my empirical material. Through this definition, devices were tools that served specific practical purposes for physicians. All definitions are exclusionary, including my own: by emphasising the mechanical nature of device, pharmaceuticals are excluded, and stressing on their professional application excludes healthcare products with wider practical application geared primarily toward laypeople, for example. Thus, my definition is not intended to be immutable, and device could be defined in other ways to include or exclude a broader range of products.

Purpose and Research Questions

Not just mere tools, medical devices can help shed light on changes in the practice of medicine. The purpose of this thesis is to examine changes in medical practice in Sweden and Denmark from 1855 to 1897 more closely by centring devices, as they were described, debated, and referred to in major medical journals in their respective countries: *Hygiea* in Sweden, and *Ugeskrift for Læger* and *Hospitals-Tidende* in Denmark. The periodisation of this thesis is not random, nor is this thesis comparative, and there is no overarching aim to juxtapose developments in either country against one another. The temporal logic is a conscious choice based on the fluid landscape of medical practice in these two countries and the technological change that took place during the latter half of the nineteenth century. In part, the involvement of makers of medical devices in medical practice and the development of knowledge has motivated this periodisation. Their unique roles will be clarified in greater detail later in this chapter. I will focus on four fields of innovation during this period: lensed instruments, orthopaedic devices, antisepsis, and asepsis. Based on this, I have formulated four primary research questions. These are:

They are articles of aide for a human being, serving some kind of support function, but not pharmaceutical products. This includes pacemakers to autoclaves and everything in between. The WHO further complicates things by stating that "products which may be considered to be medical devices in some jurisdictions but not others include: disinfection substances, aids for persons with disabilities, devices incorporating animal and/or human tissues, [and] devices for in-vitro fertilization or assisted reproduction technology". In other words, some of these items might be considered a medical device in one jurisdiction, but be excluded from this definition in another.

- In what ways do the relationships between instrument, practice, and knowledge manifest in nineteenth-century Swedish and Danish medical journals?
- What factors affected the use and proliferation of certain medical devices and technologies in the period?
- How were devices presented in relation to professional expectations and challenges?
- In what ways were devices enacted and entangled with the careers of their makers and users?

The choices I have made regarding specific areas of medical practice to study have been guided empirically. Through an initial, systematic inventory of three medical journals, *Hospitals-Tidende, Hygiea,* and *Ugeskrift for Læger,* I have identified four primary cases where devices played an important role; were discussed explicitly to such an extent they can be studied in relation to practice; and may be seen as either representative of, or important for, the development of medicine in these two Nordic countries. This has constituted four case studies, that are as follows: the introduction of new lensed and mirrored instruments in the 1850s and 1860s; Danish orthopaedic practice that came under debate locally in the 1870s and 1880s; antisepsis and the establishment of Listerism in the late 1860s and 1870s; and the advent of asepsis and the system of cleanliness that it introduced to surgical practices from the late 1880s to the early 1900s.

Previous Research

There is a wealth of Swedish and Danish research in the history of medicine, with Swedish researchers being particularly productive in the field. In 2007, Roger Qvarsell quantified general thematic trends in Swedish doctoral theses in the history of medicine written between 1970 and 2004. Outside of identifying prevailing research trends examining knowledge production and professionalisation, he encouraged research on clinical practices and studies that engage "healthcare's physical environments, therapeutic devices, and instruments".[4] Despite Qvarsell's encouragement, few studies since then have engaged with devices. This is true for Danish studies as well, that have

---

[4] Roger Qvarsell, "Historia och medicin–En studie av svenska medicinhistoriska avhandlingar 1970–2004", in *Medicinhistoria idag: Perspektiv på det samtida svenska forskningsfältet,* Eva Åhrén (ed.), 19–40, Stockholm: Nobel Museum Occasional Papers, 2007, 39. [sjukvårdens fysiska miljöer, behandlingsapparatur och instrument]

followed similar general trends. Still, these studies provide important background for my research.

The history of medicine in Sweden has been inspired by the prolific research in the critical history of medicine by the historian of ideas, Karin Johannisson. Her research has highlighted the social construction of illness and examined medicine through the lens of Foucauldian biopolitics.[5] Her work has had a far-reaching impact on the history of medicine in the country, and several Swedish researchers have followed in her footsteps and examined the history of medicine from a Foucauldian perspective grounded in power, sexuality, and/or subjectivity.[6] Studies like these have provided insight into the role of the patient and critically analysed the doctor/patient relationship in terms of power. They have given a critical perspective both on the role of medicine in society and relationships between medicine and social and structural factors. Other Swedish and Danish research has examined the question of professional development, including professionalisation, unlicensed practice, and legitimisation.[7] These studies have highlighted the discursive notions of legitimacy, the establishment of the physicians' authority, their relationships with unlicensed practitioners, and issues of gender. Illness, medical treatments, and cultural practices have also merited

---

[5] Just a few examples are Karin Johannisson. *Det mätbara samhället: statistik och samhällsdröm i 1700-talets Europa.* Stockholm: Nordstedts, 1988; Karin Johannisson. *Kroppens tunna skal: Sex essäer om kropp, historia and kultur.* Stockholm: Pan, 1997; Karin Johannisson, "Kliniken: medicinens praktik", in *Medicinen blir till vetenskap: Karolinska Institutet under två århundraden*, Karin Johannisson, Ingemar Nilsson and Roger Qvarsell (eds.), 43–83. Stockholm: Karolinska Institutet University Press, 2010

[6] Some examples are Mikael Eivergård. *Frihetens milda disciplin: Normalisering och social styrning i svensk sinnessjukvård 1850–1970.* Diss. Umeå University, 2003; Mikael Eivergård. "Frihet, makt och disciplin: om social styrning i svensk sinnessjukvård", in *Att rätt förfoga över tingen: Historiska studier av styrning och maktutövning*, Johannes Fredriksson and Esbjörn Larsson (eds.), 157–171, Uppsala: Opuscula historica Upsaliensia, 2007; Cecilia Riving. *Icke som en annan människa: Psykisk sjukdom i mötet mellan psykiatri och lokalsamhället under 1800-talets andra hälft.* Diss. Lund University, Gidlunds förlag, 2008; Annika Berg. *Den gränslösa hälsan: Signe och Axel Höjer, folkhälsan och expertisen.* Diss. Uppsala University, 2008. See also Roger Qvarsell's overview of Swedish doctoral theses in the history of medicine from 1970–2004. Qvarsell, "Historia och medicin".

[7] Signild Vallgårda. "'…Som et træ til sine grene…': specialisering af lægestanden fra slutningen af 1600-tallet til 1917", in *Historiens kultur, Fortælling, kritik, metode*, Ning de Coninck-Smith, et. al. (eds.), 81–96. Copenhagen: Museum Tusculanum, 1997; Motzi Eklöf. *Läkarens Ethos: Studier i den svenska läkarkårens identiteter, intressen och ideal, 1890–1960.* Diss. Tema Hälsa och samhälle, Linköping University, 2000; Nick Nyland. *De praktiserande læger I Danmark, 1800–1910: Træk af det historiske grundlag for almen medicin.* Odense: Audit Projekt Odense, 2000; Birgitte Rørbye. *Mellem sundhed og sygdom: Om fortid, fremskridt og virkelige læger. En narrativ kulturanalyse.* Charlottenlund: Museum Tusculanums Forlag, 2002; Ulrika Nilsson. *Kampen om Kvinnan: Professionalisering och konstruktioner av kön I svensk gynekologi 1860-1925.* Diss. Uppsala University, 2003; Sofia Ling. *Kärringmedicin och vetenskap: Läkare och kvacksalverianklagade I Sverige omkring 1770–1870.* Diss. Uppsala: Uppsala University, 2004.

attention from historians of medicine.[8] Work in this field has tended to engage questions of medical practice more directly than histories of professionalisation and legitimacy. Practice was but one of Qvarsell's recommendations to future historians of medicine. Even if they have looked closer at the everyday, these studies have paid little attention to medical devices and their relationship with practical concerns. They have not tackled the issues I deal with or engaged with a similar methodological approach by centring medical devices.[9] Others, that engage with medical devices more directly, have primarily in catalogued them.[10]

This has necessitated looking beyond Swedish and Danish research, which I will detail below, and outside the history of medicine. There are a few studies in the history of science, that examine instruments and/or their makers more directly and go beyond cataloguing to offer analytical insight. Gustav Holmberg and Johan Kärnfelt have examined instruments in the histories of astronomy and physics. These studies give better understanding of practice concerning instrument-use in Sweden and abroad.[11] Another example is Ove Amelin's doctoral thesis, which centres instrument maker Daniel Ekström. Amelin uses Ekström to explore the establishment of scientific instrument making in Sweden, and the trade's relationship with the development of

---

[8] Solveig Jülich. *Skuggor av sanning: Tidig svensk radiologi och visuell kultur.* Diss. Linköping University, 2002; Eva Åhrén. *Döden, kroppen och moderniteten.* Diss. Carlssons bokförlag, 2002; Annelie Drakman. *När kroppen slöt sig och blev fast: varför åderlåtning, miasmateori och klimatmedicin övergavs vid 1800-talets mitt.* Diss. Uppsala University, 2018; Elin Björk. *Att bota en prostata: Kastrering som behandlingsmetod för prostatahypertrofi 1893–1910.* Diss. Linköping University, 2019. Studies of medical and scientific architecture also fit in here. See Anders Åman. *Om den offentliga vården: Byggnader och verksamheter vid svenska vårdinstitutioner under 1800- och 1900-talen. En arkitekturhistorisk undersökning.* Stockholm: LiberFörlag, 1976; Hjördis Kristenson. *Vetenskapens byggnader under 1800-talet: Lund och Europa.* Stockholm: The Swedish Museum of Architecture, 1990.

[9] Both Solveig Jülich and Elin Björk engage with devices in their doctoral theses, albeit to a limited extent. Jülich's thesis does discuss roentgen machines and technology, but its primary focus is the introduction and reception of roentgen imagery in Sweden. This includes professional development in radiology as well as cultural practices around roentgen imagery. Björk relates instruments to surgical castration procedures as a treatment method for prostate hypertrophy, but this is only a cursory product of her study that centres knowledge production and the construction of the organ and its illness rather than devices. See for example Jülich, *Skuggor av sanning*, 188–192; Björk, *Att bota en prostata*, 72.

[10] Åke Meyerson. *Studier i Serafimerlasarettets instrumentsamling: Utgivna med anledning av lasarettets 200-årsjubileum.* Stockholm: Karolinska Institute's Surgical Clinic at Seraphim Hospital, 1952; Bo Lindberg. *Obstetriska instrument: en historia om gamla förlossningsinstrument i Medicinhistoriska museet i Uppsala.* Uppsala: Acta Universitatis Upsaliensis, 2020.

[11] See Johan Kärnfelt, "Vetenskapsakademiens Herschel-teleskop: En instrumentbiografi". *Slagmark.* Vol. 81, 2020, 133–154; Johan Kärnfelt, "Ett misslyckat stativ", in *Kunskap i rörelse: Kungl. Vetenskapsakademien och skapandet af det moderna samhället,* Johan Kärnfelt, Karl Grandin and Solveig Jülich (eds.), 475–481. Stockholm: Makadam, 2018. Klaus Staubermann, et. al., "Intangible Heritage: Connecting Astronomical Telescopes and Their Users". *Journal of Astronomical History and Heritage.* Vol. 24, No. 3, September 2021, 776–788.

scientific research in the country. He acknowledges the cataloguing nature of some previous research as a means of establishing a general understanding and an overview of collections and calls for more analytical research looking at scientific instruments in the future.[12] In this sense, device studies in medicine like my own are indebted to the thorough work of both catalogues and the research in the history of medicine outlined above.

There are particularities to the Swedish and Danish contexts that are important to keep in mind. Some of these involve practical medical concerns, such as the geographically specific understandings of orthopaedics and the proliferation of Listerism. However, others are more mundane, like lighting conditions during the winter months. Given the wealth of English-language research on medical devices, a closer look at these questions in the Swedish and Danish contexts is of merit. One of the prevailing problems with the dominance of English-language historical research situated largely in British, and to a lesser but still significant degree, German and French, contexts is that they risk overshadowing local specificity elsewhere. This is a problem I intend to overcome and my research positions itself alongside studies engaging medical devices more broadly, but with geographic distinction in mind.

Scientific Non-Universality?

In the concluding chapter of the anthology *Devices and Designs: Medical Technologies in Historical Perspective,* Stuart Blume poses the epistemological question of whether or not it might be possible to rethink medical practice as scientific, without being committed to universality.[13] To illustrate his point, he uses several examples of how different conclusions were drawn about the utility of medical technologies in different countries, in spite of having access to the same body of scientific results. In other words, questions of local specificity are important in the examination and proliferation of medical practices. Blume's perspective is a contemporary one; however, the relationship between local specificity and medical practice is important. In terms of historical scholarship, Frank Huisman argues that the well-funded British research infrastructure in the history of medicine has led to an imbalance, and that researchers examining other historical contexts need to highlight local histories rather than fall into the patterns developed in British and

---

[12] Ove Amelin. *Medaljens baksida: Instrumentmakaren Daniel Ekström och hans efterföljare i 1700-talets Sverige.* Diss. Uppsala University, 1999, 21.

[13] Stuart Blume, "The Politics of Endpoints", in *Devices and Designs: Medical Technologies in Historical Perspective,* Carsten Timmermann and Julie Anderson (eds.), 249–272. Basingstoke: Palgrave Macmillan, 2006, 269.

American contexts.[14] I would also include contexts from France and German-speaking regions in the asymmetrical situation that Huisman identifies. Historians examining other regions need to be mindful of this and avoid using research from these regions as universal explanations. Much like Annemarie Mol states in the introduction to *The Body Multiple: Ontology in Medical Practice,* focusing on a specific site shifts "philosophy away from formats that carry universalistic pretentions, but that in fact hide the locality to which they pertain".[15]

Books and anthologies in the history of medicine sometimes contain tidy disclaimers about the dominance of research studying British, North American, French, or German-speaking contexts, only to limit themselves to those contexts.[16] Thomas Schlich states in the introductory chapter in the anthology *The Palgrave Handbook of the History of Surgery* that the over-representation in the anthology is in part because "much of the dynamism in late modern surgery originates in these regions".[17] Even if we acknowledge Schlich's statement to be true, only part of medicine's, or surgery's, dynamism is featured in origin stories. What of dissemination and local adaptation? If anything, these might be stronger indicators of dynamism than origin stories are because they imply further activity. Several historians have more recently engaged with these questions, like Pratik Chakrabarti's study of the complex establishment of bacteriology in colonial India.[18] Chakrabarti's study, and

[14] Frank Huisman, "Transcending the Language Barrier: Medical History in a Globalizing World". *European Journal for the History of Medicine and Health.* Vol. 78, 2021, 15–20, 18–19. Huisman's point about British and American dominance is apt; however, he notes that continental European researchers should "decolonise their minds" (19) and uses decolonisation as a metaphor to encourage a wider range of historical narratives of European medicine that are context specific. To suggest that the continental European history of medicine has been colonised and might require decolonisation is a poor choice of terminology, and the metaphorical use of decolonisation is appropriative and can be weaponised to absolve guilt and complicity, as Eve Tuck and K. Wayne Yang highlight. Tuck and Yang note that "decolonization as a metaphor… turns decolonization into an empty signifier to be filled by any track towards liberation" (7). And surely, arguing for a more multifaceted history of *European* medicine is hardly truly a liberatory project in the first place, which makes the term even less meaningful in this case. See Eve Tuck and K. Wayne Yang, "Decolonization is not a metaphor". *Decolonization: Indigeneity, Education & Society.* Vol. 1, No. 1, 2012, 1–40.

[15] Annemarie Mol. *The Body Multiple: Ontology in Medical Practice.* Durham, NC: Duke University Press, 2003, viii.

[16] Some examples are Bynum, *Science and the Practice of Medicine,* xiii; Lorraine Daston and Peter Galison. *Objectivity.* New York: Zone Books, 2010, 47; Thomas Schlich, "Introduction: What Is Special About the History of Surgery", in *The Palgrave Handbook of the History of Surgery,* Thomas Schlich (ed.), 1–24. London: Palgrave Macmillan, 2018, 3.

[17] Schlich, "Introduction", 3.

[18] Pratik Chakrabarti. *Bacteriology in British India: Laboratory Medicine and the Tropics.* Rochester: Boydell & Brewer, 2012. Other examples are Ellen J. Amster. *Medicine and the Saints: Science, Islam and*

others like it, illustrate that the transfer of medical knowledge was dependent on locally specific conditions and adapted within context-specific networks.[19] As Sarah Hodges argues, the history of medicine's reliance on epistemic unity has made investigating local specificity difficult and "the global" often reproduces narratives of universality without critically engaging with these narratives.[20] Therefore, it is important that historians avoid using "the global" as a universal signifier.

As Schlich himself has shown in his studies of Listerism in German-speaking territories, an important part of these histories is how practices and technologies were adapted, or not, outside of their origins.[21] Location-based differences challenge previous assumptions in the history of medicine, making it important to underline the significance of place in the history of nineteenth-century medicine. There is a wealth of English-language histories of science, technology, and medicine that provide historical, scholarly overviews of phenomena like objectivity, Listerism, and medical science, to name a few.[22] However, many of these overviews are framed from British, German, and French perspectives, and many of them still engage in origin stories. There is a risk using these histories to speak for other, locally specific developments outside of their linguistic and geographic spheres, even if their

the Colonial Encounter in Morocco, 1877–1956. Austin: University of Texas Press, 2013; Projit Bihari Mukharji. *Doctoring Traditions: Ayurveda, Small Technologies, and Braided Sciences*. Chicago: The University of Chicago Press, 2016. See also Jennifer Johnson, "New Directions in the History of Medicine in European, Colonial and Transimperial Contexts". *Contemporary European History*. Vol. 25, No. 2, May 2016, 387–399.

[19] One example is Projit Bihari Mukharji's book *Doctoring Tradition* and how the adoption and adaptation of small devices such as thermometers and pocket watches lead to the reimagining of the body in Ayurvedic practice, in relation to and compatible with the biomedical body. Part of Mukharji's premise about how the body is reimaged in Ayurveda is developed through Annemarie Mol's notion of how the body is enacted through knowing. See for example his point on the difficulties of translating colour-based urinalysis to Bengali contexts that lexically lacked concepts for certain colours used, which lead to new ways of enacting the body for Ayurvedic doctors. Mukharji, *Doctoring Traditions*, 166–167.

[20] Sarah Hodges, "The Global Menace". *Social History of Medicine*. Vo. 25, No. 3, August 2012, 719–728, 720–722.

[21] Thomas Schlich, "Farmer to Industrialist: Lister's Antisepsis and the Making of Modern Surgery in Germany". *The Royal Society Journal of the History of Science*. Vol. 67, No. 3, September 2013, 245–260; Thomas Schlich. "Negotiating Technologies in Surgery: The Controversy about Surgical Gloves in the 1890s". *Bulletin of the History of Medicine*. Vol. 87, No. 2, Summer 2013, 170–197.

[22] For example: Daston and Galison, *Objectivity*; Bynum, *Science and the Practice of Medicine*; Michael Worboys, "Joseph Lister and the Performance of Antiseptic Surgery". *Notes and Records of The Royal Society*. Vol. 67, No. 3, September 2013, 199–209; Michael Worboys, "The History of Surgical Wound Infection: Revolution or Evolution", in *The Palgrave Handbook of the History of Surgery*, Thomas Schlich (ed.), 215–233. London: Palgrave Macmillan, 2018; Michael Worboys. *Spreading Germs: Disease Theories and Medical Practice in Britain, 1865–1900*. Cambridge: Cambridge University Press, 2000; John Pickstone. *Ways of Knowing: A New History of Science, Technology and Medicine*. Chicago: The University of Chicago Press, 2001.

authors are mindful of their limitations. Acknowledgement of the short-comings of the prevailing fixation on specific dominant narratives is clearly not enough to overcome them. This is not to say that locally specific contexts might always be significantly divergent from these broad brushstrokes. In the nineteenth century, the already-international network of exchange, propensity to travel and visit colleagues elsewhere, and a broad language proficiency of those who helped shape the fabric of local scientific and medical communities would have given practitioners similar points of reference. However, this is difficult to ascertain without deeper, local scrutiny of knowledge, its transfer and application. They might have needed to be adapted and translated to work in locally specific circumstances.

Studying local specificity does not entail an outright rejection of previous research. The nineteenth-century medical community was international. Literature from elsewhere figured prominently in Swedish and Danish medical journals. I will rely on the research Michael Worboys and William Bynum to scrutinise the general scientific developments in medicine during the period and discuss advances such as bacteriology, cellular pathology, and wound care. Here, it is important to return to the point about universality. Bynum, for example, acknowledges the limitations of his book *Science and the Practice of Medicine in the Nineteenth Century*, noting that even its Eurocentric underpinnings are Anglocentric, at least in part because broadening its scope would take him beyond his area of expertise.[23] However, Swedish and Danish journals reported on and discussed much of the science that Bynum includes in his book. This underscores the reach and importance of work by British, American, French, and German scientists and physicians even in Sweden and Denmark. Still, it necessitates that historians competent in the regions beyond the rather small "Europe" Bynum presents attend to local specificity.[24] Rather than understanding these developments as uniformly disseminated, they serve as a means to understand local specificity, as these developments relate to the use of medical devices. With the above in mind, my research is contextualised through the well-established field of

---

[23] Bynum, *Science and the Practice of Medicine*, xiii.

[24] Many have done this; however, few of these studies are in English. See for example Drakman, *När kroppen slöt sig*; Eklöf, *Läkarens Ethos*; Jülich, *Skuggor av sanning*; Nilsson, *Kampen om Kvinnan*; Nyland, *De praktiserande læger*; Schlich, "Farmer to Industrialist"; Vallgårda, "'...Som et træ til sine grene...'"; Signild Vallgårda, "Who Went to a General Hospital in the Eighteenth and Nineteenth Centuries in Copenhagen?". *European Journal of Public Health*, Vol. 9, No. 2, June 1999, 97–102; Ulrika Graninger. *Från osynligt till synligt: Bakteriologins etablering i sekelskiftets svenska medicin*. Diss. Linköping University, 1997.

Swedish and Danish history of medicine but aligned with research trends outside of Sweden and Denmark.

Practices, Devices, and Relationships

There is a wealth of research examining medical, scientific, and technological instruments, in particular within the settings outlined above. For instance, the History of Science Society's publications, the yearly edited volume *Osiris* and the scientific journal *Isis*, have had special issues dedicated to instruments.[25] Instruments have been studied in relation to knowledge production, commodification, as curatorial objects, and more.[26] The histories of instruments have also attracted widespread attention from within medicine, with many specialist journals publishing articles about the "history" of a specific device and/or category of instrument.[27] Rather than survey a field of instrument-related studies, I will outline studies that look more closely at the entanglements of devices and instruments with knowledge production, in particular tacit knowledge, commodity, and professional relationships. This section will therefore both try to place my work amongst a specific device and practice-related discourse, and highlight research that has had particular relevance to this thesis.

---

[25] Albert van Helden and Thomas L. Hankins (eds.). *Instruments*. Chicago: The University of Chicago Press, 1994; Bernard V. Lightman (ed.). *Isis*. Vol. 102, No. 4, December 2011.

[26] For medical instruments, see for example Audrey B. Davis, "Historical Studies of Medical Instruments". *History of Science*. Vol. 16, No. 2, June 1978, 107–133; Claire L. Jones, "Surgical Instruments: History and Historiography", in *The Palgrave Handbook of the History of Surgery*, Thomas Schlich (ed.), 235–257. London: Palgrave Macmillan, 2018. For engaging with instrument collections at museums see for example Ken Arnold and Thomas Söderqvist, "Medical Instruments in Museums: Immediate Impressions and Historical Meanings". *Isis*. Vol. 102, No. 4, December 2011: 718–729; Karin Tybjer, "Sharp and Telling: Surgical Collections as Instruments of Medicine, History and Culture". *Journal of the History of Collections*. Vol. 31, No. 3, November 2019, 547–562. For scientific instruments see for example Mario Biagioli, "From Print to Patents: Living on Instruments in Early Modern Europe". *History of Science*. Vol. 44, No. 2, June 2006, 139–186; Samuel J. M. M. Alberti, "Shaping Scientific Instrument Collections: A Historiography". *Journal of the History of Collections*. Vol. 31, No. 3, November 2019, 445–452. Alberti's and Tybjer's articles appear in a special issue of the Journal of the History of Collections that deals specifically with scientific instrument collections.

[27] See for example Diana K. Bowen, et. al., "Sounds and Charrière: The Rest of the Story". *Journal of Pediatric Urology*. Vol 10, 2014, 1106-1110; H. Feldmann, "Der Nasenrachenraum und die Rachenmandel in der Geschichte der Otologie und Rhinologie". *Laryngorhinootologie*. Vol. 78, No. 5, 1999, 280–289; James M. Edmonson, "History of the Instruments for Gastrointestinal Endoscopy". *Gastrointestinal Endoscopy*. Vol. 37, No. 2, March 1991, S27–S56; J. Kirkup. *The Evolution of Surgical Instruments: An Illustrated History from Ancient Times to the Twentieth Century*. Novato, CA: Norman Publishing, 2006. Kirkup has written a series of articles on the histories of medical instruments for the *Annals of the Royal College of Surgeons of England*. In addition to this, he has authored over twenty articles about specific medical instruments.

Part of this task will be in situating my study within the field of the history of science, technology, and medicine, rather than just the history of medicine. In his book *Ways of Knowing*, John Pickstone encourages the drawing together of the histories of science, technology, and medicine, because the terms left to themselves lack precision and often overlap with one another. Medicine could include any number of things, from practices to understandings of the body and its physiology to technologies.[28] A study centring medical devices would be a difficult task without looking at research that has developed in these three, distinct chronologies. As such, the research described below encompasses the histories of science, technology, and medicine and falls in line with Pickstone's more generous demarcation, but also includes studies that approach the relationships between medicine, innovation, and commerce.

The history of surgery is one such field, where the demarcations between medicine, science, and technology are flexible. Although this thesis examines more than just surgical practice, the very nature of surgery as a hands-on practice that necessitates devices makes it a fruitful area of study for the purposes of my thesis.[29] Many historians have highlighted the growing inter-relationships between nineteenth-century surgery and science.[30] Thomas Schlich repeatedly underlines that surgery itself can be understood as a technology: it is an activity; it involves tools; and it requires the application of tools and techniques.[31] Furthermore, the technical proliferation of both

---

[28] Pickstone, *Ways of Knowing*, 6.

[29] For more on surgical instruments and their relation to the nature of surgical practice see Jones, "Surgical Instruments".

[30] Gert H. Brieger, "From Conservative to Radical Surgery in Late Nineteenth-Century America", in *Medical Theory, Surgical Practice*, Christopher Lawrence (ed.), 216–231. London: Routledge, 1992; Thomas Schlich. *Surgery, Science and Industry: A Revolution in Fracture Care*. Basingstoke: Palgrave MacMillan, 2002; Thomas Schlich, "Surgery, Science and Modernity: Operating Rooms and Laboratories as Spaces of Control". *History of Science*. Vol. 45, No. 3, September 2007, 231–256; Thomas Schlich, "Asepsis and Bacteriology: A Realignment of Surgery and Laboratory Science". *Medical History*. Vol. 56, No. 3, 2012, 308–334; Owen H. Wangensteen. *The Rise of Surgery: From Empiric Craft to Scientific Discipline*. Minneapolis: University of Minnesota Press, 1978. For surgery and science in nineteenth-century gynaecology see Nilsson, *Kampen om Kvinnan*.
For relationships between medicine and science more broadly see Bynum. *Science and the Practice of Medicine*; Ingemar Nilsson, "Vetenskapen: medicinens teori", in *Medicinen blir till vetenskap: Karolinska Institutet under två århundraden*, Karin Johannisson, Ingemar Nilsson and Roger Qvarsell (eds.), 13–41. Stockholm: Karolinska Institutet University Press, 2010.

[31] Thomas Schlich and Christopher Crenner, "Technological Change in Surgery: An Introduction Essay", in *Technological Change in Modern Surgery: Historical Perspectives on Innovation*, Thomas Schlich and Christopher Crenner (eds.), 1–20. Rochester: University of Rochester Press, 2017, 1; Schlich, "Introduction", 7.

device and practice has been a topic of interest for historians of surgery.[32] Studies that examine technical innovations in medicine and their consequences for the practice over the past two hundred years offer some insight into how medicine has been transformed, professionally, practically, and politically.

Schlich's book *Surgery, Science and Industry: A Revolution in Fracture care, 1950s–1990s* examines the discipline of traumatology in medicine, primarily focusing on the development of fracture care by the *Arbeitsgemeinschaft für Osteosynthesefragen* (henceforth the AO) in the post-war period. In Schlich's study, the transfer of knowledge between sites is important, as the AO enlisted monitoring techniques for surgeons applying the method but also enlisted surgeons as collaborative parts of a network where cooperation was key to build trust.[33] Schlich's study follows how an organisation established standards and routines in the circulation of its technology, including developing its own instruments and monitoring surgeons trained in the method. Another study focused on the diffusion of technique is Sally Frampton's, on ovarian surgery in the nineteenth century. Frampton highlights the non-linearity of innovation and tactics used by surgical innovators to communicate new surgical techniques. She notes in particular that innovation in surgery was already contested in the nineteenth century because it could introduce instability in practice. Furthermore, she notes that problems arose with standardising practices that were so dependent on individual performance, because practitioners often had their own techniques and adaptations.[34]

The history of surgery is not the only sub-field of the history of medicine that studies technology, innovation, and practice. Two studies by John Pickstone and Jonathan Reinarz offer other examples of the interconnections between innovation and their practical implications. Both examine questions of labour, looking at manufacturers and professions in light of the dissemination of specific technologies in medical practice. Pickstone's study of bonesetters in Lancashire, England examines the changing forms of work from bonesetters to the production of orthopaedic prostheses: a history that stretches over two hundred years. Most relevant are the shifts from the

---

[32] See also Julie Anderson, et. al. *Surgeons Manufacturers and Patients: A Transatlantic History of Total Hip Replacement.* Basingstoke: Palgrave Macmillan, 2007.

[33] Schlich, *Surgery, Science and Industry*, 242.

[34] Sally Frampton, "Defining Difference: Competing Forms of Ovarian Surgery in the Nineteenth Century", in *Technological Change in Modern Surgery: Historical Perspectives on Innovation*, Thomas Schlich and Christopher Crenner (eds.), 51–70. Rochester: University of Rochester Press, 2017, 65.

ancillary profession of bonesetting, largely a family affair in orthopaedics passed down through generations. This profession eventually became the domain of physicians toward the late nineteenth century.[35] Jonathan Reinarz examines the acquisition and use of medical innovations in voluntary hospitals in Birmingham. Here, he urges historians to move away from linear explanations of technological diffusion in medicine.[36] While both studies are relevant, the structure of public healthcare operated differently in Sweden and Denmark than English charity hospitals. This means that the links between innovation and technological diffusion play out differently in my study.

Technology and innovation also interconnect with the development of certain sensuous faculties amongst physicians. It was not merely a matter of implementing a given technology or using a specific device: they came with tacit and perceptive challenges. Richard Kremer and Henning Schmidgen have studied the cultivation of visual perception amongst physiologists in German-speaking regions. They both underscore the importance of sense perception and the development of physiology, where experiential tasks that helped develop the visual perception of physiology students were intertwined with the expansion of physiology.[37] Part of this development was infrastructural, as Kremer highlights, where the construction of new facilities was a significant factor in the discipline's growth. Though I do not study physiology in particular, the infrastructural development was also important for the expansion of surgical practice in the two countries I do study. Here, previous research by Jeanne Kisacky on hospital architecture and the diffusion of asepsis has been important.[38] To properly implement asepsis–a germ-free environment–institutional infrastructure and environments also had to

---

[35] John V. Pickstone, "Bones in Lancashire: Towards Long-term Contextual Analysis of Medical Technology", in *Devices and Designs: Medical Technologies in Historical Perspective*, Carsten Timmermann and Julie Anderson (eds.), 17–36. Basingstoke: Palgrave Macmillan, 2006, 21–22.

[36] Jonathan Reinarz, "Mechanizing Medicine: Medical Innovations and the Birmingham Voluntary Hospitals in the Nineteenth Century", in *Devices and Designs: Medical Technologies in Historical Perspective*, Carsten Timmermann and Julie Anderson (eds.), 37–60. Basingstoke: Palgrave Macmillan, 2006, 39.

[37] Richard L. Kremer, "Building Institutes for Physiology in Prussia, 1836–1846: Contexts, Interests and Rhetoric", in *The Laboratory Revolution in Medicine*. Andrew Cunningham and Perry Williams (eds.), 72–109. Cambridge: Cambridge University Press, 2002; Henning Schmidgen, "Pictures, Preparations, and Living Processes: The Production of Immediate Visual Perception (Anschauung) in Late-19th-Century Physiology". *Journal of the History of Biology*. Vol. 37, No. 3, Autumn 2004, 477–513.

[38] Jeanne Kisacky, "Germs are in the Details: Aseptic Design and General Contractors at the Lying-In Hospital in the City of New York, 1897–1901". *Construction History*. Vol. 28, No. 1, 2013, 83–106; Jeanne Kisacky. *Rise of the Modern Hospital: An Architectural History of Health and Healing, 1870–1940*. Pittsburgh: University of Pittsburgh Press, 2017.

change, which highlights the significance of environment and its effect on practice.

Practice and device were also affected by theoretical developments in medicine, in particular the better understanding of disease aetiology and developments in wound care. Research examining the development of antiseptic and aseptic methods of wound care and surgery is also important. Ulrika Graninger's doctoral thesis studying the establishment of bacteriology in the nineteenth and turn of the twentieth century in Sweden is one example.[39] However, because of my aims, I want to get closer to practical concerns, and Graninger focuses primarily on bacteriology's theoretical positioning. In this case, the works of Michael Worboys, and yet again, Thomas Schlich, have been significant. Michael Worboy's seminal book *Spreading Germs: Disease Theories and Medical Practice in Britain, 1865–1900* examines the circulation and establishment of germ theories in nineteenth-century Britain, highlighting the multitude of different theories behind disease and infection in circulation in the nineteenth century. He has also studied the performance of Joseph Lister's method of antiseptic wound care, Listerism, and how it was communicated through text.[40] In four articles, Schlich attends to practical matters of nineteenth-century surgery and the implementation of antisepsis and asepsis where he illustrates uncertainty and incomplete diffusion of these technologies.[41] Their relevance to my study is dictated by their attention to practical concerns, and I intend on using this focus to examine how the diffusion of these methods of disinfection played out in the situations that I study.

Although I argue that the three surgical instrument makers that are important for this thesis are more than just commercial actors, it is still impossible to divorce them from their businesses, which were naturally commercially oriented. This, however, does not negate their other interests in medicine. Importantly, there have been a growing number of historians of medicine that have cautioned against and challenged the notion of a stark distinction between medicine on the one hand, and commerce on the other.[42]

---

[39] Graninger, *Från osynligt till synligt.*

[40] Michael Worboys, "Joseph Lister and the Performance of Antiseptic Surgery". *Notes and Records of The Royal Society.* Vol. 67, No. 3, September 2013, 199–209.

[41] Schlich, "Asepsis and Bacteriology"; Schlich, "Farmer to Industrialist"; Schlich, "Negotiating Technologies in Surgery"; Schlich, "Surgery, Science and Modernity".

[42] See Claire Jones, "A Barrier to Medical Treatment? British Medical Practitioners, Medical Appliances and the Patent Controversy, 1870–1920". *British Journal for the History of Science*, Vol. 49, No. 4, December 2016, 601–625; Joseph M. Gabriel, *Medical Monopoly: Intellectual Property Rights and the*

Rather, commercial influences have always been present in modern medicine. Takahiro Ueyama's book, *Health in the Marketplace: Professionalism, Therapeutic Desires, and Medical Commodification in Late-Victorian London,* studies the entanglements between physicians and medical marketers in nineteenth-century Britain. He points out the necessity of looking at nineteenth-century medicine within the frame of growing commodity culture and its role in increased commercialisation of medicine and its services.[43] This valuable work by Ueyama illustrates that commerce and medicine were not always contentious or at odds in the British case. Given the participation of surgical instrument makers in medical settings and this thesis' focus on device, some consideration of commercial questions is merited in my cases.

An additional, important aspect is the role of interpersonal relationships. Actors with commercial interests, such as device makers, formed and kept relationships with medical practitioners, and these relationships were of mutual importance. On the one hand, instrument makers actively sought to establish contact with physicians, the profession that was at the time, most responsible for purchasing their products. On the other hand, physicians benefitted from forming relationships with people who could make, modify, and repair the tools of their trade. Schlich highlights this in *Surgery, Science and Industry* as well, showing that the development of a reliable toolkit with an engineer was an important part of the method's development, and instruments and other devices could be designed according to need and specification.[44] In a study by Claire Jones, *The Medical Trade Catalogue in Britain, 1870–1914,* she notes that decisions to purchase medical instruments and devices could often be network-based. Interpersonal relationships were more important than catalogue materials.[45] The importance of these relationships is clear in both the Swedish and Danish contexts. At the same time, the pool of both surgical instrument makers and physicians was much smaller. This means that craftsmen involved specifically in surgical instrument making might have had a broader customer base in these two countries, and that

---

Origins of the Modern Pharmaceutical Industry. Chicago: The University of Chicago Press, 2014. Jones' article is from the December 2016 thematic issue of the British Journal of the History of Science on Anglo-American medicine and patent cultures.

[43] Takahiro Ueyama. *Health in the Marketplace: Professionalism, Therapeutic Desires, and Medical Commodification in Late-Victorian London.* Palo Alto: Society for the Promotion of Science and Scholarship, 2010, 283.

[44] Schlich, *Surgery, Science and Industry,* 49.

[45] Claire L. Jones. *The Medical Trade Catalogue in Britain: 1870–1914.* London: Pickering & Chatto, 2013, 21.

physicians located in the countryside would have likely also had to turn to local metalworkers and a second-hand market for medical instruments.[46]

The role location plays in the following chapters is fundamental in placing this narrative in relation to the studies outlined above. I have used Danish and Swedish studies in the history of medicine to help tackle this in my own study, and my ambition is to unite this area of research with studies of medical devices, innovation, and practices more broadly. The point is to understand the relationships devices had with knowledge and practice in nineteenth-century Swedish and Danish medicine in association with the larger developments in medicine, science, and technology, but through a locally specific lens. My hope then is to contribute to greater sophistication in the historical narrative of nineteenth-century European medicine. This is also an argument for why this thesis is written in English rather than a Scandinavian language.

Empirical Material

One of the points I want to underline in this thesis is that medical journals can be rich sources of information beyond theory. Articles in the primary Swedish and Danish medical journals examined, *Hygiea*, *Ugeskrift for Læger* (The Journal of the Danish Medical Association) and *Hospitals-Tidende* (Hospital Courier), tell the reader more about medical practice than might meet the eye. As other historians have highlighted, medical journals could be polemic or otherwise used as rhetorical instruments by practitioners, and it is important to keep this in mind when studying them.[47] All three journals had national coverage; however, there is likely some geographical discrepancy given the centralisation of each country's respective society of medicine to the capitols. For instance, meetings for the Swedish Society of Medicine were held in Stockholm, which, given the distance and logistical challenges involved in travel, would have prioritised individuals located in the Swedish capitol. Despite these geographical considerations, many journal articles

---

[46] This is an area that requires more thorough investigation. The COVID-19 pandemic that took place from 2020 to 2022 negated my ability to directly investigate the provenance of museum collections of surgical instruments. One area of interest could be the further development and specialisation of the metal trades in the nineteenth century, in particular after the deregulation of the guild systems in 1846 in Sweden and in 1862 in Denmark. Regarding the Swedish context, Måns Jansson has examined metal trades in the eighteenth century. See Måns Jansson. *Making Metal Making: Circulation of Workshop Practices in the Swedish Metal Trades, 1730–1775*. Diss. Uppsala University, 2017.

[47] See for example, Drakman, *När kroppen slöt sig*, 28; Roy Porter, "The Rise of Medical Journalism in Britain to 1800", in *Medical Journals and Medical Knowledge: Historical Essays*. William F. Bynum, Stephen Lock and Roy Porter (eds.), 6–28. New York: Routledge, 2019.

focus on technologies and matters of practice and were long, instructive texts to help guide practitioners in implementing a new technique or technology.[48] Texts like these would have been helpful for subscribing practitioners in rural locations. More to the point, rhetorical tensions aside, journals can be rich sources of practical information if we read their contents as communicating practical knowledge, that of performance, rather than as a mere tool of theoretical matters in medicine. In addition to this, solid theoretical foundations were not a prerequisite for practical adoption, as many of my empirical cases show.[49] As I will detail in the following chapters, articles on how to implement a technology practically were important pieces of publication at the time, and in many cases the clinical implications of practice were more important in their proliferation and use. Because my primary sources are in Swedish and Danish, the translations in this book are my own. I have provided the original citations in the footnotes for comparison.

Medical Journals

The primary bulk of my empirical material consists of published medical journals, in particular the Swedish Society of Medicine's former publication *Hygiea* (1839–1938), the Danish Medical Association's publication *Ugeskrift for Læger* (1839–present), and the Danish medical periodical *Hospitals-Tidende* (1858–1938). Aside from language, there are some important differences: *Hygiea* was a monthly, included minutes from the Swedish Society of Medicine's meetings in some volumes, and was bound in both year and half-year volumes. *Ugeskrift* was a weekly–*uge* being the Danish word for week–

---

[48] Michael Worboys highlights this in the case of Joseph Lister, whose antiseptic method of wound management was often considered to be convoluted and difficult to understand with an unclear theoretical basis by historians. Worboys, "Joseph Lister and the Performance of Antiseptic Surgery".

[49] Ulrika Graningers thesis *Från synligt till osynligt* argues that bacteriology did not become widely accepted in Sweden until the end of the nineteenth century. And, while that might be true theoretically, articles discussing practical concerns that related to the eventual establishment of bacteriology in Sweden were plentiful from the 1870s onward. See Graninger, *Från osynligt till synligt*. Compare with, for example: [Anon.], "Forgiftning med Karbolsyre: Efter Dr. Machin (Brit. med. journ. Marts 1868.–L'un. méd. 1868. Nr. 108)". *Ugeskrift for Læger*. Series 3, Vol. 6, No. 20, 17 October 1868, 295–296; [Anon.], "Om Anvendelsen af Karbolsyren i Chirurgien". *Hospitalds-Tidende*. Vol. 12, No. 21, 26 May 1869, 82–83; [Anon.], "Kloral som antisepticum. Efter Dujardin-Beaumetx og Hirne (L'un. méd. 1873. Nr. 62 og Nr. 63)". *Ugeskrift for Læger*. Series 3, Vol. 16, No. 12, 6 September 1873, 177–181; [Anon.], "Vatforbinding. Efter Hervey (Arch. gén. de méd. Dcbr. 1871–Juni 1872)". *Ugeskrift for Læger*. Series 3, Vol. 15, No. 11. 1 March 1873, 161–172; Jacques Borelius, "Antiseptiken på Listers afdelning på Kings College Hospital i London". *Hygiea*. Vol. 51, No. 11, November 1889, 665–669; Jacques Borelius, "Den aseptiska sårbehandlingen". *Hygiea*. Vol. 55, No. 4, April 1893, 415–429; Oscar Hecksher, "Om Mangler ved Indpakningen af sterile Forbindstoffer". *Hospitals-Tidende*. Vol. 38, No. 4, 23 January 1895, 113–115.

and was primarily bound in half-year volumes. *Hospitals-Tidende* was also a weekly and was bound in yearly volumes and included excerpts from meetings of the Danish Medical Society from 1888 onward.[50] Otherwise, they are written in their respective national languages, with a combination of original articles, translated articles, translated overviews and summaries, published (and sometimes translated) lectures, commentaries, excerpts from travel diaries, and more. All three were published for the benefit of members or physicians proficient in the local languages but were available for purchase and subscription for the general public as well.

Devices are most prominently featured in the journals as compliments to descriptions of new technologies and techniques. Sometimes the author notes modifications made to a device to accommodate the technique or method in question.[51] They seldom seem to have warranted articles themselves.[52] Explicit focus on a device is relatively rare, and articles are, perhaps unsurprisingly, often about devices that served a specific function in a practice or method. Outside of articles, they also figure as elements of discussion in meeting commentary. In Sweden, instrument makers who were given membership to the society often presented their instruments at meetings, especially if they were new or in another way remarkable (foreign acquisitions included). Sometimes commentary from physicians follows, other times instruments appear in brief, one-sentence notices, sometimes they are not even named specifically. A few exceptions to these cases exist and are discussed in greater detail in the chapters that follow.

I have chosen to work systematically. This means I have studied each volume more or less in its entirety once, made notes and subsequently returned to articles that examined a device more closely or described a

---

[50] At present, the Danish Medical Association is also a trade union and an umbrella organisation for three other trade unions, the Association of Junior Doctors, General Practitioners Organisation and Association of Medical Specialists. The Swedish Society of Medicine is strictly a professional organisation, not a trade union.

[51] See for example Ivar Svensson, "Från kirurgiska afdelningen af Sabbatsbergs sjukhus". *Hygiea*. Vol. 43, No. 7, July 1881, 321–381, 330–2; F. Westermark, "Om vaginofixation af den retroflekterade uterus". *Hygiea*. Vol. 56, No. 2, Feburary 1894, 159–170, 166; Ivar Svensson, "Om punktion af pleuritiska exsudat". *Hygiea*. Vol. 57, No. 8, August 1895, 122–153, 125; F. Kjellman, "Om operationen af näspolyper". *Hygiea*. Vol. 43, No. 6, June 1881, 281–286, 284–5.

[52] See for example F. A. Cederschjöld, "Ett nytt Perforatorium". *Hygiea*. Vol. 12, No. 9, September 1850, 531–534; Sigfred Levy, "Om Kjæderbrokbaand (Efter Emil Edel. Arch. f. klin. Chir. XXII. 3)". *Ugeskrift for Læger*. Vol. 26, No. 28, 14 December 1878, 433–435; Jacques Borelius, "Om Hennebergs desinfektor för sterilsering af förbandsmaterial m. m". *Hygiea*. Vol. 52, No. 9, September 1890, 677–680; S. Lindström, "En ny medicinsk möbel". *Hygiea*. Vol. 56, No. 4, April 1894, 364–366; Max Stille, "Operationsbord för laparotomier och gynekologiska operationer". *Hygiea*. Vol. 59, No. 2, February 1897, 289–290.

technology that implicated one or more devices.[53] Additional re-reads were undertaken following the establishment of the thesis' four cases, which are described in more detail at the end of this chapter. These themes have been established based solely on journal readings, not the other material categories examined. The articles are primarily written for an audience–that of physicians, with specific training and understanding of the body and its illnesses and diseases. This can be challenging for a layperson. The language is attuned to this audience, and jargon, while necessary, is common. In addition to this, decoding the language of nineteenth-century medicine takes some time. Even after building up a technical vocabulary, nineteenth-century medical journals figure in different historical circumstances, which requires some measure of social, scientific, and political decoding to interpret their contents. This is especially true when confronted with articles describing or analysing devices that we are familiar with today, like stethoscopes, microscopes, etc., which might mislead one into presuming their use has always been unproblematic for practitioners. Furthermore, because this thesis is written in English, translation of terminology has occasionally required some extra footwork to use a relatable English term with historical bearing.

Ugeskrift, Hygiea, and *Hospitals-Tidende* provide significant amounts of material on their own, with yearly volumes amounting to between four and eight hundred pages each early in the period and over one thousand toward the turn of the century. This means that some journals have been left out, such as the Swedish journal *Eira* (1877–1903), which was the journal for the Swedish Society for Provincial Doctors. The Swedish-based journal *Nordiskt medicinskt arkiv* (Nordic Medical Archive, 1869–1919) is also excluded due to the pan-Nordic nature of the publication. Neither of these publications cover the entire scope of the thesis' timeframe in the way *Hygiea, Ugeskrift* and *Hospitals-Tidende* do. *Eira,* for example, covers a small timescale, starting relatively late in the examined period and continuing for a mere twenty-six years. It is difficult to imagine figures regarding readership; however, given that *Hygiea* and *Ugeskrift* were the organs of professional societies, their readership was likely considerable amongst the profession. Additionally, despite a forum like *Eira,* provincial doctors read and contributed to *Hygiea.*[54] Furthermore, this is a study of device, knowledge, and

---

[53] This process is slightly reminiscent of the one Latour describes in *The Pasteurization of France* where he states that he does "not [confine himself] to a particular science but [records] all the references made by the authors". See Bruno Latour. *The Pasteurization of France.* Trans. Alan Sheridan and John Law. Cambridge, Massachusetts: Harvard University Press, 1988, 9.

[54] Drakman, *När kroppen slöt sig,* 44.

practice more generally, so I have not delved into material aimed solely at medicine's specialisations.

Trade Catalogues, Archive Material, and Newspapers

These three, material categories may seem odd to put together, but they all serve as complementary material. One way to obtain an overview of the devices produced by surgical instrument makers is through their trade catalogues. The few trade catalogues I have localised, the bulk of which have been found at the National Library of Sweden and Hagströmer Library, both in Stockholm, have been well-preserved. Claire Jones, whose 2013 book *The Medical Trade Catalogue in Britain, 1870-1914* is one of the few comprehensive resources in the history of medicine examining trade catalogues, defines them as "a book-like publication" that could vary in length and form, but was a form of advertising directed towards practitioners of medicine.[55] In this sense, they could both be relatively simple, no more than a list of prices with images of select products; or more complex, offering detailed explanations, numerous images, and in some cases instructions for usage. Jones notes that physicians influenced the contents of some of these publications. For example, catalogues might have included detailed information about how to use the devices and the differences between similar products at the request of physicians.[56] The Swedish and Danish language catalogues available to me are primarily of the simpler type. Both trade catalogues and price currents are forms of advertisement, with price currents being the most basic, listing names and prices, sometimes with images of select products. However, regardless of exhaustiveness, it is important to be mindful of their purpose: to market and sell devices.

While they are important to mention, trade catalogues and price currents have not been relied on in this thesis, with one exception: Danish surgical instrument maker Camillus Nyrop's medical trade catalogue *Bandager og Instrumenter*. *Bandager og Instrumeter* is different to the other, simpler catalogues and price currents I have recovered from Swedish and Danish instrument makers. It was first published in 1864 and republished four times.[57] Unlike the simpler variety, listing only names and prices, *Bandager og Instrumenter* offers lengthy descriptions of a select number of devices with images, a price current, and addendums with new instruments. Many of the

---

[55] Jones, *The Medical Trade Catalogue in Britain*, 1.

[56] Ibid., 19.

[57] The final edition was published in 1884 by two of Nyrop's, Johan Ernst and Louis Nyrop. The other editions were published in 1869 and 1877.

descriptions in *Bandager og Instrumenter* include practical information tailored to the use of the devices that Nyrop chose to profile. The catalogue itself will be discussed in greater detail throughout this thesis; however, it is noteworthy here for its uniqueness in comparison to the other catalogues and price currents attributed to instrument makers from these countries. While it is difficult to say definitively whether this is the only catalogue of the more lavish type produced in these two countries, it is the only one I have been able to recover.

The unpublished material located in archives in Sweden and Denmark primarily includes institutional archives from healthcare and education, but also two, sparse archives for instrument makers. The archives, which have been relatively unproblematic in their presentation, institutional composition, and thoroughness, will not be discussed in detail. Hospital and medical school archives are often thorough and well-preserved. I have made use of material, primarily ledgers, inventory, and annual reports in these archives, when available. These include Seraphim Hospital, Sabbatsberg Hospital and the Karolinska Institute in Stockholm, Sweden; Uppsala University Hospital and the Faculty of Medicine at Uppsala University in Uppsala, Sweden; and private hospital and former school for the education of nurses, Sophia-hemmet in Stockholm, Sweden. This list is not exhaustive. This is due to the COVID-19 pandemic during 2020–2022 and the border closures, travel restrictions, and limited institutional accessibility that have characterised the pandemic. This means that the archives have been Swedish and localised to the capitol region. However, this material has had little bearing on the primary results of this thesis. Archival material elsewhere in Sweden and Denmark merits investigation in the future.

Archives of individuals or private business are not nearly as thoroughly preserved as those of public institutions. Indeed, few instrument makers have archives. The two exceptions are the small archives of instrument makers Camillus Nyrop at the Danish State Archive in Copenhagen and Alb. Stille/Stille-Werner AB in the Science Museum's archives in Stockholm.[58] Nyrop's archive includes a massive ledger covering the years 1857–1863, as well as two letters. The Stille archive includes some pictures, a price current and an anniversary book. The materials in the Stille archive mostly cover the years following the turn of the century with no older material. I have had to

---

[58] The archives of Camillus Nyrop and Albert Stille have not been utilised in this book. 07809. Rigsarkivet, Nyrop, Camillus, instrumentmager, bandagist; F F956. Tekniska museet, Handlingar rörande Albert Stille, Kirurgisk Instrumentfabrik, AB Stille-Werner, Stockholm, Teknik- och industrihistoriska arkivet.

look elsewhere to develop a better understanding of the trade, how it changed, and the relationships between surgical instrument makers and physicians during the period. In this case, newspaper articles and a book by Camillus Nyrop's son of the same name on his father's work–*Camillus Nyrop og det kirurgiske Instrumentmageri I Danmark* (Camillus Nyrop and surgical instrument making in Denmark) have assisted in forming a more complete image of their work and relationships to medicine, at least in the Danish case.

Newspaper articles have also served to complement material from medical journals and trade catalogues/price currents. I have relied on both keyword searches and more systematic read-throughs of newspaper materials available digitally through the Swedish newspaper database Svenska dagstidningar (Swedish Daily Press) available through the National Library and the Danish Royal Library's service Mediestream. These searches have primarily involved information about both Swedish and Danish instrument makers and corroborate other information from medical journals, which means my searches and read-throughs have been guided by approximate dates from medical journals rather than a systematic look at all newspaper material between 1855 and 1897.

Characteristics of Medical Journals and Surgical Instrument Makers

The three medical journals that form the bulk of my empirical material is from require some further explanation. *Hygiea* was an organ of the Swedish Society of Medicine and is no longer published but was active between 1839 and 1938. *Ugeskrift for Læger*, founded in 1839, is still published and is the Danish Medical Society's general medical journal. *Hospitals-Tidende* was published between 1858 and 1938. While all three are similar in some respects, they differ in others. *Hygiea* and *Ugeskrift for Læger* published original works, translated summaries and commentary on foreign publications. Many of *Ugeskrift*'s articles have a strong, theoretical focus. *Hospitals-Tidende* published much of the same; however, its subheading says it all: "optegnelser af praktisk Lægekunst fra Ind- og Udlandet", which translates to "domestic and foreign records of practical medicine".[59] Many of the articles here are of a practical, clinical character, and theoretical commentary is often

---

[59] The introductory article in the first issue highlights this, stating that *erfaringskilder*, personal experiences (i.e., case studies), were the primary point of reference for the periodical. [Anon.], "Forord". *Hospitals-Tidende*. Vol. 1, No. 1, January 6, 1858, 1.

interwoven with practical implications and understandings and clinical experiences.

A large number of articles are unsigned, in particular early in the period that I have examined, throughout the 1850s. While *Hygiea*'s articles are more often attributed to an author, this is not always the case. Articles in *Ugeskrift for Læger* and *Hospitals-Tidende* are more often unattributed: a trend that continues throughout the period examined, though dropping off toward the turn of the century. Summaries of articles in the foreign medical press are more likely to be unattributed. This could have been because the translator attempted to stay as true as possible to the original article, and no attribution was necessary because a reference to the original article was already present. However, they could have also been translated by the editor. In some cases, these articles were still signed by the responsible translator, and in some cases, the translator provided commentary.[60] It is difficult to determine if there was a general praxis in this respect, but this is also outside of the scope of this thesis. Counting or otherwise attempting to determine authorship has also been out of the scope of this thesis; however, it merits further study.[61]

Many of the original articles in the journals consist of technical details that speak to an in-group, suggesting that although they were also likely read outside of medical circles, their primary purpose was communication within these circles. Although Danish and Swedish physicians would be competent in French and German–modern languages were a requirement in the pre-university educations–the translated summaries of articles published in foreign languages do not always speak to their reach outside of medical circles either. In many cases, they were not direct translations of foreign articles. In this sense, they were likely intended to communicate scientific and clinical information to physicians who might not have been able to access the period-icals they were published in directly. This would have been an important service for provincial doctors [*provinsialläkare/provinsiallæger*] and

---

[60] See for example G. Böttiger, "Om Etherisationen. Tal, hållet vid franska Wetenskaps-Academiens Årssammankomst d. å., af VELPEAU. Medd. Af D:r G. Böttiger". *Hygiea*. Vol. 12, No. 6, June 1850, 350–364; continued in the following issue, Vol. 12, No. 7, July 1850, 411–415; Harald Philipsen, "Om antiseptisk Forbinding. Efter Prof. Joseph Lister i Glasgow («The Lancet», 21de Septbr. 1867)". *Ugeskrift for Læger*. Series 3, Vol. 4, No. 25, 23 November 1867, 381–390; M. Sondén, "Diskussion om antiseptica, Berliner kiln. Wochenschr. N:o 17. 1878". *Hygiea*. Vol. 40, No. 5, May 1878, 254–255; Carl Rossander, "Sonnenburg: Zur Diagnose und Therapie der Carbolintoxicationen. Deutsche Zeitschrift für Chirurgie. Band. 9, sid. 356". *Hygiea*. Vol. 40, No. 9, September 1878, 499–501.

[61] Roy Porter discusses this in the British context. He notes that attribution was not seen as appropriate in some social circles, like the gentry; however, this is irrelevant to my case because unattributed articles were common in both the Swedish and Danish press more broadly. Porter, "The Rise of Medical Journalism in Britain to 1800".

physicians otherwise located outside of larger centres, who likely would have limited ability to access to foreign journals.[62] Medical societies were more easily able to purchase subscriptions to a variety of publications and the collective labour of members could assist in the dissemination of relevant works through, for example, translated summaries. The journals' enrolment in medicine as well as technical and theoretical discussions and debates argues against their laity as primarily popular organs for communicating medical scientific information.

This point is important in relation to the three surgical instrument makers discussed most often in this thesis. Although a less generous reading might categorise these instrument makers as "laypeople", I am adamant that they are not. It is clear that all three read these journals in at least a cursory fashion. But beyond journals, they worked closely with physicians, were well-read on matters of medical science and practice, and participated in the development of a body of medical scientific knowledge related to the use of medical devices. This included practical matters involving the use of medical devices.[63] This will be discussed in greater detail in following chapters; however, I stress that the instrument makers mentioned most frequently in this thesis were active participants in the production of scientific knowledge. I will give a short biographical presentation of these men in order to provide better understanding of their relationships with physicians and their positions within their trade. Fundamentally, they were accepted members of the medical community and their contributions should be understood as such. They worked in close contact with physicians, both within their own borders and internationally.[64] This does not mean that there were not contentions. I will discuss some of these in chapter three. I use the designation "surgical instrument maker" because it is the professional title used in my empirical materials [*kirurgisk instrumentmakare/kirurgiskinstrumentmager*].

---

[62] A similar point is made by Roy Porter when he points out that provincial physicians and medical societies in smaller centres in Britain were keen subscribers of medical serials in the eighteenth century. Porter, "The Rise of Medical Journalism in Britain to 1800", 19. See also Ana Carneiro, et. al., "Shaping Doctors and Society: The Portuguese Medical Press (1880–1926)". *Media History*. Vol. 25, No. 1, 2019, 23–50, 28.

[63] David LeVay makes a similar point, noting that in the British and French contexts, one-on-one contact between physicians and "appliance makers" was common and were often acknowledged publicly. See David LeVay. *The History of Orthopaedics: An Account of the Study and Practice of Orthopaedics from the Earliest Times to the Modern Era*. Lancashire: The Parthenon Publishing Group, 1990, 79 & 237.

[64] I analyse some of these relationships in an article. Kristin Halverson, "Medical Technologies and the Social Strategies of Two Surgical Instrument Makers in Denmark and Sweden, 1870–1900". *Acta medico-historica Rigensia*. Vol. 14, 2021, 101–117.

To be clear, these men constructed a variety of medical devices beyond surgical instruments: from beds, to masks, to orthopaedic devices.

Swedish surgical instrument maker Albert Stille (1814–1893) and Danish surgical instrument maker and bandagist[65] Camillus Nyrop (1811–1883) were active around the same time and had similar career trajectories. Nyrop's career began as a turner and metalworker before travelling abroad to study surgical instrument making, and Stille received a stipend to undertake training in surgical instrument making abroad.[66] Both Nyrop and Stille spent time in Paris working under the renowned master cutler and surgical instrument maker Frédéric-Beniôt Charrière. Nyrop, due to a personal conflict with Charrière, ended up studying under surgical instrument maker Amatus Lüer as well, who was also based in Paris.[67] Upon returning home from their stays abroad, Nyrop and Stille quickly established themselves as surgical instrument makers in their respective capitols, Stockholm and Copenhagen. In 1841, Stille began working as the medical school Karolinska Institute's surgical instrument maker, and the same year Nyrop became the Danish Surgical Academy's instrument maker. Here, the two men took slightly divergent paths, with Stille's primary focus continuing to be surgical instruments. Nyrop additionally interested himself in the construction and use of orthopaedic devices to treat patients with musculoskeletal problems, and disorders like scoliosis. He worked together with at least three physicians, J. C. A. Bock, C. Jessen, and A. Friedenreich, on orthopaedic treatments with braces, bands, and trusses in particular (see figure 1).[68] Although Stille did not take interest in the direct treatment of patients like Nyrop did, he still worked closely with physicians to construct and modify instruments. Albert Stille seemed to have taken a particular interest in ovariotomies and attended the first one performed in Sweden by Swedish gynaecologist Sven Sköldberg in

[65] Bandagist is the Danish name for the profession most similar to present-day orthotists and is a modern, regulated profession. However, it is also the term used in my historical sources for a category of unregulated medical practitioners that primarily busied themselves with the construction and application of mechanical braces, bands, trusses, and bandages for patients with musculoskeletal disorders such as scoliosis and hernias. "Truss maker" is one professional equivalent but does not capture the full range of practice nineteenth-century Danish bandagists undertook. They do not seem to have systematically engaged in mechanical manipulation of the joints, unlike bonesetters. The French term *bandagiste* is closer, referring to makers of medical appliances and mechanical devices, and much like some of their Danish counterparts, collaborated with physicians. I will discuss Danish bandagists in more detail in the third chapter. See also LeVay, *The History of Orthopaedics*, 237.

[66] C. Nyrop. *Slægten Nyrop: Nogle biografiske oplysninger*. Copenhagen, Nielsen & Lydiche, 1908, 87; [Anon.]. "Inrikes". *Najaden*. 31 January 1840.

[67] C. Nyrop. *Camillus Nyrop*, 62. Charrière apparently did not look upon Nyrop's work favorably.

[68] Jul. Petersen, "Camillus Nyrop". *Dansk biografisk Lexikon*. Copenhagen: Gyldendalske Boghandels Forlag, 1898, 359.

1866.[69] He was elected a member of the Swedish Society of Medicine in 1868, and while Nyrop was never a member of the Danish counterpart, he published extensively in *Ugeskrift for Læger* and *Hospitals-Tidende*. Nyrop attended at least one ovariotomy as well, with one of his sons.[70] He also was awarded the title of professor for his work in 1860. Two of Nyrop's sons Johan Ernst and Louis Nyrop took over his business after his death in 1883.[71] In the case of Albert Stille's workshop, his son Max began working as a foreman in 1880 and took over the business after Albert fell ill in 1884.

Behandling af Rygradskrumninger.

Det tør vel antages, at den Tid er forbi, da den horizontale **Strækning** var det meest fremherskende mekaniske Middel mod ovennævnte svagelige Udvikling. Den nyere Tid har, og det sikkerlig til stor Gavn, fremkaldt en stor Deel forskjelligartede lette **portative Trykapparater,** der foruden mange andre aabenbare Fordele have den, at de skaane den unge **Patient** for det ofte ikke heldigvirkende **lang**e Leie. I en Række af Aar har jeg arbeidet paa at frembringe hensigtssvarende mekaniske Midler mod Rygradsdeformiteter, og har foruden de daglige Beviser paa, at min Stræben i denne Retning har været heldig, havt den Tilfredsstillelse at see **mit Princip, hvorved Brystkassen aldeles intet Tryk er udsat for**, under mit Navn optaget og benyttet i to af Udlandets større orthopædiske Helbredelsesanstalter.

Den af mig i Forening med Hr. Distriktslæge Jessen (Stormgade Nr. 8 i Stuen) for flere Aar siden begyndte orthopædiske Virksomhed fortsættes som hidtil. Skriftlige og mundtlige Anmeldelser af Patienter modtages saavel af Hr. Dr. Jessen, som af

Camillus Nyrop,

Professor, Universitetsinstrumentmager,
St. Kjøbmagergade Nr. 46 i Kjøbenhavn.
Kjøbenhavn, i Mai 1865.

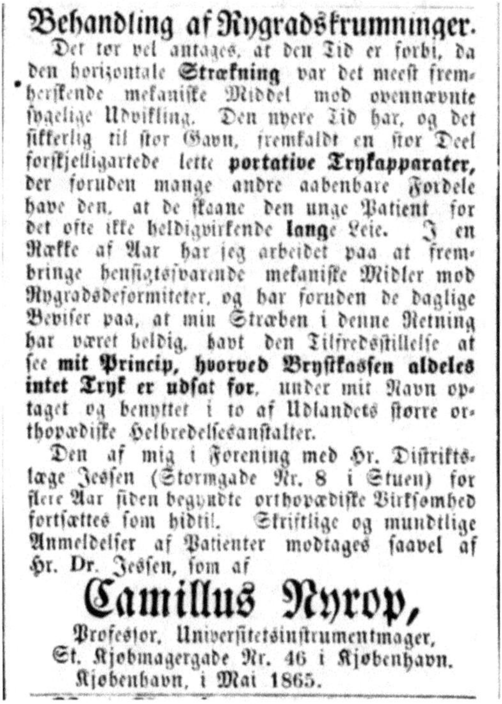

Fig. 1. A newspaper advertisement signed by Nyrop and published in 1865 advertising the treatment of scoliosis. Potential patients could contact either physician C. Jessen or Nyrop himself. Note the prominence of Nyrop's name, pictured at the bottom of the advertisement along with his address. No contact information is provided for C. Jessen. Camillus Nyrop. [Advertisement]. *Fredriksborgs Amts Tidende og Adressavis*. 16 May 1865.

[69] Sven Sköldberg, "Fall af Ovariotomi, III". *Hygiea*. Vol. 29, No. 11, November 1867, 479–481; Sven Sköldberg, "Fall af Ovariotomi, VIII". *Hygiea*. Vol. 31, No. 7, July 1869, 316–318.

[70] F. Howitz, "Et Tilfælde af Ovariotomi". *Hospitals-Tidende*. Vol. 7, No. 12, 23 March 1864, 45–47

[71] Johan Ernst Nyrop spent some time learning the trade under his father, as well as with the Stilles in Stockholm and, like his father, Lüer in Paris. See C. Nyrop, *Camillus Nyrop*, 115.

Max Stille (1853–1906) is one of very few people without medical training to publish an article in *Hygiea*.[72] His career offers insight into both the expansion of industry in Sweden, changes in how medical instruments were made, and shifts in the profession of surgical instrument making as a whole. Like his father Albert, Max was also a member of the Swedish Society of Medicine, elected in 1887. Max spent time abroad in France, Germany, and England to practice under surgical instrument makers and to learn his trade. However, rather than start working immediately, he attended the Royal Central Gymnastics Institute [*Kungliga Gymnastiska Centralinstitutet*], which was founded in 1813 by Swedish physical education pioneer Pehr Henrik Ling.[73] Under Max's leadership, the Stille firm grew from just 25 workers to 100 by the time of his death in 1906.[74] Unlike his father, Max also patented a total of eight devices: a lift mechanism for operating tables; a stretcher; a mechanical device for operating chairs and a modification to the earlier patent a year later; an instrument for cutting into the skull and removing plaster bandages; a mechanical arrangement for devices used to break or set limbs; a bag for transporting sterilised equipment; and a combined oven and rinsing apparatus for instruments.[75] Devices for surgery, especially in conformation to the exacting requirements of aseptic sterilisation techniques, seemed to attract most of Max's interest and gave him the most recognition. As I will discuss in greater detail in the fifth chapter, his showroom/model surgical suite and operating tables were well-known both in Sweden and abroad.

[72] Stille, "Operationsbord".

[73] John Berg, "Minnesteckning: Max Stille". *Hygiea*. Vol. 68, No. 4, April 1906, 358–363, 358–9.

[74] Berg, "Minnesteckning", 360. Newspaper articles about a lock-out at Stille's workshop in 1895 also provide some detail about employment. Workers were locked-out after removing a foreman whom they perceived as a tyrant, from the premises in a wheelbarrow. Press coverage of the lock-out mentions 46 workers involved in some way; whereby, three where fired for refusing to apologise for their actions. See [Anon.], "Lock-outen hos fabrikör Stille". *Upsala Nya Tidningen*. 21 August 1895; [Anon.], "I sista minuten". *Upsala Nya Tidningen*. 21 August 1895; and [Anon.], "Lockouten kos [sic] Stilles". *Social-demokraten*, 23 August, 1895.

[75] A. M. (Max) Stille, "Lyftinrättning vid operationsbord, sjuksängar m.m.". 1893. Swedish patent SE4720C1, filed 5 July 1893, issued 18 November 1893; A. M. Stille, "Bårsäng". 1894. Swedish patent SE5351C1, filed 8 March 1894, issued 11 August 1894; A. M. Stille, "Anordning vid operationssoffor". 1895. Swedish patent SE6315C1, filed 15 January 1895, issued 7 September 1895; A. M. Stille, "Instrument för uppklippning af hufvudskålsbenen, gipsbandage och dylikt". 1895. Swedish patent SE6729C1, filed 8 November 1895, issued 21 March 1896; A. M. Stille, "Anordning vid operationssoffor". 1896. Swedish patent SE6756C1, filed 23 December 1895, issued 11 April 1896 [modification of SE6315C1]; A. M. Stille, "Anordning vid apparater för afbrytande eller rättställande af lemmar à menniskokroppen". 1896. Swedish patent SE7872C1, filed 1 December 1896, issued 15 May 1897; A. M. Stille, "Anordning vid väskor för transport och förvaring af desinfektions- eller steriliseringskärl". 1897. Swedish patent SE7470C1, filed 11 February 1896, issued 16 January 1897; A. M. Stille, "Kombinerad instrumentkokare och sköljkanna". 1897. Swedish patent SE8415C1, filed 1 April 1897, issued 30 October 1897.

Max Stille's obituary in *Hygiea*, written by surgeon John Berg, gives insight into the value of his work for Swedish physicians. Motzi Eklöf points out in her doctoral thesis that eulogies in professional, medical journals served to form professional ideals. Though Eklöf examines the eulogies of physicians, she notes that not all physicians were bestowed the honour of an obituary written by a colleague published in a medical journal and that they were typically reserved for colleagues of a particular, honourable status.[76] Neither Camillus Nyrop nor Albert Stille were eulogised in the examined journals like Max Stille was, at most receiving a small notice in the section where deaths were reported at the end of each issue.[77] Given Eklöf's more thorough look at eulogisation in medical journals and the eulogy's relationship with status, it is particularly noteworthy that Max Stille was worthy of the distinct honour in *Hygiea*. Although his father Albert's death was marked with a notice in *Hospitals-Tidende*, Max's was not mentioned in either *Ugeskrift* or *Hospitals-Tidende*. Nyrop's death was noted in both Danish periodicals, but it was not mentioned in *Hygiea*.

All three men were still exceptions, in that they occupied relatively privileged positions in their trade. In medical journals, the work of other surgical instrument makers is much less visible. Two slight exceptions are Swedish surgical instrument maker Ch. O. Werner and Danish bandagist Anton Rasmussen. Werner, who, like Albert and Max Stille, was also elected a member of the Swedish Society of Medicine in 1894. Rasmussen published occasionally in *Ugeksrift for Læger* and was otherwise mentioned in articles. Both Werner and Rasmussen were much less prominent figures than the Stilles and Nyrop were. The workshops of Stille and Werner merged to form Stille-Werner AB in 1910. The firm was bought out by Mo and Domsjö AB and Sanna Holding. Sanna Holding declared bankruptcy in 1993, but the Stille name was saved from the estate and Stille AB exists to this day. In the case of Anton Rasmussen, he was initially trained as a glover, but later spent time in Berlin training as a bandagist with August Lutter. When he returned to Copenhagen in 1854, he was affiliated with an orthopaedic institute and Frederiks Hospital.[78] In addition to this, he operated a public bathhouse,

---

[76] Eklöf, *Läkarens Ethos*, 269.

[77] See [Anon.], "Officielt". *Hospitals-Tidende*. Vol. 26, No. 52, 26 December 1883, 1248; [Anon.], "Dødsfald". *Ugeskrift for Læger*. Series 4, Vol. 9, No. 1, 5 January 1884, 23; [Anon.], "Dødsfald i Udlandet". *Hospitals-Tidende*. Vol. 36, No. 45, 8 November 1893, 1116.

[78] C. Nyrop, "Rasmussen, Anton Gustav Casimir". *Dansk biografisk Lexikon*. C. F. Bricka (ed.). 503. Volume 8. Copenhagen: Gyldendalske Boghandels Forlag, 1899.

which he advertised in *Ugeskrift for Læger*.[79] Much like even the more prominent Stilles and Nyrop, there is some degree of difficulty uncovering biographical information about these men and their work.

To claim there was a large cadre of surgical instrument makers in either
country would be incorrect. Archival and other records show that there were
around nine surgical instrument makers in Sweden and approximately
twenty-five surgical instrument makers and/or bandagists in Denmark. It is
unlikely that these men were solely occupied with the construction of medical
devices.[80] These numbers might not be entirely representative either, as
cutlers and other makers of fine instruments might have made medical
devices, but not been classified as "surgical instrument makers" in land
records for taxation [*mantal*], census data [*folketællinger/folkräkningar*], and
other records of commerce.[81] Even Nyrop, with a comparatively prominent
position as surgical instrument maker for Copenhagen University's medical
school, also worked as a cutler and with other kinds of metalwork into the
1880s (see figure 2).[82] Two Swedish surgical instrument makers based in
Uppsala, Johan Rabén and Anders Nyman began repairing and constructing
velocipedes in the 1880s, for example. Rabén had previously received
financial compensation from Uppsala University's Faculty of Medicine,
which abruptly stopped in 1863 after a large acquisition of medical instruments and curiosities from physician C. M. Retzius.[83]

---

[79] Frederik Trier, "A. Rasmussens medikopneumatiske Anstalt i Kjøbenhavn". *Ugeskrift for Læger*. Series
2, Vol. 41, No. 10, 27 August 1864, 152–158; Anton Rasmussen, "Bekjendtgjørelse". *Ugeskrift for Læger*.
Series 3, Vol. 3, No. 12, 12 March 1867, 183. Trier was the editor of *Ugeskrift* when he wrote the article
about Rasmussen's bathhouse. Trier noted that even though it might raise eyebrows that Rasmussen's
bath house was not run by a physician, but that Rasmussen's skill spoke for itself. He also mentioned
that physician Oscar Storch worked at the facility (154).

[80] See Nyrop, *Camillus Nyrop*, 119–121; Peter Gullers. *Verktygsmakare & operatörer: några aspekter på
den kirurgiska instrumenttillverkningens svenska historia*. Report 37. Stockholm: Arbetslivscentrum,
1982. Gullers misses at least two in his report, Johan Rabén and Anders Nyman, who were both based
in the city of Uppsala just north of Stockholm. See also SE/SSA/0099 Stockholm stadsarkiv, Hall- och
manufakturrätten, B 3: Fabriksberättelser, 53–56.

[81] This is further confirmed in C. Nyrop, *Camillus Nyrop*. He notes two workshops, one run by I.C. and
A. Cotzand, and a man with the surname Fleron. Both predated Nyrop's workshop; however, neither
exhibited their instruments, nor carried stock. Rather, their surgical instruments were made to order.
I.C. and A. Cotzand were the brother and nephew respectively of A.W. Cotzand, who took over the
workshop of perhaps Denmark's first surgical instrument maker, a cutler named Descottes. Descottes
had travelled to England and France to study surgical instrument making in 1765 at the behest of King
Fredrik V of Denmark.
See *Udsigt over Udstillningen af indenlandske Industrie-Producter*. Bianco Lund & Schneider, 1837, 32.

[82] Camillus Nyrop. [Advertisement]. *Fædrelandet*. 7 December 1881, 294. Nyrop is advertising table
knives of his workshop's construction.

[83] Uppsala University, Medicinska fakulteten, G I: Räkenskaper.

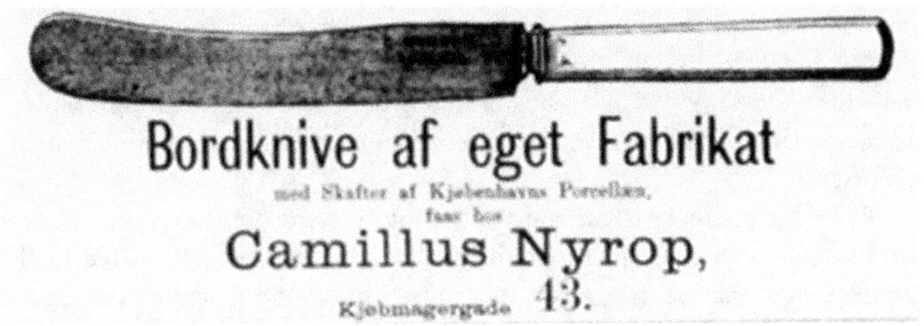

Fig. 2. A newspaper advertisement for table knives constructed at Camillus Nyrop's workshop, 1881. Camillus Nyrop, [Advertisement]. *Fædrelandet*. 7 December 1881.

The construction and sale of medical devices during the period studied was not a trade with endless demand in either of these two countries. Camillus Nyrop offered tips on how to both store instruments correctly and repair them in his trade catalogue *Bandager og Instrumenter*. I will discuss this in greater detail in the following chapters; however, it is important to underline that the concept of single-use items, something that we might associate as a characteristic of medicine and its devices now, had not yet taken hold. Physicians were generally responsible for their own instruments, as well as other, simpler items such as bandages. Instrument sets could be, and were, resold, as is the case with a collection of medical devices and other items sold by C. M. Retzius to the Medical Faculty at Uppsala University.[84] Simon Werrett details similar trends in his book *Thrifty Science*. He notes in particular that the era of disposable goods was interconnected with the role of sanitation and the risk of germs.[85] Archives and journals from the period offer commentary on repairing and sharpening instruments and what kinds of bandage materials could be reused and what should be discarded. For example, one article in *Hygiea* detailed the circumstances dictating whether dressings could be reused, noting that they should be discarded if the wound was septic.[86] Furthermore, many physicians made some items, like bandages and suture material, themselves.[87] Later in the period, toward the turn of the

[84] Uppsala University, Medicinska fakulteten, D II: Inventarie- och arkivförteckningar; Uppsala University, Medicinska fakulteten, G I: Räkenskaper.

[85] Simon Werrett. *Thrifty Science: Making the Most of Materials in the History of Experiment*. Chicago: The University of Chicago Press, 2019, 186.

[86] A. Wiborgh, "Om antiseptisk förbandstyg". *Hygiea*. Vol. 40, No. 8, August 1878, 413–416, 414.

[87] Wiborgh, "Om antiseptisk förbandstyg", 413; Ivar Svensson, "Från kirurgiska afdelningen af Sabbatsbergs sjukhus". *Hygiea*. Vol. 43, No. 7, July 1881, 321–381, 342–343.

century, when physicians could purchase things like pre-packaged gauze and other bandage materials, the safety and sterility of these kinds of items was called into question.[88] This indicates that even if other, premade alternatives were available, physicians might have still preferred to prepare these items themselves.

These factors make it difficult to account for some of the everyday objects that I discuss in subsequent chapters: they were not always visible in the archival material of institutions because they were bought and traded individually. Furthermore, the COVID-19 pandemic of 2020–2022 made it difficult to look closely at museum collections to better understand the provenance of medical instruments and devices and how they changed hands during the latter half of the nineteenth century. This is an issue that could merit some further research when collections are more easily accessible again, or perhaps by enterprising curatorial staff interested in better exploring the networks of ownership behind these more "everyday" medical objects.

Toward the turn of the century, the number of physicians in both countries increased and, as I will discuss in the fifth chapter, systems of cleanliness best exemplified with asepsis shifted the responsibility for the procurement and maintenance of certain kinds of medical devices and articles from individuals to institutions. This is an important demarcation in the periodisation of my thesis. The contact surgical instrument makers had with physicians was a unique part of nineteenth-century medicine and the shifting responsibility for procurement, from individual physicians to institutions, likely changed this relationship. Furthermore, this is part of the logic behind focusing closely on everyday objects. Institutions procured more valuable instruments throughout the period. For example, although archival material is not always easy to discern, some ledgers show examples of institutional procurement. This is particularly the case for more valuable devices such as microscopes.

Although physicians are frequently mentioned throughout this thesis, I will only provide biographical information about them in a few exceptional cases. Rather than occupying space in this introductory chapter, I will do this as the few exceptions appear. While their work has unquestionably been important to the proliferation and use of medical devices, and indeed, devices have been constructed and modified on request, the technicians and their

---

[88] Oscar Heckscher, "Om Mangler ved Indpakningen af sterile Forbindstoffer". *Hospitals-Tidende*. Vol. 38, No. 4 23 January 1895, 113–115, 114.

work occupy a much less studied position in Sweden and Denmark. Their relationships with physicians challenges the notion of fixed professional demarcations in this region, and highlights the participation of unlicensed practitioners in the production of medical knowledge in the nineteenth century. Furthermore, given the numerical upper hand physicians have in contrast to surgical instrument makers, the task of upturning biographical information for physicians would be laborious.

Method and Theory

Studying medical devices in historical materials offers some challenges. For example, they are often taken for granted; appear only briefly in otherwise long articles about a particular technology[89]; or, they are figures in ledgers, accounting only for quantity and prices.[90] Sometimes they are described more thoroughly in journal or newspaper articles, but with the pretext that the article is usually about the instrument maker behind them or the practice they are meant to assist.[91] Throughout the research process, I have asked myself how it is possible to study devices as dynamic participants in history and how to make sense of their relationships with others.

I have already provided an overview of previous research and positioned myself alongside international research of a more practice-oriented character, with a particular emphasis on the importance of local specificity. Unlike these studies, however, actor-network theory (henceforth ANT) is the methodological and theoretical framework for my study. This means that while my study might share some characteristics with previous research in the histories of devices and technologies in medicine, there will also be some degree of diversion. For example, I have focused less on contextualising developments alongside questions of professionalisation and healthcare

---

[89] See for example Kjellman, "Om operationen af näspolyper"; Borelius, "Om Hennebergs desinfektor"; Svensson, "Om punktion af pleuritiska exsudat".

[90] See SE/SSA/0252/A Riksarkivet, Sabbatsbergs sjukhus administrativ arkiv, D 2: Inventarie-förteckningar, G 1 B: Inventariehuvudböcker, G 2: Kassaböcker; Uppsala University, Medicinska fakulteten, D II: Inventarie- och arkivförteckningar; Uppsala University, Medicinska fakulteten, G I: Räkenskaper; SE/RA/420251 Riksarkivet, Serafimerlasarettet, G 1 A: Huvudböcker 1850–1900, G 6 BC: Månadsräkenskaper redovisade kontovis; SE/RA/740111 Riksarkivet, Sophiahemmet, G 1 A: Huvudbok 1883–1899; 07809. Rigsarkivet, Nyrop, Camillus, instrumentmager, bandagist.

[91] See for example *Förhandlingar vid Svenska läkarsällskapets sammankomster*, 18 February 1895, 8 October 1895, 12 November 1895; [Anon.], "Inrikes"; [Anon.], "En mönster-operationssal". *Dagens Nyheter*. 28 February 1894; [Anon.], "Erkännande från Amerika åt svensk industri". *Smålandsposten*. Feburary 9, 1894; [Anon.], "Stilles operationssal vid läkarkongressen i Rom". *Stockholms Dagblad*. April 22, 1894.

politics moving through the nineteenth century.[92] Fundamentally, ANT can be an effective means to explore the concept of scientific non-universality. Additionally, it can be a rewarding method for conducting historical research on phenomena that are well-studied elsewhere. As Kristin Asdal points out, ANT "may serve to fruitfully problematize a conventional contextualizing approach [...] hence open the past and *multiply* the possible versions of how to approach issues and compose collectives" (emphasis in original).[93] Rather than provide an overview of ANT's history below, I will discuss two of the method's key concepts that have been relevant to my work. These are fluidity and enactment, which are most clearly developed in the work of Annemarie Mol. This means that I am less interested in "classic" ANT, best exemplified by the early work of Bruno Latour, and more in what might be called After-ANT, which concerns itself with a different degree of complexity and tends to be less concerned with situations that have involved scientific conflict and controversies.[94] I will also discuss the ways that ANT can be helpful in historical studies.

Actor-Network Theory, Fluidity, and Enactments

The fundament to ANT as it relates to my research is to not define the world beforehand, but rather to trace the actors' own moves in world-making. In the introductory chapter of Bruno Latour's book, *The Pasteurization of France*, Latour asks the following questions: "What will we talk about? Which actors will we begin with? What intentions and what interest will we attribute to them?"[95] These questions set the stage for the research process. The point is that the researcher cannot know in advance the makeup of the world, and that one rather should follow actors' transformations in world-making.[96] He explains the research process further as recording all references made to the phenomena in question, across disciplines, and trying to understand how actors relate to one another without defining beforehand their composition and status in relation to one another.[97] This sense of not operating within an

---

[92] Some examples of this are Nilsson, *Kampen om kvinnan*; Pickstone, "Bones in Lancashire"; Kremer, "Building Institutes for Physiology in Prussia"; Ueyama, *Health in the Marketplace*.

[93] Kristin Asdal, "Contexts in Action–And the Future of the Past in STS". *Science, Technology, and Human Values*. Vol. 37, No. 4, April 2012, 379–403, 398.

[94] For more information on some of the problems identified with "classic" ANT, see John Law, "After ANT: complexity, naming and topology", in *Actor Network Theory and After*, John Law and John Hassard (eds.), 1–14. Oxford: Blackwell Publishing, 1999.

[95] Latour, *The Pasteurization of France*, 9.

[96] Ibid., 10.

[97] Ibid., 11.

a priori construction of the world is a helpful tool in exploring local specificity and is how I have approached my research process and empirical materials. For instance, this has been particularly important in understanding the dynamic relationships between surgical instrument makers and physicians, in circumstances when their professional difference was actually of little consequence and a few instrument makers were active participants in the formation of medical knowledge.

In fact, professional demarcations revealed themselves to be rather fluid. Fluidity is one of the key actor-network concepts with relevance to my work. It is best explained as a critique of the tendency to create binarisms, firm boundaries, and label phenomena in such a way that it makes the world more rigid and clearly defined than it actually is.[98] These rigid definitions and fixed boundaries have been used in the history of medicine for phenomena like Listerism, for example. They lead one to believe that they refer to specific, clearly defined phenomena, but, as I will discuss in the fourth chapter, this is often a hastily drawn conclusion and ignores local specificities and adaptations.[99]

Fluidity emphasises the complexity of technical and cultural systems and pushes back against the notion of entities having single states of being. This concept becomes most clear on the level of practice. In my case, looking closely at how journal articles detailed for instance Listerist performance gives clues on how it was adapted locally, and the complexities and tensions contained within terms like "antisepsis" or "Lister's method", rather than working from *a priori* assumptions. In practice, objects can differ, in particular when they exchange sites, even when they share a common name.[100] So, although followers of Lister coordinated their practices through the use of similar terminology, close readings of clinical descriptions in journals make it clear that wound management unfolded in practice in many different ways. Or, using a term coined by Annemarie Mol, Listerist wound management was "enacted" in different ways in practice. The terms "enacting" and "enactment" highlight how objects and phenomena unfold on the level of practice, rather than focusing on their theoretical basis.[101] Because these terms imply activity, the circumstances involved in the objects' enactment become

---

[98] Mol, *The Body Multiple*, in particular 119–150; Marianne de Laet and Annemarie Mol, "The Zimbabwe Bush Pump: Mechanics of a Fluid Technology". *Social Studies of Science*. Vol. 30, No. 2, April 2000, 225–263.

[99] In the British context, Michael Worboys highlights this in his book *Spreading Germs*, although not an actor-network study.

[100] Mol, *The Body Multiple*, 84.

[101] Ibid., 83.

more important than outside conditions. By thinking with enacting and enactment, practice is foregrounded and illustrates the ways objects are handled differently between sites. This underscores what Annemarie Mol highlights, that "objects have local identities" and that they can shift when the circumstances around them change.[102]

ANT, Context, and History

As others have argued, because of ANT's anti-context approach, it can be an empirically driven tool for historical research that helps move beyond sets of preconceived notions about structures and contexts.[103] My intention is not to work against context in the same way. However, one problem with context is that it can often be, as Rita Felski notes, a "box"; a fixed, static container that research objects are contained in and related to.[104] This "boxing" limits the ways in which phenomena can be understood and analysed and it closes off the potential for other, perhaps unexpected, possibilities to appear. Along these lines, Kristin Asdal and Ingunn Moser highlight that, because of this "boxing", context and contextualisation can be restricting and obfuscate the richness of historical materials and research objects.[105] My intention here is not to cast aside context completely. Rather, it is to avoid preconceived notions and maintain an openness for the possibility that contexts might be different on the level of practice, and ANTs stress on how objects are enacted in practice is helpful in this regard. This entails recontextualisation rather than decontextualisation. On the level of practice, assuming the actions of actors were influenced or otherwise situated in an outside context might be incorrect, empirically. For example, presuming that discussions about anti-septic wound care were situated within a contextual frame involving what we now understand as bacteriology is both incorrect and teleological. By focusing on how circumstances unfolded in practice, I have better been able to attend to the range of actors involved in my case studies and how multiple actors participated in the enactment of phenomena.

---

[102] Ibid., 55.

[103] See for example Rita Felski, "Context Stinks!". *New Literary History*. Vol. 42, No. 4, Autumn 2011, 573–591; Asdal, "Contexts in Action"; Kristin Asdal and Helge Jordheim, "Texts on the Move: Textuality and Historicity Revisited". *History and Theory*. Vol. 57, No. 1, March 2018, 56–74; Peter Skagius. *Den offentliga ohälsan: En historisk studie av barnpsykologi och psykiatri i svensk media, 1968–2008*. Diss., Linköping University, 2020.

[104] Felski, "Context Stinks", 577.

[105] Kristin Asdal and Ingunn Moser, "Experiments in Context and Contexting". *Science, Technology, and Human Values*. Vol. 34, No. 4, July 2012, 291–306, 295.

In my case, I have primarily examined medical journals and the relation between ANT, context, and textual materials bears mention here. Asdal notes that in the historian's use of ANT, texts should not be reduced to their contexts as models of explaining what actors "really" mean, but rather be interpreted more literally.[106] Clinical texts about Listerist antisepsis are one example where the few theoretical diversions indicate that the method's positive results seemed to have been more important for physicians than the theoretical basis of the method. One of the other interpretive possibilities here is understanding the situation where an utterance may occur. Annemarie Mol highlights that different situations imply different kinds of utterances. For example, she underlines that facts can be presented in a way that makes them seem controversial in medical journals, when that may not be the case in practice.[107] Some of my examples illustrate this, and keeping medium in mind has been a helpful tool in presenting a more nuanced image of the history of medicine.

This approach to text is additionally important given the circumstances involved in many of the texts in nineteenth-century medical journals. As Kristin Asdal and Helge Jordheim argue, texts are not static; they are on the move.[108] Perhaps the most explicit examples of this in my materials are the frequently published translated articles or summaries of articles. These texts have been published elsewhere, translated to the local vernacular, and published either in their entirety or summarised. But "move" also operates on a more subtle level. Asdal and Jordheim underline that because texts move, through space, time, but also can be emotionally moving, "they are not just mobile, but mobilizing".[109] They can enact change; for example, by inspiring the practitioners to test new optical devices, or mobilise practitioners. For this study, ANT has been useful in examining Swedish and Danish histories of device, practice, and knowledge in relation to previous research, but without placing my research objects in boxes consisting of preconceived notions. For instance, the richness and fluidity of the nineteenth-century Danish orthopaedic landscape can be better explained and understood by looking more closely at practice and practical concerns. In this sense, the actors and the intentions behind their actions cannot be explained by, or reduced to, a contextual framework that they do not have access to them-

---

selves. Rather, the inquiry involves the active process of world-making, which may open up and broaden the possibilities of historical inquiry.[110]

In addition to ANT, I will introduce three concepts in the following chapters that help explain some of the phenomena that this method has illuminated. Though not concepts within ANT as such, they serve to help clarify some of the practical problems encountered by practitioners for researchers. They also shift away from knowledge binarisms that, in some previous research, have tended to prioritise the importance of theoretical knowledge rather than practice-based knowledge. The first concept is that of the mindful hand, and it serves as general theme throughout my thesis. It is introduced in the book *The Mindful Hand* where Lissa Roberts and Simon Schaffer write how the separate categorisation of *epistemē* and *technē* has involved treating work of the head and the hand as distinct categories of knowledge. What they identify as "hierarchies of the hand and head" have "left us with a historical map shaped by oppositional and hierarchically ordered pairs: scholar/artisan, science/technology, pure/applied and theory/practice".[111] As my research shows, this distinction is not clear-cut. Surgical instrument makers were agents in the production and consumption of medical knowledge, even under so-called scientific terms. Though ANT does not seem to have been a guiding light in *The Mindful Hand*, I have found this hesitancy toward binarism to be a rewarding frame for my research.

The other two concepts are Michael Polanyi's tacit knowledge and Ludwik Fleck's thought-collectives. I will extrapolate on these in more detail in the subsequent empirical chapters, in particular chapter two. But, briefly, tacit knowledge according to Polanyi is difficult to communicate, in his well-known statement that "we can know more than we can tell".[112] This means that communicating and transferring knowledge built up through practice or other sensual means is difficult. This is also an important piece of the puzzle when relying on textual sources to understand practice. Articles indeed communicated practice and offered explanations about techniques or how to use devices. This helps account for the complexity of some medical texts that communicate this form of knowledge. Fleck's thought styles are interesting for me insofar as they help shed light on some of the difficulties that practitioners faced putting devices to use in practice. Thought styles are bodies of

---

[110] Asdal, "Contexts in Action", 397.

[111] Lissa Roberts and Simon Schaffer, "Preface", in *The Mindful Hand: Inquiry and Invention from the Late Renaissance to Early Industrialisation*, Lissa Roberts, et. al. (eds.), xiii–xxvii. Amsterdam: Edita KNAW, 2007, xiv.

[112] Michael Polanyi. *The Tacit Dimension.* Garden City, New York: Doubleday & Company, 1966, 4.

knowledge that are the result of collective processes.[113] Lensed devices for examining the body's internal structures and Fleck's distinction between looking and seeing are important here, in that these structures appear interesting only in relation to the formation of a thought style, a body of knowledge that explains why they are important, what to look for, and the distinctions between disease and healthy structures.

Chapter Outline

The chapters in this thesis are arranged thematically, with each focusing on a specific category of medical device. These overarching categories are mirrored and lensed instruments, orthopaedic devices, antiseptic practice and devices, and devices in relation to the transition from antiseptic practice to asepsis. Although the disposition does not follow a strict chronological order, there is some temporal logic behind their arrangement. Chapters two and three study the period between approximately 1855 and 1883, while chapters four and five examine developments between around 1865 to 1897. Each category of device corresponds with a period where their presence in journals was contentious or new and where practitioners were trying to figure out and motivate the use of instruments in these categories.

Following this introductory chapter, the second chapter centres lensed and mirror instruments, in particular ophthalmoscopes, laryngoscopes, rhinoscopes, and endoscopes. It engages with articles published about these devices, which were mainly of a practical character, teaching would-be users how to use them. All these instruments offered a look into the body and its many cavities, but there were both practical and knowledge-based tensions here. In some cases, the issue was not that the instruments themselves were problematic, but that practitioners needed to know what they were looking at, why it was important, and hone their visual perception. Medicine's relationship with theory and growing entanglements with science are engaged in greater detail, as I highlight that the sometimes-muddled waters of theory were not seen as insurmountable challenges, nor did they negate practical introduction.

The third chapter focused on the orthopaedic work of Camillus Nyrop as a case for highlighting the fluidity of Danish medicine. Nyrop and his work are difficult to place as that of solely a technician and his career is one of fluidity, which simultaneously weaves together technical knowledge and his

---

[113] Ludwik Fleck, "To Look, To See, To Know", in *Cognition and Fact: Materials on Ludwik Fleck*. Robert S. Cohen and Thomas Schnelle (eds.), 129–151. Dordrecht: D. Reidel Publishing Company, 1986.

hands-on work in orthopaedics. But professional boundaries between physicians and unlicensed medical practice were not strictly demarcated at this time, and they would remain so through the period of study. As such, Nyrop's work in orthopaedics and his participation in discussions in *Ugeskrift for Læger* were relatively unproblematic, even if he did meet critique. This fluid medical landscape will be examined through the lens of coexistence, where differences were tolerated to some degree, even if tensions could arise between licensed and unlicensed practitioners.

The fourth chapter looks at the advent of antisepsis, where I will continue with the contentious relationships between theory and practice. Here, I will frame the introduction of Listerist wound care around a practical problem, amputation, and attempts to develop safe and functional alternatives. Infection mitigating wound care, in this case Listerism, was important in this process, and often discussed together with practical issues in exploring alternatives to amputation. Furthermore, while Listerism has often been related to the development of bacteriology and germ theory, practitioners were more concerned with the method's practical implications. Many of the journal articles on antisepsis were practical guides rather than overviews or interventions on bacteriological theory. Because of the surgeon's relationship with device technologies in practice, many of these articles also included recommendations and ruminations on the relationship between Listerist practice and device.

This discussion leads into the fifth chapter where I will continue with microbes and look at the development of aseptic practice as a system of cleanliness. Listerism and asepsis were used concurrently, but aseptic practices increasingly required more consideration over space and object than Listerism did. This lends itself to a closer look at surgical venues toward the turn of the century in relation to aseptic practice and how the implementation of this system of cleanliness increasingly required institutional support. This chapter highlights that shifts in medical practice involved surgical instrument makers and that they were even active participants in the development of medical knowledge. For instance, Swedish instrument maker Max Stille opened a model surgical suite in 1894, which projected an ideal. It was his ideal, but one that was rooted in surgical practice and developments in wound care like asepsis. This will then lead into a study of Stille's work on examination and surgical tables, which were modified to conform with aseptic hygiene.

In the sixth and final chapter, I will summarise the results of this thesis. Following this conclusory summary, I will comment briefly on potential ways the actor-network approach might contribute to further studies that engage practical concerns and the importance of attending to the local when studying the proliferation and spread of medical knowledge. Finally, I will provide two suggestions for future research that engage some of themes that I highlight in the following empirical chapters.

2. Making the Once Invisible Visible:
Lensed Instruments and the Expansion of Diagnostics

In 1865, an unattributed article in *Ugeskrift for Læger* declared that physicians were now "living in the age of direct examination".[114] After this declaration, the article continued, stating that an "often heard statement to physicians, [that] 'They can't see inside us!', [was] losing ground and rightly so, as [several physicians] have taken the opposite standpoint and proven their assertations".[115] They could indeed see inside patients. A year earlier, Danish surgical instrument maker Camillus Nyrop wrote in the 1864 edition of his trade catalogue *Bandager og Instrumenter*, that "the idea of a reflector casting the reflection of sunlight or artificial light into and on various organs deep in the body, and thereby driving away the darkness, so that they could, to a larger extent than otherwise, be seen, and that a doctor can make diagnoses with a greater degree of certainty, has offered the physician and the manufacturer of these objects a great deal of territory to work and research in, in order to invent useful apparatuses".[116] Nyrop carried on, noting in particular that "recent years have produced an extraordinarily large number of various new creations in the form of lighting devices and mirrors for the pharynx, nose, ear, eye, urethra, large intestine, etc.".[117] Darkness had been driven away and physicians could look inside their patients: enter the age of direct examination. But driving away darkness was dependent on other factors than just the technological. This chapter will focus on mirrored and lensed instruments for the throat, nose, and eye in particular, laryngoscopes, rhinoscopes, and ophthalmoscopes, and the practical developments related

---

[114] [Anon.], "Endoskopien". *Ugeskrift for Læger*. Series 2, Vol. 42, No. 29, 17 June 1865, 449–458, 449. [Vi leve I de direkte Undersøgelsesmethoders Tid.]

[115] [Anon.], "Endoskopien", 449. [den almindelige, ofte hørte Udtalelse till Lægen: »De kan dog ikke see ind i oss!« taber stedse mere Terræn og det med Rette; thi Auenbrügger, Laennec, Récamier, Helmholtz, Garcia, Türck og Flere have været af den modsatte Mening og bevist deres Paastand.]

[116] Camillus Nyrop. *Bandager og Instrumenter afbildede og beskrevne med en tilføi et Prisfortegnelse.* Copenhagen: G.E.C. Gad, 1864, 149. [Den Tanke ved en Reflector at indkaste Gjenskin af Sollyset eller af kunstigt Lys i og paa forskjellige dybtliggende Organer og derved forjage Mørket, saa at disse i en høiere Grad end ellers kunne blive tilgængelige for Synet, og Lægen altsaa med mere Sikkerhed kan stille Diagnoser, har givet baade Lægen og Fabrikanten af deslige Gjenstande et stort Terrain at arbeide og forske i for at udfinde hensigtssvarende Apparater.]

[117] Nyrop, *Bandager og Instrumenter*, 149. [De senere Aar i Særdeleshed have derfor ogsaa fremkaldt en overordenlig stor Mængde forskjelligartede nye Skabninger i Form af Belysnings-Apparater og Speile for Svælget, Næsen, Øret, Øiet, Urinrøret, Masttarmen o.s.v.]

to the use of these devices from approximately 1850 until around 1860, with the above statements in mind.

The transitory nature of medicine around the mid-nineteenth century is clear in Danish and Swedish medical journals. Articles about weather phenomena[118] and animal migration[119] and their subsequent effects on health appeared alongside others on cellular pathology[120] and complex physiological functions[121]. The 1850s and 1860s in particular were indicative of overlap of different and fluid understandings of health and the cause of disease. This is illustrated in the following quote from an article from 1859, and is a key premise for this chapter–that medical practice and the understanding of illness was fluid. An anonymous physician remarked on the growing interest in so-called scientific medicine in an article in *Ugeskrift*, stating that "there is hardly anyone who would deny that the majority of physicians today, in the actual pursuit of their art, follow the teachings of the older schools in particular. Even the most exacting pathologist and the greatest physiologist and anatomist, will not be able to avoid receiving council from that [older] school and substantially stand by this point of view at the hospital bedside".[122] In other words, rather than merely examining cells to determine the cause of illness, physicians also looked at the bigger picture, because, according to the same article, "man is influenced by cosmic and local conditions, dependent

[118] See Alfred Hilarion Wistrand, "Sammandrag af års-rapporterna från Kongl. Allmänna Garrisons-Sjukhuset i Stockholm för åren 1846–1850, jemte summarisk redogörelse för Sjukvården å Sjukhusets medicinska afdelning under loppet af år 1850". *Hygiea*. Vol. 16, No. 7, July 1851, 385–414. Wistrand lists factors such as temperature and wind.

[119] See for example Gerhard Snellman, "Beskriftning öfver den i Kemi Socken Terwola Capell gångbara Skått-Sjukan". *Hygiea*. Vol. 12, No. 1, January 1850, 39–47; [Anon.], "Om de specifiske fremkaldende Aarsager til Epidemier". *Ugeskrift for Læger*. Series 2, Vol. 20, No. 20–21, 20 May 1854, 295–323. See also Annelie Drakman. *När kroppen slöt sig och blev fast: varför åderlåtning, miasmateori och klimatmedicin övergavs vid 1800-talets mitt*. Diss. Uppsala University, 2018. Her fourth chapter (72–98) in particular discusses notions of the body's relationship with its environment, including weather phenomena and temperature.

[120] See for example [Anon.], "Om Anæmie foraarsaget ved Formindskelse af Blodets Æggehvideholdighed og deraf följgende Vattersot". *Ugeskrift for Læger*. Series 2, Vol. 13, No. 7, 17 August 1850, 97–110; C. A. Rosborg, "Hjertats fettsjukdomar af Richard Quain, M.D.". *Hygiea*. Vol.15, No. 1, January 1853, 32–46; Sten Stenberg, "Kemisk undersökning af leucocythæmiskt blod". *Hygiea*. Vol. 20, No. 2, February 1858, 83–89.

[121] See for example [Anon.], "Om Hjerteforkamrenes Funktion". *Ugeskrift for Læger*. Series 2, Vol. 18, No. 17, 30 April 1853, 249–260; A. A. Langell, "Bidrag till läran om auskultationen af fel i hjertats valver och mynningar", *Hygiea*. Vol. 19, No. 10, October 1857, 683–700.

[122] [Anon.], "Pathologisk Physiologi–Cellularpathologi". *Ugeskrift for Læger*. Series 2, Vol. 31, No. 13–14. 12 March 1859, 193–202, 193–4. [Der er neppe Nogen, som vil nægte, at Flertallet af Nutidens Læger i den egentlige Udøvelse af deres Konst især følger ældre Skoles Lærdomme; selv den mest exakte Patholog og den største Physiolog og Anatom vil ikke kunne undgaae, dersom han kommer til Sygesengen, at hente Raad fra denne Skole og væsentlig stille sig paa dennes Standpunkt.]

on his parents, on food, on his spiritual and corporeal activities [and] on his mental state".[123] These quotations illustrate the overlap and tensions between different kinds of medical practice and illness. The "older schools", involving environmental conditions and its relationships with the body and illnesses was being augmented, as the first quotation above suggests, or as viewed by some, replaced, by one that more closely resembled practice in the natural sciences.[124]

These ideas prevailed concurrently during the 1850s and 1860s with other means of diagnostics and understandings of disease, even as interest in the function of the body's smaller structures, like cells and their roll in disease became a more common characteristic of journal articles.[125] This is contrary to the typical categorisations of medicine that appear in some of the popular Swedish literature on the history of medicine. Karin Johannisson states for example that the latter half of the nineteenth century introduced a medical monolith, erasing the previous multitude ways to understand illness.[126] Additionally, Gunnar Broberg highlights that Swedish medicine can be divided into nine distinct periods.[127] Broberg identifies the period between the late eighteenth-century and around 1850 as that of "romantic medicine", while the subsequent period, "industrial medicine", runs approximately from the mid-1860s to just prior to the first world war. Here, he connects the "romantic period" with the clinical and spiritual, while the "industrial" period is characterised by science, new illnesses, and a stronger medical profession. Most of the 1850s and the 1860s fall into a gap between romantic and later industrial medicine.[128]

While diagnosing and understanding illness became increasingly focused on microscopic origins, empiricism, and generalisation, as Johannisson highlights, this did not happen immediately, nor precisely around mid-

---

[123] [Anon.], "Pathologisk Physiologi", 200. [Mennesket er stillet under Indflydelse af kosmiske og lokale Forhold, er afhængig af sine Forældre, af Næringsmidlerne, af sin aandelige og legemilge Virksomhed, af sjælelige Tilstande]

[124] See for example William F. Bynum. *Science and the Practice of Medicine in the Nineteenth Century.* Cambridge: Cambridge University Press, 1994, 94.

[125] See Drakman, *När kroppen slöt sig* for a study that examines nineteenth-century understandings of diease in Sweden in greater detail.

[126] Karin Johannisson. *Kroppens tunna skal: Sex essäer om kropp, historia and kultur.* Stockholm: Pan, 1997, 189.

[127] The other periods Broberg discusses are *vikingatiden* [the Viking Age], *medeltiden* [the Middle Ages], *reformationen* [the Reformation], *barocken* [the Baroque], *upplysningen* [the Age of Enlightenment], *folkhemmet* [Folkhemmet, "the people's home"], and *postmodernismen* [postmodernism]. See Gunnar Broberg, "Liten svensk medicinhistoria", in *Til at stwdera läkedom: Tio studier i svensk medicinhistoria,* Gunnar Broberg (ed.), 9–50. Lund: Sekel, 2008.

[128] Broberg, "Liten svensk medicinhistoria", 22–23.

century when looking at Danish and Swedish medicine in particular.[129] And, although Broberg does note that periodisation entails problems, perhaps we need to be better attuned to what is at stake with the choices behind a linear periodisation of medicine and what it might leave out.[130] The multitude of different medical practices and ideas about diagnostics during these two decades seems to resist concise periodisation. Perhaps what we might understand as contradictions, as Broberg notes in reference to the Swedish physician Pehr Gustaf Cederschjöld, who was pioneer in obstetrics in Sweden as well as a dedicated adherent of animal magnetism, are just different elements of the totality of medicine at the time.

With the fluidity of medical practice during the 1850s and 1860s in mind, I will tackle some of the practical challenges that practitioners referenced in *Ugeskrift for Læger*, *Hygiea*, and *Hospitals-Tidende* in relation to the use of laryngoscopes, rhinoscopes, and ophthalmoscopes. Medicine was undergoing theoretical and technical changes, which had bearing on the use of these devices. An important characteristic of these types of instruments was that they made structures once difficult or impossible to see with the naked eye, visible. Although lensed instruments had existed for centuries, the practical use of these devices was related to new understandings of illness, and with reference points to other devices such as microscopes. These features altered the physician's relationship with clinical work and diagnostics. Experiential possibility did not in and of itself delineate the role they would play as diagnostic instruments; they were also instrumental in accumulating bodies of knowledge of both practical and scientific characters in order to propagate for their utility. The age of direct examination and the devices that illuminated the dark recesses of the body were dependent on one another.

---

[129] Annelie Drakman examined this extensively in her doctoral thesis, *När kroppen slöt sig*. She examines the shift from an understanding of illness that, according to her, worked from "flows", both bodily and environmental, to one defined by "boundary protection". This latter principle entails the body requires protection from harmful matter that can cause disorders. She notes that this shift occurred around 1865. She contests that this change was dependent on the introduction of bacteriology and is clear in pointing out that these two thought styles existed simultaneously, with boundary protecting medicine gaining influence around mid-century. She also highlights the overlap between these two understandings practically–they did not completely replace each other–rather, when boundary protecting medicine became the dominant type, physicians who were more convinced by flows found other contexts to practice in.

[130] Annemarie Mol points out that categories imply exclusion. What does not fit is left out and put somewhere else. In the case of the above periodisation, it is simply left out. Annemarie Mol. *The Body Multiple: Ontology in Medical Practice*. Durham, NC: Duke University Press, 2003, 135–136.

Physicians needed to know and understand what they were looking at. Developments in medical microscopy, both in terms of examining cellular structures in the body as well as practical developments in optics, were important. This will set the stage for this chapter. Ludwik Fleck's thought styles and Michael Polanyi's tacit knowledge will provide some analytical help here. Physicians had to both know what they were looking at and *why* it was meaningful, but they also required tacit knowledge, the knowledge of a sensual type that is difficult to convey verbally. Fleck distinguishes between the acts of looking and seeing, stating for example that "in order to see one has to know what is essential and what is inessential [...] otherwise we look but do not see, we look intently at too many details without grasping the observed form as a definite entirety".[131] A thought style is a shared body of knowledge developed within a collective body, like in the medical or scientific communities.[132] For the purpose of this chapter, it is the requisite knowledge in order to use the lensed instruments discussed as diagnostic tools. In the case of tacit knowledge, it can be likened to the knowledge required to use these devices seamlessly in practice. When one knows how, these activities are carried out automatically. But bringing awareness to them and conveying specific movements can be challenging, and key parts of a performance must be identified in order to transfer this kind of knowledge.[133] Both tacit knowledge and thought styles underscore the importance of theory and practice in the use of these devices, and the marrying of these two forms of knowledge.

Following this frame of reference, I will examine discussions about laryngoscopes, rhinoscopes, and ophthalmoscopes in medical journals and the relationships between theory and practice with regards to their use. On the one hand, being able to see inside patients was a novelty. On the other hand, practitioners needed to know what they were looking at and navigate the device's use in order to motivate the practical application of these devices, meaning both theoretical knowledge and the training of perception and practice were key factors in their use. But "seeing inside", when theory and practice were better aligned, was not always particularly practical even after physicians had a better grasp of the visual information presented before them. Physicians were also met with lighting challenges, as I will illustrate over the final pages of this chapter. This required them to adapt to the

---

[131] Ludwik Fleck, "To Look, To See, To Know", in *Cognition and Fact: Materials on Ludwik Fleck*. Robert S. Cohen and Thomas Schnelle (eds.), 129–151. Dordrecht: D. Reidel Publishing Company, 1986, 130.

[132] Fleck, "To Look, To See, To Know", 148.

[133] Polanyi uses the phrase "silencing the noise". Michael Polanyi. *The Tacit Dimension*. Garden City, New York: Doubleday & Company, 1966, 14. For knowledge transfer specifically, see pg. 30.

simultaneous use of a myriad of lighting apparatuses alongside their examinations in order to assist their trained and training eyes, which might subsequently be altered in order to promote ease of use. Importantly, changes in diagnostic practice were made possible by different understandings of the body, and the equipment that made new diagnostic methods possible.

Making Diagnosis

In terms of the clinical work involved in making diagnosis, the period indicates a change in focus from larger structures in the body, such as organs, to smaller structures and a shift in the relationship between the clinical presentation of a disorder and its origin. William Bynum uses scurvy as an example, which would present clinically as bleeding of the gums or as blood under the skin, but this did not necessarily mean that the site of the primary illness was in the blood.[134] This understanding developed concurrent to other understandings of illness, dependent on environmental factors, humoral medicine, miasma, and others.[135] Although the shift in focus might not have immediately overtaken other clinical understandings, it added to the fluidity of medical practice around mid-century. Journals filled a normative function here in publishing work that was focused on locating the origin of disease in the small structures of the body, such as cells.[136] However, connected to their normative function, journals were important in the establishment of a thought style involving the body's less visible and cohesive structures.

In their surveys of the history of medicine, both William Bynum and John Pickstone make similar points about the growing opportunity for carrying out scientific work, in terms of both career prospects as well as scientific understandings of the origin of disease.[137] Even if this was the case in the context they examine, the majority of physicians in Sweden and Denmark were still private generalists. However, medical journals followed scientific

---

[134] Bynum, *Science and the Practice of Medicine*, 124.

[135] See Drakman, *När kroppen slöt sig*, in particular chapters 4 and 5 where she details some of the characteristics of the medical systems she discusses: the earlier based on "flows" and the latter focused on barriers from one's surroundings. See also the summary in fn 129 in this chapter.

[136] See Roy Porter, "Introduction", in *Medical Journals and Medical Knowledge: Historical Essays*. William F. Bynum, Stephen Lock and Roy Porter (eds.), 1–5. New York: Routledge, 2019. Porter highlights in the case of *The Lancet* for example, that the periodical likely helped set the tone for norms in medical practice. I discuss this in a little more detail in the first chapter of this thesis, where norms outside of Sweden and Denmark might have also helped in their establishment in these two countries due to the prevalence of translated overviews. See pg. 33ff.

[137] Bynum, *Science and the Practice of Medicine*, 94; John Pickstone. *Ways of Knowing: A New History of Science, Technology and Medicine*. Chicago: The University of Chicago Press, 2001, 111.

developments and published both original articles and translated overviews from foreign medical journals on them.[138] Many of these explored topics involving cellular chemistry, physiology, and pathology. Some examples include articles on the blood's coagulation and chemical composition, and other topics such as arrhythmias in the heart, nerve endings in amputated limbs, and tumours.[139] Integrated approaches between medicine and other scientific disciplines, like chemistry, became increasingly relevant in the techniques involved in carrying out analytical work, which principally drew medicine closer to the natural sciences. Furthermore, this work, although distant from the realities of most physicians, provided a new basis of understanding the body on the cellular level. In Karin Johannisson's book *Kroppens tunna skal*, she states that the developments in medical science after the 1850s changed the visibility of disease, where it "moved from the body's visible exterior to an interior space where only the physician had a key".[140] But, how were they able to see into this interior space?

Devices like microscopes and other lensed devices, like the ophthalmoscope, rhinoscope, and laryngoscope, will be discussed in more detail later. However, they highlight the physical repertoire physicians could include in order to do diagnostic work on the body's microscopic structures, and the necessity of technological tools to practically assist this origin-seeking type of medical understanding. This stands in contrast to the body's relationship to environmental factors and humoral medicine for instance. In the quote above, Johannisson identifies a significant change; however, she attributes it largely to bacteriology, pathological anatomy, and illness conceptualised

---

[138] In the Swedish context see for example Broberg, "Liten svensk medicinhistoria"; Drakman, *När kroppen slöt sig*, 39–41 in particular; Motzi Eklöf. *Läkarens Ethos: Studier i den svenska läkarkårens identiteter, intressen och ideal, 1890–1960*. Diss. Tema Hälsa och samhälle, Linköping University, 2000. In the Danish context see Signild Vallgårda, et. al. *Sundhedsvæsen og sundhedspolitik*. Copenhagen: Munksgaard, 2010; Nick Nyland. *De praktiserande læger I Danmark, 1800–1910: Træk af det historiske grundlag for almen medicin*. Odense: Audit Projekt Odense, 2000.

[139] See for example Rosborg, "Hjertats fettsjukdomar"; Langell, "Bidrag till läran om auskultationen"; Stenberg, "Kemisk undersökning af leucocythæmiskt blod"; O. A. Svalin, "Om den fibroplastiska tumören; diskussion rörande diagnostiken af svulster, hvilka blifvit ansedde som kräftartade". *Hygiea*. Vol. 15, No. 1. January 1853, 24–32; [Anon.], "Om de paa Nervestammernes Ender ved amputerede Lemmer forekommende Knuder Prof. Wdel. Zeitschr. d. k. k. Gellesch. D. Aertze zu Wien. Jan. 1855". *Ugeskrift for Læger*. Series 2, Vol. 25, No. 5, 26 January 1856, 65–73; [Anon.], "Claude Bernards nyere Undersögelser om Blodets Egenskaber (Af et Brev fra Paris.)". *Ugeskrift for Læger*. Series 2, Vol. 28, No. 18, 10 April 1858, 265–277; [Anon.], "Om Blodets Koagulation (B. Richardson: The cause of the coagulation of the blood anm. i The brit. and for. med. chir. review. Juli 1858)". *Ugeskrift for Læger*. Series 2, Vol. 29, No. 6, 31 July 1858, 74–84.

[140] Johannisson, *Kroppens tunna skal*, 190. [sjukdom flyttades från kroppens synliga yta till ett inre rum dit bara läkaren hade nyckeln.]

around cause rather than symptom.[141] She does not mention the role of devices, which although they would not completely open the door themselves, using her key metaphor, they might unlock the deadbolt. Seeing devices as the sole catalysts for change would be both reductive and deterministic. Still, the overemphasis on analytical work and theory mitigates the point of practicality: looking into the interiors of the body also aligned with technological developments, even if they were not specific catalysts. As Lissa Roberts and Simon Schaffer emphasize in their introduction to *The Mindful Hand*, the focus on mental labour has given us a historiography shaped by oppositional hierarchies, like that of theory and practice.[142] Rather, they highlight the hybridity of knowledge production. This is clear when devices are acknowledged in these processes, where theory and practice together were important in order to make use of them and gauge their usefulness.

Many examinations were made possible in part by technological developments, including the advent of the microscope, improvements in lenses, and the introduction of other mirrored and lensed instruments used for analytical and diagnostic work in medicine. While microscopes had been around for centuries, the achromatic lenses, invented in the 1830s, minimised chromatic and spherical aberration. This brought red and blue light into a common focus and reduced distortion and coloured haloes in the field of vision, which made microscopic images more reliable.[143] Although it is unlikely all physicians were interested in or capable of carrying out microscopic examinations, similar devices, that made the invisible visible, became much handier for the everyday practitioner. The ophthalmoscope, laryngoscope, and rhinoscope are examples of this. The ophthalmoscope was introduced in 1851 by German physiologist Hermann von Helmholtz. In 1854, Manuel García, a Spanish vocal pedagogue, published observations of his vocal cords and larynx, seen with a provisional laryngoscope made with two mirrors and

---

[141] Ibid., 190.

[142] Lissa Roberts and Simon Schaffer, "Preface", in *The Mindful Hand: Inquiry and Invention from the Late Renaissance to Early Industrialisation*, Lissa Roberts, et. al. (eds.), xiii–xxvii. Amsterdam: Edita KNAW, 2007, xiv.

[143] See for example Brian Bracegirdle, "J. J. Lister and the Establishment of Histology". *Medical History*. Vol. 21, No. 2, April 1977, 187–191. J. J. Lister designed some of the first achromatic lenses and was the father of surgeon Joseph Lister, who will be discussed in greater detail in the next chapter in relation to antiseptic surgery. Bracegirdle also notes that French pathologist Xavier Bichat did not trust the microscope and worked without one. He was still able to distinguish a number of tissue structures and is widely referred to as the founder of modern histology (the study of the microscopic anatomy of biological tissues). For the French context see for example Ann La Berge, "Medical Microscopy in Paris, 1830–1855", in *French Medical Culture in the Nineteenth Century*, Ann La Berge and Mordechai Feingold (eds.). 296–326. Amsterdam: Editions Rodopi, 1994.

using reflected sunlight.[144] The technique used for examinations of the nasal cavity developed during this same period operated on similar principles as laryngoscopy, with a mirrored device looking from the throat into the nasal cavity (posterior rhinoscopy), and was largely developed by Austrian physiologist Johann Nepomuk Czermak in 1860 from the principles of laryngoscopy. These devices helped relate clinical presentation with the origin of a disorder by aiding physicians in looking inside the body while being minimally invasive.

Lensed and mirrored devices like these opened up cavities that were previously invisible to the naked eye, allowing physicians to "look inside" as the quote that opens the chapter highlights. This helped them to "observe [...] different constitutions and also judge the condition of the muscles and their associated nerves".[145] The Swedish physician Carl Sundberg echoes this sentiment in a book from 1920 about the history of medicine and its societal importance in the nineteenth century. Sundberg stated that "for cavities that were not directly available for the eye to see, such as the oesophagus, bladder, and the urinary tract, etc., tube-formed instruments were put together with mirrored apparatuses and small, electrical lights inside, that could be inserted in these cavities and also made them visible for the eye".[146] But making these cavities visible was not the only factor in the use of these instruments. They had to be handy, practitioners had to know how to use them, and they had to develop techniques to work with the multitudes of patient-bodies they were confronted with. These devices assisted in the development of a thought style of illness that allowed physicians to analyse what they saw and contributed to the tacit knowledge necessary to carry out these examinations. In other words, physicians had to know what they were looking at and why it was meaningful, and they had to be able to use the devices discussed in this chapter with some utility. Both these problems related to one another, as we shall see in the following sections.

[144] Regarding Helmholtz and the ophthalmoscope, see F. A. Ekström, "Ögonspegelns bruk vid diagnosen af sjukdomar i ögats inre delar". *Hygiea*. Vol. 16, No. 11, November 1854, 649–656, 652.
Regarding the laryngoscope see H. Hülphers, "Om luftstrup-spegeln, laryngoskopet". *Hygiea*. Vol. 20, No. 8, August 1858, 469–474. On the rhinoscope, see [Anon.], "Rhinoskopi: Efter Szermak [sic] (W. Wschr. 16de Febr. 1861)". *Ugeskrift for Læger*. Series 2, Vol. 34, No. 15, 23 March 1861, 225–231.
[145] Carl Sundberg. *Läkarvetenskapen och dess samhällsbetydelse under det nittonde århundradet*. Stockholm: P.A. Nordsted & Söners Förlag, 1920, 101. [Genom iakttagelsen av... olika utseende också bedömandet av de musklers och dem tillhörande nervers tillstånd.]
[146] Sundberg, *Läkarvetenskapen och dess samhällsbetydelse*, 101. [För sådana rum och kanaler, som ej voro direkt tillgängliga för ögat, såsom matstrupen, urinblåsan och urinvägarna m. m., sammansattes rörformade instrument med spegelanordningar och små elektriska lampor i deras inre, vilket allt infördes i dessa hålrum och kanaler och gjorde också dessa tillgängliga för ögat].

The Microscope and Visual Perception

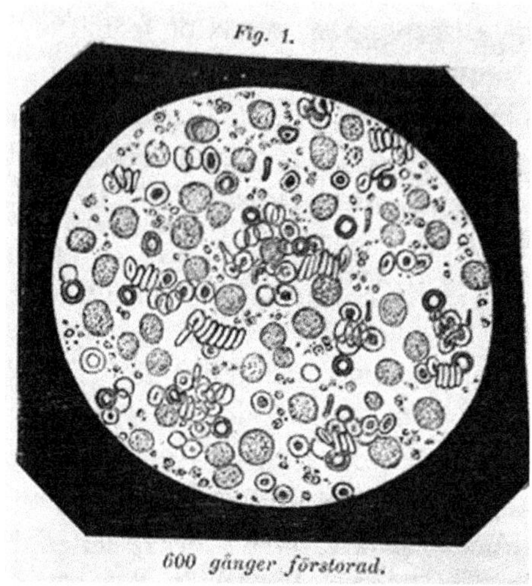

Fig. 3. From a blood sample taken from a patient. Magnus Huss, "Sällsyntare sjukdoms-fall". *Hygiea*. Vol. 18, No. 8, August 1856, 525–555, 529.

Ponder over the image above and what it illustrates for a moment. In an article in *Hygiea* from 1855, physician Magnus Huss detailed the diagnosis of several patients who presented at Seraphim Hospital in Stockholm. Included in this article were several drawings of the microscopic analyses used to diagnose the patients, including figure 3. The image above is a 600x enlargement of blood from a patient who presented with a nosebleed. Huss has drawn blood after cutting the patient's arm and analysed it under a micro-scope. The "blood disks"–*bloddiskerna*, his terminology, blood cells would be ours–are the objects with the light rings and dark centres as well as the objects with the dark rings and light centres. Huss analysed and compared the blood from the nosebleed and the scratch in order to help reach his diagnosis after observing physical signs in the patient, which was *leucocythæmia splencia* (splenic leukaemia), based on the differences in white blood cells–*ofärgade korpusklerna* "white corpuscles" in his terms–observed in the sample from the cut.[147] The patient in question fell ill as a young boy and had health problems since then. He arrived at Seraphim Hospital in Stockholm with pain in his sacrum and lower extremities, bleeding, and painful blisters filled with blood.[148] Huss examined the patient, took his pulse, had a colleague do

---

[147] Magnus Huss, "Sällsyntare sjukdomsfall". *Hygiea*. Vol. 18, No. 8, August 1856, 525–555, 529.
[148] Huss, "Sällsyntare sjukdomsfall", 527.

a urinalysis, and examined the blood. The clinical diagnosis of splenic leukaemia stemmed from these examinations, in particular the microscopic blood analysis. This is an illustration of how, with the help of a device such as a microscope, physicians could better connect clinical presentation with the origin of the patient's disorder.

There are two important points that this article and its accompanying image illustrate. Firstly, it highlights the kinds of analytical work done with microscopes in order to diagnose patients, and how this worked alongside other methods of diagnosis. Secondly, it illustrates the looking/seeing conundrum exemplified by Fleck. Visual perception was an important aspect of medicine's growing subdisciplines. According to Henning Schmidgen in a study on the production of visual perception in nineteenth century physiology, Czermak, the physiologist who developed the rhinoscope, underscored the importance of visual perception in the development of physiology.[149] Other studies, like Richard Kremer's work on Prussian physiology, also highlight the importance of cultivating the visual perception of physiologists and its relationship with the development of physiology in Prussia.[150] Both Kremer and Schmidgen use the German word *Anschauung*, meaning roughly sense impression and the process of making these sense perceptions conscious.[151] This concept has similar implications as Fleck's thought styles and differentiation between looking and seeing.[152] Furthermore, *Anschauung* was best cultivated through experiential tasks rather than descriptive ones, as Kremer and Schmidgen point out. The relationship between clinical presentations and disease origins needed to be substantiated with a body of knowledge, as well as supported through the practitioners own developed visual perception, which in the case of my study, was supported with the help of lensed devices and journal articles detailing their practical use.

Another important factor for the use of the microscope, as well as the other lensed and mirrored instruments discussed below, was skill and the effort it took to build up technique. Like training visual perception, this kind

---

[149] Henning Schmidgen, "Pictures, Preparations, and Living Processes: The Production of Immediate Visual Perception (Anschauung) in Late-19th-Century Physiology". *Journal of the History of Biology*. Vol. 37, No. 3, Autumn 2004, 477–513, 483.

[150] Richard L. Kremer, "Building Institutes for Physiology in Prussia, 1836–1846: Contexts, Interests and Rhetoric", in *The Laboratory Revolution in Medicine*. Andrew Cunningham and Perry Williams (eds.), 72–109. Cambridge: Cambridge University Press, 2002.

[151] Kremer, "Building Institutes for Physiology in Prussia", 94; Schmidgen, "Pictures, Preparations and Living Processes", 283–284.

[152] See also Nicola Mößner, "Scientific Images as Circulating Ideas: An Application of Ludwik Fleck's Thought Styles". *Journal for General Philosophy of Science/Zeitschrift für allgemeine Wissenschaftstheorie*. Vol. 47, No. 2, September 2016, 307–329.

of sensual knowledge was difficult to transmit textually, and even though many articles detailed how to use microscopes and other instruments in the medical journals, at least some of the know-how was in building up one's own technique. Michael Polanyi states that "we can know more than we can tell".[153] This dimension of knowing highlights the difficulties in transferring some kinds of knowledge that are built up through experience or other, more sensual means. Kremer also makes this observation in physiological pedagogy, where education needed to be intuitive and practical, as "only then could the gap between medical theory and praxis be bridged".[154] Similarly, the use of the microscope, as described above, and the uses of the ophthalmoscope, rhinoscope, and laryngoscope, were discussed in terms of both theory and praxis. Aside from the tacit knowledge required in order to use a microscope, users were required to decipher what they were looking at and sorting, analysing, and making sense of the information provided. Making use of this information was also a tool of delegation. Physicians delegated the task of observation, at least to some degree, to the microscope itself, which aided and amplified the eye's ability to observe miniscule structures of the body. In this way, data obtained with the help of a device, the microscope, became an important tool in medicine.[155]

Though the microscope had been around in different forms for several centuries, both *Hygiea* and *Ugeskrift* are testaments to the expansion of medical microscopy throughout the 1850s and the growing value of the microscope as a tool.[156] Bynum highlights the importance of the microscope for nineteenth century medicine, stating that technical developments in microscopy was enabling better analysis and becoming an important scientific tool.[157] He additionally states that microscopy began to function as a symbol for the scientific authority of medicine and that, through the work of Rudolf Virchow around mid-century, "microscopes encouraged doctors to think about the dynamics of disease, about the genesis of lesions rather than their gross, end-stage structures".[158] Indeed, physicians in both these

---

[153] Polanyi, *The Tacit Dimension*, 4.

[154] Kremer, "Building Institutes for Physiology in Prussia", 100.

[155] Stuart Blume. *Insight and Industry: On the Dynamics of Technological Change in Medicine.* Cambridge, Mass.; MIT Press, 1992, 13.

[156] See for example Charles Singer, who offers examples of microscopic examination of ulcers from the seventeenth century, including Athanasius Kircher's work on the composition of blood and the nature of infection. Charles Singer, "Notes on the Early History of Microscopy". *Proceedings of the Royal Society of Medicine.* Vol. 7, 1914, 247–279.

[157] Bynum, *Science and the Practice of Medicine*, 100.

[158] Ibid., 123.

countries received information about Virchow's work through medical journals. For example, in 1858 Virchow lectured on cellular pathology in Berlin, later published in English in the volume *Cellular Pathology*, stating *omnis cellula e cellula*: every cell originates from another cell.[159] This statement was referenced in articles on cellular pathology in *Ugeskrift* and *Hygiea* the following year, 1859.[160] Swedish and Danish physicians who read their local medical journals would have been familiar with Virchow and other new information from the field, and were even active disseminators of foreign publications and lectures.

Journals provide other examples of interest in studies in cellular pathology from abroad, which helped establish a requisite thought style to dutifully carry out examinations with the device. One example, an article by O. A. Svalin in *Hygiea* from 1853, compiled French research into diagnosing tumours through microscopy. By looking at French work, Svalin encouraged surgeons in particular to, "with all the forces of [the profession's] influence work towards the diffusion of the use of microscopic studies in diagnosing tumours".[161] After illustrating the possibilities of using microscopy to identify and classify common types of growths, Svalin stated that "as soon as surgeons become more comfortable with this means of examination, compile and compare observations amongst each other, they will without question have no difficulties making diagnoses, without needing to examine growths themselves under microscopes".[162] Articles such as Svalin's could have additionally assisted practitioners in cultivating the necessary sensual knowledge in order to carry out analysis with the device by providing both analytical and practical frames of reference.

Local studies attracted attention as well. The Karolinska Institute's then-professor of anatomy, Anders Retzius, was an active participant in the Swedish Society of Medicine's meetings, presenting results, for example,

---

[159] Rudolf Virchow. *Cellular Pathology*. Trans. Frank Chance. London: John Churchill, 1860, 27.

[160] [Anon.], "Pathologisk Physiologi"; Christian Lovén, "Om Begreppen Retning och Retbarhet, af Prof. Rudolf Virchow (Archive für pathologishe Anatomie und Physiologie und für klinische Medicin Bd. XIV (neue Folge Bd. IV) Hft. 1 ausgegeben in August 1858.)". *Hygiea*. Vol. 20, No. 5, May 1859, 277–294.

[161] Svalin, "Om den fibroplastisak tumören", 29. [Åt detta sällskap skall, som jag hoppas, hedern blifva förbehållen att med hela kraften af dess inflytande medverka till utbredandet af de mikroskopiska studiernas användning på diagnostiken af tumörerna.]

[162] Ibid., 31. [Så snart chirurgerna blifvit mera förtrogne med detta undersökningsmedel, och hunnit samla samt sinsemellan jemföra en hel följd af iakttagelser, skall det utan tvifvel blifva för dem lätt att genast fastställa diagnosen, utan att de först behöfva undersöka svulsterna sjelfva under mikroskopet.]

from microscopic studies of tissues, organs, and pathologies.[163] These microscopic examinations, according to surgeon H. Santesson, were "particularly worthy of attention".[164] Attention that they received: microscopy was part of the surgical module for medical students at the medical school the Karolinska Institute from 1855, and much like microscopy, the ophthalmoscope, the aforementioned handheld lensed device for examining the eye, was also part of this module. Richard Kremer notes that students at German-language universities had already built their teaching around students' competency in basic microscopic analysis by the mid 1840s.[165]

The growing use of the microscope in medicine is also clear in the Karolinska Institute's archive. The earliest inventory list in this archive is from 1859, so material acquired earlier than so might remain unaccounted for. A microscope makes its first appearance in archival records in 1860 in the chemical laboratory's inventory, as well as two microscopes in one of the Institute's rooms labelled *Norra Rummet* (the North Room).[166] Although records are unavailable between 1861 and 1873, device related acquisitions, or at least inventories, increased, including a number of new departments that did not appear in the records from 1860. In 1881 and 1882 for example, five microscopes are listed in inventories from eight different departments.[167] These records do not provide information about use or sharing but the growing number of microscopes at the university over the years indicates that any previous actions of communal distribution and/or use likely would have become more limited, with departments acquiring their own instruments and adapting them to their specific needs. In conjunction with this institutional development, a drop-off in the number of articles in *Hygiea* detailing microscope usage and technical details began in the 1860s, where articles mentioned microscopic analysis, but no longer went into detail about how it

---

[163] See for example *Förhandlingar vid Svenska läkarsällskapets sammankomster*, 7 September 1851; 14 September 1851.

[164] *Förhandlingar vid Svenska läkarsällskapets sammankomster*, 7 September 1851. [förtjena en särskild uppmärksamhet]

[165] Kremer, "Building Institutes for Physiology in Prussia", 100. For the module for students at the Karolinska Insitute, see [Anon.], "Berättelse om Undervisningen vid Kongl. Carolinska Medico-Kirurgiska Institutet Under år 1855". *Hygiea*, Vol. 18, No. 1, January 1856, 3–15, 8.

[166] SE/RA/420128/02 Riksarkivet, Karolinska institutet 1813–1980, D I 1: Inventarieförteckningar 1859–1892.

[167] SE/RA/420128/02 Riksarkivet, Karolinska institutet 1813–1980, D I 1: Inventarieförteckningar 1859–1892.

was done.[168] In this sense, the 1850s can be understood as a period of development, instructing practitioners how to undertake this kind of analytical work and working out a functional thought style, and subsequent articles presumed the reader might already have the requisite tacit knowledge to conduct the work themselves.[169]

There is an important practical distinction to be made here: all physicians likely did not use microscopes as part of their everyday work or understood it as a useful device. They were expensive. In the Karolinska Institute's archive, one of the earliest microscopes to appear in their inventory in 1860 was valued at 384.60 riksdaler riksmynt (rdr rmt). For the sake of comparison, a city physician [*stadsläkare*], who was employed by the district they worked in, made 700 rdr rmt per year in 1865.[170] These devices might have been out of reach for regular physicians not engaged in research. Interestingly, there was little direct critique towards the use of tools to augment the sense in *Ugeskrift*, *Hygiea* or *Hospitals-Tidende*. This stands in contrast to other research that notes a broader scepticism toward their introduction.[171] In contrast, the devices I discuss below, the ophthalmoscope, rhinoscope, and laryngoscope, are all hand-held devices that were used in the direct examination of patients. Rather than being the domain of hospital or university physicians, they could be adopted to a greater extent by generalists to assist with their clinical work, especially with the analytical and practical knowledge required for their successful use. Furthermore, they were less costly. An ophthalmoscope in Camillus Nyrop's *Bandager og Instrumenter* was priced at 7 rigsdaler and a laryngoscope at just 1 rigsdaler and 3 marks. For the sake of comparison, Nick

---

[168] See for example *Förhandlingar vid Svenska läkarsällskapets sammankomster*, 6 November 1860 on a case of extrauterine pregnancy whereby a microscopic analysis of the different tissues, including a tumour and the placenta were conducted. J. Björkén, "Bentumör i sinus frontalis". *Hygiea*. Vol. 26, No. 1, January 1864, 17–27; [Anon.], "Koppernes pathologiske Anatomi". *Ugeskrift for Læger*. Series 2, Vol. 40, No. 28–29, 18 June 1864, 433–449.

[169] Annelie Drakman highlights that in Sweden, for example, instruction in medical school was largely based on texts from the period of classical antiquity up until approximately the 1850s, but became more empirical from the 1870s onward. She notes that in the 1870s a degree in medicine included instruction in anatomy, histology, physiology, medical and physiological chemistry, general pathology, obstetrics, general surgery, the history of medicine and physiological obstetrics. Drakman, *När kroppen slöt sig*, 43.

[170] See Lars O. Lagerqvist. *Vad kostade det? Priser och löner, från medeltid till våra dagar*. Lund: Historiska Media, 2011, 140.

[171] In *Objectivity*, Lorraine Daston and Peter Galison note regarding French physician Alfred Donné's *Cours de microscopie complémentaire des études médicales*, an atlas from 1845 that used photographs, that the author's inclusion of photographs was in part due to his colleagues' mistrust of microscopic images, seeing them as illusions. Lorraine Daston and Peter Galison. *Objectivity*. New York: Zone Books, 2010, 235. The French pathology Xavier Bichat is one example. See also Bracegirdle, "J. J. Lister and the Establishment of Histology".

Nyland notes that in the period between 1847 and 1870 a district physician [*distriktslæge*] earned around 950 rigsdaler per year.[172]

Practice Makes Perfect

The growing importance of the microscope in medicine served as a frame for the use of other lensed instruments during the period, in spite of their practical differences. Not only did it help visualise internal structures such as cells, it also provided a descriptive reference for physicians, a means of comparison that the reader would likely have been familiar with. Both the ophthalmoscope and microscope were part of the Karolinska Institute's surgical module from 1858. Additionally, when the ophthalmoscope was discussed as a new tool for ophthalmologists, the microscope was invoked as a means of reference. In 1852, an overview in *Ugeskrift* of ophthalmological literature from outside the country used the microscope as a reference, stating that the ophthalmoscope was "quite like a microscope [...] where one would be able to achieve a higher degree of enlargement".[173] Aside from the similarities in creating enlargements of small structures, this invocation could be analytically understood in Fleck's terms as well: it offered a referential thought style that the readership of medical journals would have been familiar with.[174] Furthermore, with the correct technique, one could eventually see the retina with ten times the enlargement of the naked eye.[175] Technique was important for being able to see anything anyway. The inventor of the ophthalmoscope, Hermann von Helmholtz, found, in developing the instrument, that the direction of the light source was a determining factor in being able to see into the eye at all, and that the observer must look into the patient's eye in the same direction the light is cast, for example.[176]

Still, cellular pathology in general and Virchow's work specifically needed to acquire practical relevance. Other scholars have pointed out that the bevy of new and sometimes contradictory scientific information circulating at the

---

[172] Nick Nyland. *De praktiserande læger I Danmark, 1800–1910: Træk af det historiske grundlag for almen medicin*. Odense: Audit Projekt Odense, 2000, 186.

[173] E. Paulli, "Undersögelsen af Nethinden i det levende Öie". *Ugeskrift for Læger*. Series 2, Vol. 17, No. 23, 4 December 1852, 353–364, 358. [som Ganske ligner et Mikroskop ... man vilde være istand til at opnaae en höiere Grad af Forstörrelse]

[174] Fleck, "To Look, To See, To Know", 144.

[175] Paulli, "Undersögelsen af Nethinden", 360.

[176] Ekström, "Ögonspegelns bruk", 652.

time might have made practitioners approach with caution.[177] However, it was practice, not theory that seemed most acute for Swedish and Danish physicians. Looking inside patients with these instruments was challenging, and physicians needed to understand the significance of what they were looking at and the variations observed. Technical issues, such as learning to use the instrument and knowing what to look for were problems, as was the weather. Additionally, early lensed devices might not help much with visualisation, with the previous overview of ophthalmological literature from 1852 stating that the object of examination appeared "quite unclear and small" with one device.[178] There were different attempts at producing a better image in order increase the use of the device, and the article mentions a number of different devices by Helmholtz and other Germans Rüete and Meyerstein, and the French Follin, as well as technical experiments with light in order to produce better images.

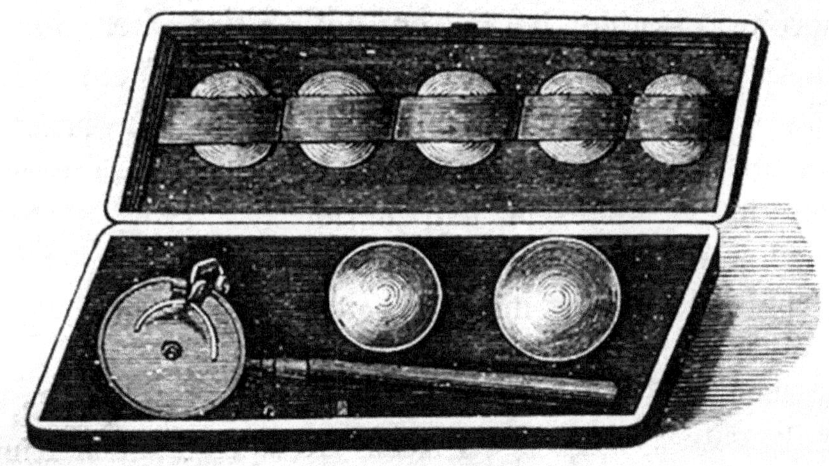

Fig. 4. An ophthalmoscope set with concave mirrors and lenses of different strengths. This particular ophthalmoscope's design is attributed to German ophthalmologist Richard Liebreich. Camillus Nyrop. *Bandager og Instrumenter afbildede og beskrevne med en tilføi et Prisfortegnelse.* Copenhagen: G.E.C. Gad, 1864, 161.

---

[177] Daston and Galison, *Objectivity*, 213. Solveig Jülich also points this out in relation to the introduction of x-ray apparatuses in Sweden, where their practical use was questioned initially, and the hopes of, for example surgeons, were somewhat dashed by the quality of images the early apparatuses actually produced. See Solveig Jülich. *Skuggor av sanning. Tidig svensk radiologi och visuell kultur.* Diss. Linköping University, 2002, 267.

[178] Paulli, "Undersögelsen af Nethinden", 361. [ganske utydelig og meget formindsket]

The first Swedish physician in the period to praise the ophthalmoscope in an original article, F. A. Ekström, stated in 1854 that he hoped "that the instrument would have a future, as it has many positive qualities [...]. It is quite simple, so that even one of our optical instrument manufacturers should be able to make it for a small sum [...] and additionally rather easy to use".[179] The article from 1852 in *Ugeskrift* mentioned in the previous paragraph came to a similar conclusion, in spite of the technical problems encountered: "[this] has opened a new and thus far unknown way to diagnose the most important illnesses of the eye".[180] Perhaps as a testament to its perceived usefulness and successful amalgamation into practice, the Karolinska Institute's outpatient training for medical students in surgery also included training in ophthalmoscopy by 1858, as "examination with the ophthalmoscope has been necessary".[181] In terms of research, a Danish thesis in medicine from 1857 looked at ophthalmology and studied the use of the ophthalmoscope in particular.[182] In 1858, H. Hülphers argued in *Hygiea* that "from being overlooked or disliked in the beginning, it is currently seen as one of the most important discoveries in recent times for the development of ophthalmology and an irreplaceable addition to every eye doctor's armamentarium, and additionally completely necessary for every close examination of the organ of sight".[183] The technical development of this device allowed physicians to visualise the inner structures of the eye, with developments along the way to project better images. But in order for it to be a useful tool for ophthalmology, physicians had to first understand what they were looking at and associate it with a body of knowledge. By the time Hülphers

---

[179] Ekström, "Ögonspegelns bruk", 656. [Vi hafva således all anledning hoppas, att instrumentet skall få en framtid, helst som det äger de många fördelarne att vara... ytterst enkelt, och således äfven af våra optiska instrument-fabrikanter bör kunna förfärdigas till billigt pris... och dessutom är temligen lätt lärdt att använda.]

[180] Paulli, "Undersögelsen af Nethinden", 364. [har saaledes aabnet en ny, hidtil ukjendt Vei for Bedömmelsen af Öiets vigtigste og betydningsfuldeste Sygdomme.]

[181] [Anon.], "Berättelse om Undervisningen vid Kongl. Karolinska Mediko-Kirurgiska Institutet: Under läsåret 1857–58". *Hygiea*. Vol. 20, No. 9, September 1858, 513–520, 517. [Härunder har en särskild uppmärksamhet fästats vid de fall, der undersökning med *ögonspegeln* varit behöflig.]

[182] [Anon.], "Disputats". *Ugeskrift for Læger*. Series 2, Vol. 27, No. 16, 3 October 1857, 248, 248; see, Edmund Hansen [Grut]. *Kort Fremstilling af den i praktiske Øiemed anvendelie Undersøgelse med Øienspeilet og af de ved denne Undersøgelse indvundne Resultater*. Diss. Copenhagen University, 1857.

[183] Notably, he did not specifically name any sceptics or detractors of the ophthalmoscope, nor were there any articles published in *Hygiea* criticizing it. Hülphers, "Om luftstrup-spegeln", 469. [Från att i början hafva varit förbisedd eller föraktad är den numera erkänd såsom en af nyare tiders vigtigaste upptäckter till oftalmologiens utbildning, såsom ett oumbärligt tillbehör i hvarje ögonläkares armamentarium och såsom alldeles nödvändig för hvarje noggranare undersökning af synorganet.] Hülphers does not criticise the device on the basis of García's non-medical background, nor have I uncovered any critique due to this in the Swedish or Danish literature.

sang the praises of the device in 1858, the work on a knowledge bank that physicians working in this field could recall during and/or after examinations was underway.[184]

The primary focus of Hülphers' article was not the ophthalmoscope though; it was another lensed device, this time for examination of the throat: the laryngoscope. The inventor of the device, Manuel García, used a combination of light and mirrored devices to observe his own vocal cords and larynx. However, García was a vocal pedagogue, not a physician, and his use of the device served different purposes related to the musical use of the voice and the formation of sound. Hülphers presented the laryngoscope by using the described successes of the ophthalmoscope in practice, and its alleged irreplaceability after years of technical practice. After noting his own physiological examinations with the laryngoscope, he saw potential in the device for "practical physicians" due to the variety of structures in the throat it made visible. He encouraged practitioners to give it a try and most of all develop technique before dismissing the device, urging that "one should not, through a few possible unsuccessful tests, immediately be put-off from using the instrument".[185] Staying the course required the development of tacit knowledge on how to properly use it, but some forms of knowledge could not be properly articulated through journal articles alone.

---

[184] For example, well-known Prussian ophthalmologist Albrecht von Graefe founded the journal *Archiv für Ophthalmologie* in 1854. His work was referenced at least ten times in *Hygiea* during the period. See "Graefe" in *Hygiea: Register öfver banden elfva (1849)–Tjugutvå (1860)*. P.A. Norstedt & Söner, 1863, 65; and, *Hygiea: Register öfver banden XXIII (1861)–XXXII (1870)*. Stockholm: P.A. Norstedt & Söner, 1874, 65. In *Ugeskrift for Læger*, Graefe is only mentioned directly three times between 1844–1860 according to their register. See "Gräfe"in *Ugeskrift for Læger: Sag- og Navneregister til Ugeskrift for Læger. Första Række I–X Bind og anden Række I–XXXI Bind (1839–1860)*. Copenhagen: C. A. Reitzels Forlag, 1860, 64. The German spelling of his name is Gräfe, which accounts for the differences in the two indexes. However, there are over thirty articles on the eye, its anatomy and physiology and illnesses. See "ophthalmologi", "øienoperationer" and "Øiet" in Sag- og Navnregister, 38, 58–59. *Hygiea* also published several articles on illnesses of the eye and its anatomy during the 1850s, see "ophthalmatrik", "ögon", "ögonlinsens fördunkling", "ögonsjukdom" in Register öfver banden elfva (1849)–Tjugutvå (1860), 65, 99; and, "ögonsjukdom", "ögonlockens anatomi" and "ögats formförändring" in Register öfver banden XXIII (1861)–XXXII (1870), 56. In terms of the throat, See "Stammen" in Sag- og Navnregister, 47; and "pharyngealpolyp" in Register öfver banden XXIII (1861)–XXXII (1870). For the nasal cavity, see "næseaabninger", "næsen", "næsepolypers Fjærnelse" and "næsesvælgpolyper" in *Ugeskrift for Læger: Sag- og Navneregister til Ugeskrift for Læger. Anden Række XXXII–XLIII Bind og Tredje Række I–XXVIII Bind (1860–1879)*. Copenhagen: C. A. Reitzels Forlag, 1880, 42; and "polyp, naso-pharyngeal" in Register öfver banden XXIII (1861)–XXXII (1870), 39. *Hygiea*'s index is largely categorized after disorder and pathology, while *Ugeskrift* indexes after article title and subject. With that in mind, relevant references might have been missed from the above overview.

[185] Hülphers, "Om luftstrup-spegeln", 473. [man icke skall, genom några möjligen misslyckade försök, genast låta afskräcka sig från bruket af ett instrument]

The comparison with the ophthalmoscope offered an example of a similar device that took time to be able to use with good results. A commentary in *Ugeskrift* from January 1859 on an Austrian article highlighted problems using the device on patients with strong gag reflexes and, much like with the ophthalmoscope, "one quickly realises that prior to anyone using this instrument with any utility, one must acquire some skill in handling it".[186] In addition to this, its use should be motivated in scientific terms: what did it offer practitioners in making diagnoses? In an article in *Ugeskrift* from 1859 referencing the aforementioned Austrian article, one physician questioned whether or not the instrument would actually stand a chance in attaining a practical place in medicine. This author criticises the original article for not motivating the laryngoscope's use in pathological terms, and references other Austrian articles that do, citing that "other physicians have used the laryngoscope for the diagnosis of pathological conditions in the throat and at the base of the tongue".[187] The author stated further that motivating the practical use of this instrument should reference its usefulness on these terms, rather than just detailing how it could be used.[188] What this article illustrates is that one both had to know how to properly use these instruments, and that techniques were not always easy to learn, but also that the device's medical use had to be scientifically motivated in clinical terms.

Another article in *Ugeskrift* from the same year confirmed the practical issues physicians may have encountered with the laryngoscope from the Austrian article above, stating that "it is important to avoid contact with the base of the tongue, as gagging will soon occur".[189] In addition to avoiding the patients tongue, physicians were recommended to get patients to widen their tongues and stretch them downward; encourage them to take deep, slow breaths; use sunlight to see the necessary parts of the throat; different techniques of where the physicians hand should be placed; and tools or techniques to minimise light reflecting in the physician's eye.[190] This article confirmed a number of points in the Austrian article, including placement of

---

186 [Anon.], "Om Speculum laryngis og dets Anvendelsesmethode". *Ugeskift for Læger*. Series 2, Vol. 30, No. 5, 22 January 1859, 66–9, 69. [Det indsees lettelig, at Enhver, før han med nogen Nytte kan anvende dette Instrument, maa erhverve sig en vis Færdighed i at handtere det, hvorved de forskjellige Kunstgreb ville frembyde sig af sig selv.]

187 [Anon.], "Erfaringer om Brugen af Strubespeilet". *Ugeskrift for Læger*. Series 2, Vol. 30, No. 18, 9 April 1859, 273–280, 273. [andre Læger have benyttet Strubespeilet saavel til Diagnosen af pathologiske Tilstande i Struben og paa Tungeroden]

188 [Anon.], "Erfaringer", 274.

189 Ibid., 274 [Ved Anbringelsen af Instrumentet er det af Vigtighed at undgaae Berøring af Tungens Basis, thi derved opstaae strax Kløgninger]

190 Ibid., 275–6.

the tongue and the use of sunlight, with the summary of the Austrian article pointing out the practicalities of conducting the examination "when the sun is high", with another recommending a variety of different screens to help illuminate the throat during examination.[191] Articles like these provided a frame for physicians to gauge how to use them, and fundamental aspects of their use, which likely assisted in their adaptation.[192]

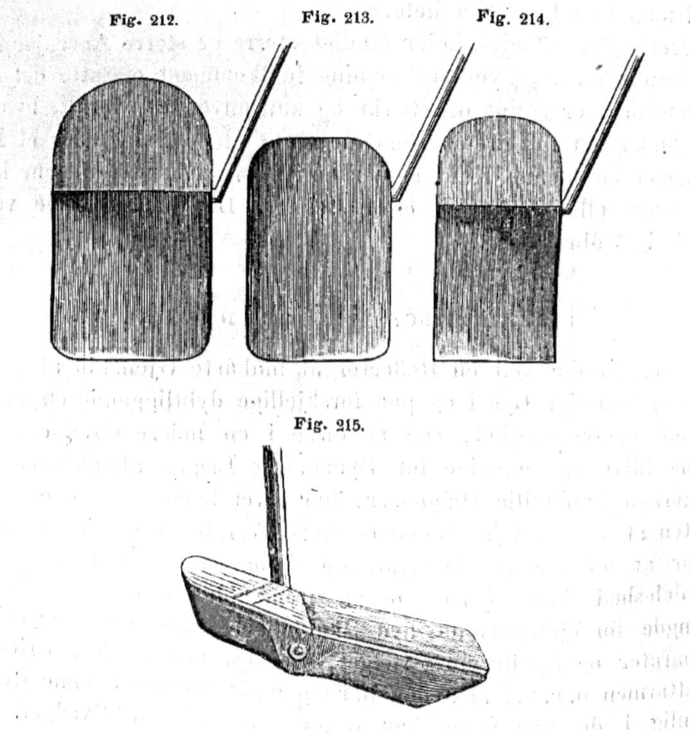

Fig. 5. Professor Wintrick's laryngoscope as pictured in Camillus Nyrop. *Bandager og Instrumenter afbildede og beskrevne med en tilføi et Prisfortegnelse.* Copenhagen: G.E.C. Gad, 1864, 150.

The learning curve involved in using some of these new devices required instruction and practice, and physicians were encouraged to hold out instead of initially dismissing a device–a point that underlines the time it could take for a new device and technology to break through. Nevertheless, sometimes

[191] [Anon.], "Om Speculum laryngis", 67. [naar Solen stod høit paa Himlen]
[192] See Polanyi, *The Tacit Dimension*, 30.

merely describing how to do something was not enough: practitioners needed to conduct examinations with these devices themselves and work on their own technique. To encourage practitioners to build up skill, one article in *Ugeskrift* from 1861 on examination of the nasal cavity, rhinoscopy, stated that "the problem lies in one's own lack of practice, and does not delineate that the method itself is useless or impractical".[193] Also, because of the learning curve, instruments could be used incorrectly, which could cause problems. An article in *Hospitals-Tidende* from 1859 called the ophthalmoscope dangerous due to the constant dilation of the pupil and irritation caused by the light source.[194] One summary in *Ugeskrift* from 1858, which looked at French recommendations, noted that "no one should try to use this instrument [a handheld ophthalmoscope] for examining the patient's eye before one has developed skill [in using it]".[195] This device required practice in order to develop correct techniques and the article recommends practice on someone other than the patient. Although not explicitly mentioned, this could have been an example of physicians practicing on themselves or their colleagues. Furthermore, physicians had to understand the perspective of the patient and how much they could withstand in one sitting, as well as be able to regulate lighting and other, practical nuances, and this could take time.[196]

Building up skill could also lead to uncovering techniques that made usage easier, which were shared in the two journals. The commentary on and summary of an Austrian article from *Ugeskrift* from 1859 also mentioned some practical tips for usage. This included coating the mirror in oil in order to ensure it did not fog up while in the patient's mouth, which would inhibit the physician's examination. It also stated that physicians should encourage patients to "continue to breathe and rinse their mouths from excessive secretions in advance".[197] These procedures could be trying on patients. One article from 1860 noted that patients should be given time to rest, due to the challenges of maintaining the correct position during examination.[198] This might indicate the length of these examinations at this time, if the patient

[193] [Anon.], "Rhinoskopi", 226. [Feilen ligger i ens egen Mangel på Øvelse, ikke i at selve Methoden er værdiløs eller upraktisk.]

[194] [Anon.], "Om farlige Følger af den ophthalmoscopiske Ungersøgelse [sic] af Øiet". *Hospitals-Tidende.* Vol. 2, No. 32, 10 August 1859, 127–128, 127.

[195] [Anon.], "Om uforsigtig Anvendelse af Ophtalmoskopet (Desmarres i Gazette des Hôpiteaux. 1859. Nr. 67.)". *Ugeskrift for Læger.* Series 2, Vol. 32, No. 21, 5 May 1860, 325–327, 327. [Ingen bør forsøge paa at undersøge nogen Patients Øie med det, før man har opnaaet en saadan Færdighed.]

[196] [Anon.], "Om uforsigtig Anvendelse af Ophtalmoskopet", 326.

[197] [Anon.], "Om Speculum laryngis", 67. [Under Undersøgelsen maa Patienten vedblive at aande og i Forveien rense Munden for overflødige Sekreter.]

[198] [Anon.], "Om uforsigtig Anvendelse af Ophtalmoskopet", 326.

needed time to rest during examination. Instructive articles like these provided a backbone for tackling practical problems and offered a forum for sharing the performance of these diagnostic examinations.

Seeing and Picturing Patient Difference

Physicians confronted problems directly with the laryngoscope. Though they had to build up technique to handle these instruments, they also needed to instruct patients in proper behaviour whilst being examined. Fundamentally, patients were also very different, perhaps in following directions, but also physiologically. This meant that practitioners needed to recognise the individual qualities of a patient that might inhibit ease of use. One article from 1859 notes that while patients with large throats responded well to examinations with the laryngoscope, others experienced problems. Once again, gagging was common for many, though proper technique was not the only factor in limiting this reflex. Practitioners could encourage patients to open wider, use a smaller scope, or "after inserting the instrument, compressing the tongue with a small instrument".[199]

One way of acquiring these skills would be using the device on patients and, over time, finding out what techniques work under what circumstances. Another way, suggested in the case of rhinoscopy, was practicing on corpses. One article recommends that "prior to undertaking examinations on living people, one should become familiar with the conditions in drawings and on corpses".[200] Switching to patients should be done cautiously. One tip was to "choose people with little sensibility and wide throats".[201] Anaesthetics could also be used on patients during the course of the examination. However, this could potentially be risky, since, although there were options such as chloroform, ether, and bromide of ethyl, there were no entirely safe options for the palate and throat at the time.[202] Suggestions like these would be helpful for practitioners, because they detailed what they should be able to see, and different techniques, like how to illuminate different parts of the given cavity. The article on rhinoscopy from *Ugeskrift* from 1861 also included examples from four successful cases, detailing modifications and other tools used.[203] It

---

[199] [Anon.], "Om Speculum laryngis", 68; [Anon.], "Erfaringer", 276.
[200] [Anon.], "Rhinoskopi", 226. [Førend man giver sig til at undersøge paa levende Mennesker, bør man have gjort sig fortrolig med Forholdene paa Tegninger og paa Kadaveret]
[201] Ibid., 227. [da vælge Personer med et lidet sensibelt og vidt Svælg.]
[202] Ibid., 227.
[203] Ibid., 230.

additionally included illustrations to guide practitioners, which offered an illustrated cross-section with a clearly labelled map of relevant parts.

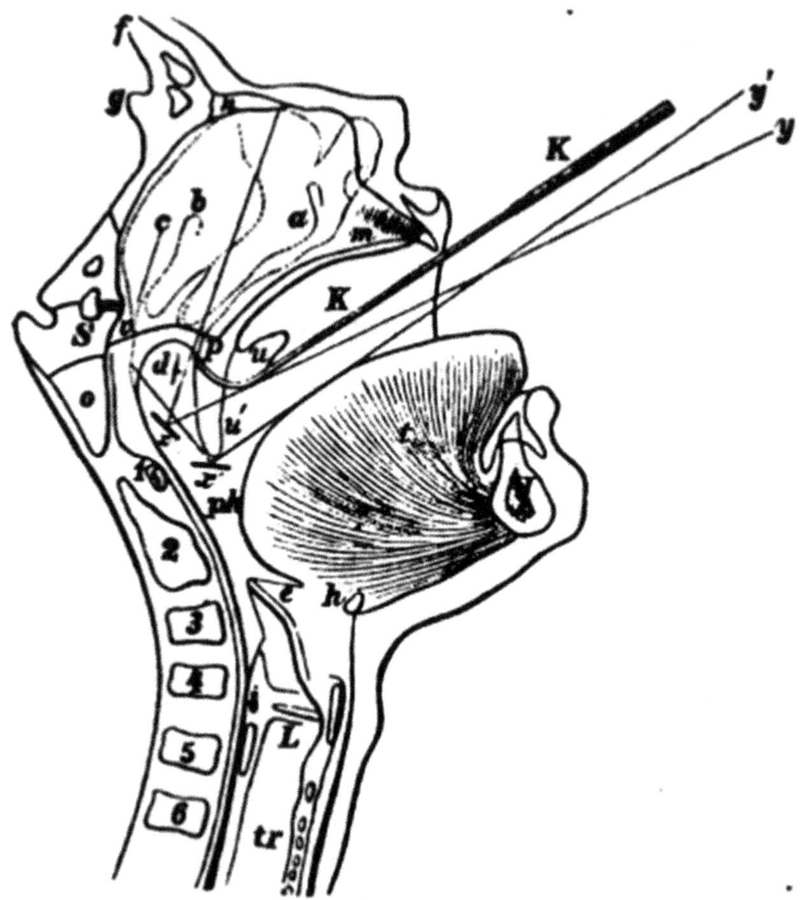

Fig. 6. A cross section of the relevant areas for rhinoscopy with a mirrored instrument. [Anon.], "Rhinoskopi: Efter Szermak [sic] (W. Wschr. 16de Febr. 1861)". *Ugeskrift for Læger*. Series 2, Vol. 34, No. 15, 23 March 1861, 225–231, 227.

The image in figure 6 shows the relevant area for rhinoscopic examination, including labels that corresponded with an additional key, not included above. Following the key was a relevant description of how the head was tilted, where the tongue was, and why it was in that position: "the head is bent dramatically backwards… [and] the tongue is placed at a sufficient depth".[204] This illustration, in conjunction with the corresponding key and text in the article, instructs the physician in how to manipulate the patient's, or the corpse's, body in order to conduct an examination with a rhinoscope. The article used the key to describe the individual parts the physician was looking at. It also described in detail what the cross-section showed, but also highlighted what was necessary to be able to carry out this examination successfully. Importantly, by using the position pictured in the illustration above, "the base of the skull is bent strongly backward […] the tongue is sufficiently deep, and thus, the mouth, pharynx and nasal cavities are in completely free relation to one another".[205] For those physicians who were uninitiated in these kinds of examinations previously, the description in conjunction with the illustration and its key would have helped in carrying out an examination with a rhinoscope.

Part of the purpose of the illustration was to inform the physician what he would be looking at during an examination. Even if the head should be in the recommended position, the device itself could be moved depending on what structure(s) the physician needed to see. The article listed different techniques and positions of the related parts, referring back to figure 6, and noted different structures based on mirror angle and position. For example, "if the mirror is deeper, more horizontal and approximately at x', and the direction of vision and illumination is at $y'x'$, then the posterior and upper walls of the pharynx are illuminated and reflected", referring to the different angled lines in the image.[206] The illustration itself was not enlightening insofar as it depicted the structures of the throat or nasal cavity, or a pathological condition: it was instructional. In this case, it was not instructing the physician what to see, but rather *how* to see, or, at least, offering advice on how to see. Outside of the illustration and instructional text following it, the author included four cases where observations and diagnoses were made with the help of the instrument.[207]

The newness in encountering some of the interior areas of the body, and with some degree of detail and magnification made "the inner parts of the body available to the eye", according to Carl Sundberg, writing in 1920 about

---

[204] Ibid., 228. [Hjerneskallen bøiet stærkt tilbage mod Halsen… Tungen staaer tilstrækkelig dybt]
[205] Ibid., 228. [Hjerneskallen bøiet stærkt tilbage… Tungen staaer tilstrækkelig dybt, og saaledes staae Mund-, Svælg- og Næsehule i fuldkommen fri Forbindelse med hverandre.]
[206] Ibid., 228–9. [Ligger Speilet dybere, mere vandret, omtrent ved x', og er Syns- og Belysningsretningen $y'x'$, saa bliver den bagre og øvre Væg af Svælget belyst og afspeilet]
[207] Ibid., 230–1.

the history of medicine.[208] But merely making these devices available was not enough. Fleck points out that "the use of an apparatus is always the expression of applying a certain developed thought style".[209] Fleck also underlined the importance of an observation's relation to a body of scientific knowledge.[210] But again, as the articles on the lensed instruments show, part of the problem was that background scientific knowledge had not always been compiled and the knowledge they had at their disposal around mid-century had been based on other scientific observations and relationships. Physicians had only recently been able to look at these structures in enough detail, and the background to enable them to see them was still under development, and they were often working from a different understanding of disease.

Physicians were also confronted with the tacit dimension of use. Merely describing (or even illustrating) how to employ a technique was not always enough: practitioners needed to understand the important pieces of carrying out these examinations. Fundamentally though, carrying out examinations even as trials called for a requisite human to practice on. The previously mentioned suggestion of practicing on corpses comes into play here, where technique could be built up prior to enlisting a warm body for the purpose.[211] But still, physicians would have had to experience work on a living human body in order to learn how to mitigate reactions such as coughing, gagging, or perhaps vomiting, and how to handle physiological and anatomical differences and different degrees of sensitivity in patients. This challenge is reflected in one of the Swedish Society of Medicine's meetings in 1856, where three physicians concurred that in order to judge the future of the ophthalmoscope more experience with it was required: the device needed to be used.[212]

One characteristic of the articles involving these new devices, is that many of them mention sceptics and scepticism. A translated article in *Ugeskrift* from 1859 mentioned practitioners experiencing "great difficulty" with laryngoscopes.[213] An article that was in part a reply acknowledged the difficulties, but provided tips to practitioners based on experience.[214] While it is true that even if it may have taken time to properly build techniques, not all physicians might have been willing to experiment with them or learn them. However, there is little direct evidence in journals for sceptical relationships

---

[208] Sundberg, *Läkarvetenskapen och dess samhällsbetydelse*, 100.
[209] Fleck, "To Look, To See, To Know", 144.
[210] Ibid., 147.
[211] See [Anon.], "Rhinoskopi", 226.
[212] *Förhandlingar vid Svenska läkarsällskapets sammankomster*, 6 May 1856.
[213] [Anon.], "Om Speculum laryngis", 66. [store Vanskeligheder]
[214] [Anon.], "Erfaringer".

to these technologies. This could be for at least two reasons. Firstly, given the mention of scepticism, it might be reasonable to presume that examinations that required pathological knowledge and other, unfamiliar skills, challenged practice in a way that made it problematic. These include gauging lens quality and its impact on imaging.[215] This question is not just related to Fleck's looking/seeing dilemma and relationships with thought styles or bodies of knowledge. Rather, it challenged previously established corpuses of medical scientific knowledge. Secondly, few of these problematisations actually appear in medical journals. This does not mean that sceptics did not exist, but rather that medical journals were not necessarily a forum for published scepticism. Journals established norms, and as other researchers have pointed out, many texts in the nineteenth century medical press are polemic, often with the intention of winning over readers.[216] Along these same lines, scepticism might have also been overstated, given the forum.[217] By pointing out scepticism and working polemically against it, practitioners could have been trying to both win over the not-yet converted as well as argue for the rational adoption of these devices. Giving instruction in how to use these devices in relation to real, physical contact with patients was an additional piece of the puzzle and a greater degree of help could have meant that physicians were more likely to try them out.

Driving Away Darkness

It is not strange that the use of these devices might have been difficult to motivate practically at first. They were complicated, required technical refinements and care, physicians needed to know how to process the visual information, and the images seen through the lenses were not always of great quality. Furthermore, they could require a bevy of other, additional devices in order to aide in perception, the looking/seeing dilemma notwithstanding. Just one instrument, purported to make examination of the throat easier, might have required several additional apparatuses to aide examination, or at the very least improve use. The recommendation that examinations be carried out when the sun is high, or even using sunlight at all, was limiting, both with regards to weather as well as time. This is especially true in the Nordic countries, where daylight hours during the winter are limited, if the

---

[215] See Blume, *Insight and Industry*, 71, 195.
[216] Drakman, *När kroppen slöt sig*, 28; Porter, "Introduction", 1–5; Sally Frampton and Jennerifer Wallis (eds.). *Reading the Nineteenth-Century Medical Journal*. New York: Routledge, 2021.
[217] See Mol, *The Body Multiple*, 116.

sun rises at all in the most northerly parts, and dreary, cloudy weather and storms would have further limited usage and required visual aids in order to be useful at all during less forgiving and sunny seasons. Under these circumstances, another light source and a curved mirror to reflect the light on the area of examination would be required in order for mere looking to be possible, let alone the perceptive work involved in seeing and the attention it would require.

Indeed, in all three journals, articles offering insight into practices used by other physicians often included recommendations for additional apparatuses in order to assist examinations. For example, one translated summary of a French article in *Ugeskrift* from 1860 outlined the French physician Desmarres' techniques whilst using an ophthalmoscope. These included making use of a wax candle for light, held by the patient on their shoulder, belladonna to enlarge the pupil, and letting the patient rest, because the position required could be tiring for them.[218] Belladonna or any substance for enlarging the pupil would also require accommodation, as too much light would damage the patient's eye. Physicians also needed to be mindful of irritation caused by illuminating the eye with light. An article in *Hospitals-Tidende* from 1859 cautioned physicians against conducting long examinations with light, and if they knew the examination would take a considerable amount of time, to not use agents to dilate the pupils, as they otherwise risked causing their patient serious eye damage.[219] Once again, the learning curve for these instruments could be complex: physicians were required to not only understand and analyse the visual information gleaned from examination and how to use the instruments themselves, they also needed to multitask. They had to know how to best use the instruments on patients with specific physiologies, instruct patients on proper behaviour during examinations, understand when they might need to take a break, when and how to use apparatuses to aide examination and be mindful of the use of light.

These light-related problems were not left without comment or aide. Camillus Nyrop listed "Magnium lamps" (magnesium), typically used for photography, for purchase through his firm in *Bandager og Instrumenter* and referenced an article from 1865 by physician Eugene Ibsen in *Ugeskrift for Læger*.[220] The employment of photography lighting in medicine illustrates that devices not specifically developed for use in medicine could be repurposed for medical use. Ibsen's article on the usage of these lamps for

---

[218] [Anon.], "Om uforsigtig Anvendelse af Ophtalmoskopet", 326.
[219] [Anon.], "Om farlige Følger", 127.
[220] Nyrop, *Bandager og Instrumenter*, 83.

laryngoscopy highlights this. This French developmaent was supposed to "cast light onto the mirror on the upper part of the pharynx, which is of course reflected further down the throat and trachea".[221] The light itself was alleged to be quite strong, with Ibsen stating that it was as strong as sunlight.[222] This would have been a practical necessity during the dreary winter months, especially further north, but could have also been otherwise advantageous, in rooms with generally poor lighting, sunlight or otherwise.

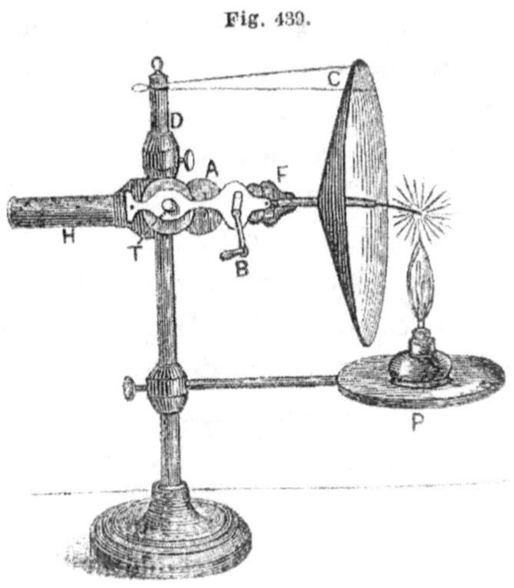

Fig. 7. A magnium lamp as pictured in Camillus Nyrop. *Bandager og Instrumenter afbildede og beskrevne med en tilføi et Prisfortegnelse*. Copenhagen: G.E.C. Gad, 1864, 84.

According to Ibsen, these lamps offered advantages that previous alternatives did not. Ibsen compared them to limelight and electric light, stating that "with limelight one must first develop oxyhydrogen each time, and with electric light one had the inconvenience of first connecting 50–60 elements, that, with filling, takes an afternoon [to do]".[223] Nyrop noted in *Bandager og Instrumenter* that photographs taken with magnesium light were "just as beautiful as with sunlight" and that Ibsen was the first in Denmark to have

---

[221] Eugen Ibsen, "Om Magniumlysets Anvendelse ved Laryngoskopi". *Ugeskrift for Læger*. Series 2, Vol. 43, No. 24, 18 November 1865, 392–394, 392.

[222] Ibsen, "Om Magniumlysets Anvendelse", 393.

[223] Ibid., 393. [Ved Kalklyset skulde man jo nemlig først hver Gang udvikle Brint og Ilt, og ved det elektriske Lys havde man den Uleilighed hver Gang først at sammenkjæde en 50–60 Elementer, hvilket med Fyldingen god tog vel tager en Eftermiddag.] The type of lighting in the second part of Ibsen's statement is probably carbon arc-lighting, which required liquid batteries to operate.

his portrait taken with magnesium light.[224] Outside of this lamp, Nyrop also listed "Wintrick's [sic] lighting apparatus", alongside a laryngoscope of physician Anton Winterich's design.[225] The lighting apparatus was powered by petroleum, with a glass ball to reflect light and its height was adjustable.[226] In the pages following Winterich's devices in the same edition of *Bandager og Instrumenter*, Nyrop describes several other illumination devices that could be used in examinations of the cavities of the head. Still, nothing seemed to compare to magnesium light, as Nyrop detailed examinations done by a French physician where "with the help of mirrors and lenses, images of the throat could be projected on a screen and he [the physician] was able to perform a laryngoscopy for an entire auditorium".[227] In *Bandager og Instrumenter*, the magnesium lamps listed were largely hand-held, which offered some advantage to those mounted on stands. One hand-held lamp gave the user control over the combustion process, which could conserve fuel. Additionally, because it was hand-held, the user was in control of the direction of the light source and could move it when necessary.[228] Yet, hand-held devices still meant the physician needed to use his free hand to hold and move the light or employ an assistant to help.

[224] Nyrop, *Bandager og Instrumenter*, 85. [Portraiter tagne ved Magniumlys have vist sig at kunne blive ligesaa smukke som ved Sollys.]

[225] "Wintrick" was Anton Winterich, who wrote a treatise on diseases of the respiratory organs, "Die Krankheiten der Respirationsorgane", which was part of the volume *Handbuch der speciellen Pathologie und Therapie* edited by Rudolf Virchow. Nyrop mentions this text in *Bandager og Instrumenter* on page 152, which corroborates this assumption in spite of the spelling variation. The book *The Principles and Practice of Laryngoscopy & Rhinoscopy in Diseases of the Throat and Nasal Passages* by Antoine Ruppaner also substantiates this claim. On page 21, Ruppaner mentions a lighting apparatus attributed to Winterich. Antoine Ruppaner. *The Principles and Practice of Laryngoscopy & Rhinoscopy in Diseases of the Throat and Nasal Passages*. New York: A. Simpson & Co., 1868.

[226] Nyrop, *Bandager og Instrumenter*, 151.

[227] Ibid., 86. [ved Hjælp af Speile og Lindser kunnet kaste Billedet af Struben hen paa en Skjærm, hvorved det altsaa er lykkedes ham at laryngoscopere for et helt Auditorium.] Though outside the scope of this chapter, both studies mentioned earlier by Kremer and Schmidgen reference the importance of such projections in the development of physiologists' visual perception and as a pedagogical tool. See Kremer, "Building Institutes for Physiology in Prussia"; Schmidgen, "Pictures, Preparations, and Living Processes".

[228] Nyrop, *Bandager og Instrumenter*, 84.

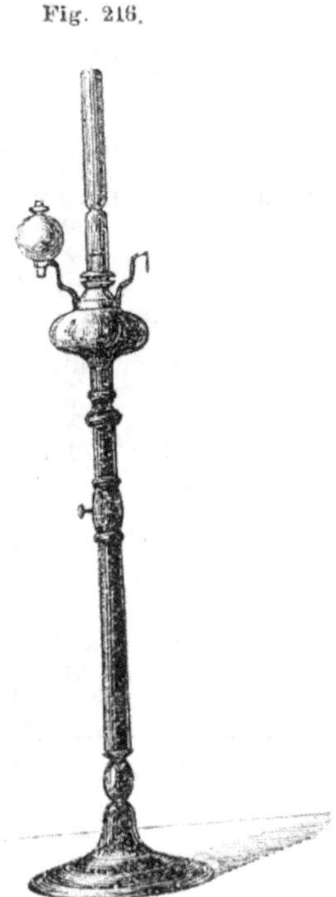

Fig. 8. "Wintrick's lighting apparatus". Camillus Nyrop. *Bandager og Instrumenter afbildede og beskrevne med en tilføi et Prisfortegnelse.* Copenhagen: G.E.C. Gad, 1864, 151.

Larger apparatuses and beautiful light aside, Nyrop also described a mirrored apparatus to be worn on the head for the purpose of illumination, which could be used in conjunction with the aforementioned lighting apparatus by Winterich. Albeit cautiously, he attributed this device to Winterich as well.[229] The mirrored headband would reflect light from the glass ball, providing light for the laryngoscope and examination. This would naturally free up the physician's hands, but Nyrop also mentioned that both eyes were freed up for examining the throat with the scope as well.[230] In addition to freeing up various body parts, the physician was also able to maintain at least some kind of distance between himself and the patient. Maintaining distance would have offered the physician some measure of protective advantage, in the instance the patient was ill. Nyrop does not mention this in *Bandager og Instrumenter*;

---

[229] He stated in a footnote that there were some uncertainties if attribution was correct. See Ibid., 151.
[230] Ibid., 152.

however, a book by American physician Antoine Ruppaner, *The Principles and Practice of Laryngoscopy & Rhinoscopy in Disease of the Throat and Nasal Passages* from 1868 pointed out the practical advantages of being able to remain at a distance, or at least be mobile. In reference to a similar forehead-mounted device Nyrop mentioned, Ruppaner stated that:

> with this reflector on the forehead, its position capable of being changed in an instant, both hands of the operator remain free [...] In cases of diptheria [sic] and scarlatina especially, an examination can be made in a more thorough manner [...] without obliging the patient to raise the head from the pillow. There being more or ess [sic] risk of inhaling the patient's breath under such circumstances, and of having some morbid secretions coughed into the face, the physician is thus less exposed to infection than otherwise.[231]

Regarding the practical problems raised earlier and the techniques to mitigate some of them, for instance when patients were prone to gag, this device would have also offered practitioners an advantage, both protective and practical.

Another example of hands-free lighting is offered in an endoscope accredited to French physician and so-called "father of endoscopy", Antonin J. Desormeaux. This device was designed to insert in the urinary tract, but could also be used to examine the prostate. Desormeaux' endoscope was detailed in *Bandager og Instrumenter* as well. Nyrop referred back to another scope by Desormeaux–an urethroscope–that allegedly lacked satisfactory diagnostic results. This endoscope was different: "I have heard statements of the opposite nature from our most respected physicians [...] and a more detailed description of it [the endoscope] could be of interest".[232] In order to illuminate his readers on the potential merits of this device, Nyrop copied an article from *Ugeskrift* from June 1865. What makes this endoscope interesting from the perspective of lighting is that it had a built-in lighting apparatus. The apparatus was connected to the instrument, whereby a mirror reflected the light through a lens. The lighting apparatus was a camphine lamp with a small chimney-like tube to redirect smoke, keep a controlled source of oxygen, and ensure the device did not get too warm.[233]

---

[231] Ruppaner, *The Principles and Practice of Laryngoscopy & Rhinoscopy*, 19.

[232] Nyrop, *Bandager og Instrumenter*, 61. [nu har jeg hørt Udtaleser i modsat Retning af vore mest ansete Læger... og en mer i det Enkelte gaaende Beskrivelse kan vist derfor være af Interesse.]

[233] [Anon.], "Endoskopien". *Ugeskrift for Læger*. Series 2, Vol. 42, No. 29, 17 June 1865, 450–458; see also Nyrop, *Bandager og Instrumenter*, 61.

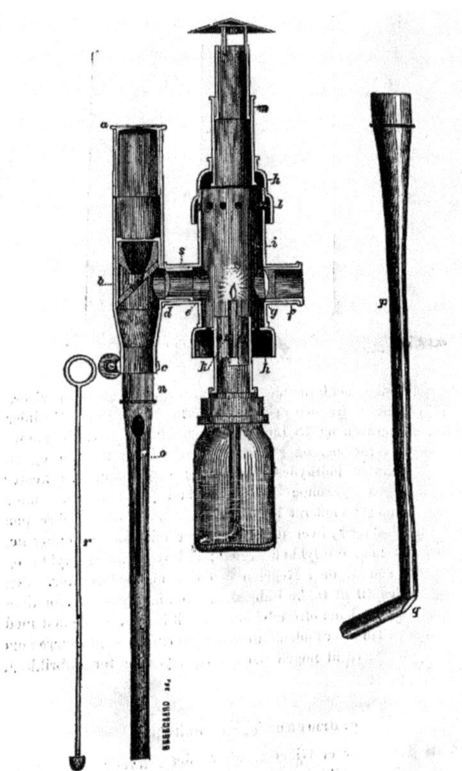

Fig. 9. Desormeaux's endoscope, as illustrated in *Ugeskrift for Læger*. Camphine lamp and chimney device, centre. The tube on the bottom left was designed to be inserted in the urinary tract, whilst the attachment to the left could be used to examine the prostate. [Anon.], "Endoskopien". *Ugeskrift for Læger*. Series 2, Vol. 42, No. 29, 17 June 1865, 450–458, 451.

With lighting issues addressed, either through the built-in solution in the above endoscope or external apparatuses, practitioners were better equipped to see inside and examine patients. In the article about the endoscope in *Ugeskrift*, the author noted that Desormeaux had presented a version of the instrument to the French Academy of Sciences in 1852; however, the value of the instrument was difficult to see then.[234] This reconnects with the previous discussion regarding Virchow and cellular pathology. It is important because the nexus of theoretical knowledge and practical application had not converged to make examining inside a patient with an instrument valuable.

---

[234] [Anon.], "Endoskopien", 449.

In other words, the practical possibility of looking inside the patient was one thing; however, seeing the interior structures of the body and being able to connect them to an established database of knowledge was quite another, to return to Fleck's thought styles. Furthermore, the article's author was clear to note that "it is not endoscopy's task to make well-known methods of examination obsolete, but rather to supplement them".[235] Once practitioners had a knowledge bank to refer to and the practical means to assist them, looking inside could be argued as a supplementary means of diagnosis alongside the "older schools", as the author above did in *Ugeskrift* regarding the endoscope.

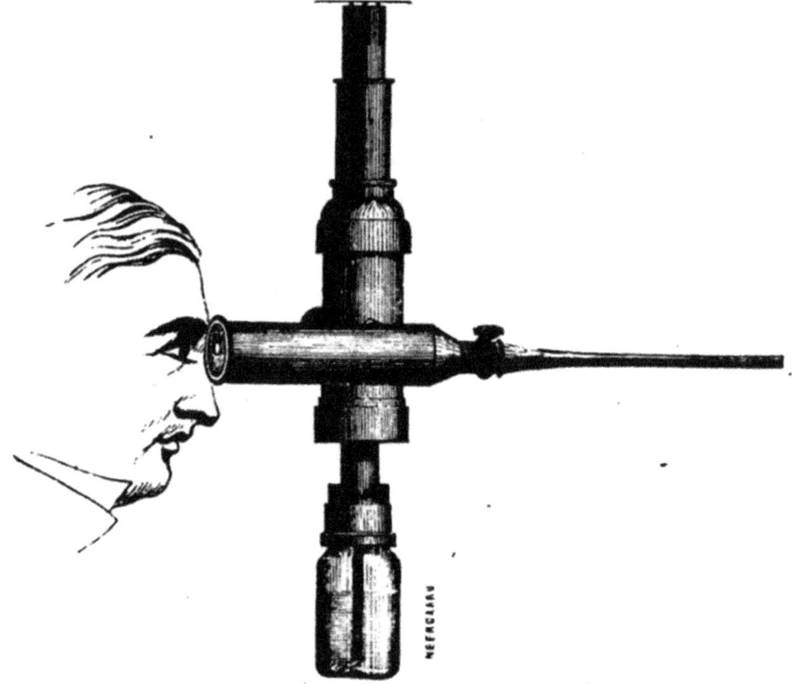

Fig. 10. Another illustration of the aforementioned endoscope. It is hard to gauge size from this image alone and how a physician would maneuver it. It was not a hand-held device and would have likely been placed on a flat surface. *Ugeskrift for Læger* 1865. [Anon.], "Endoskopien". *Ugeskrift for Læger*. Series 2, Vol. 42, No. 29, 17 June 1865, 450–458, 452.

[235] Ibid., 455. [Det er ikke Endoskopiens Opgave at gjøre de bekjendte Undersøgelsesmaader overflødige, men at supplere dem.]

Concluding Remarks

In this chapter, I have shown that the use of laryngoscopes, ophthalmoscopes, and rhinoscopes was connected with the establishment of both thought styles and tacit knowledge. Physicians needed to know what they were looking at and why it was significant from a clinical point of view, and they needed to be able to handle these instruments with some utility in order for them to be useful. The novelty of being able to look inside the dark recesses of the body was not enough to motivate their use practically, in particular during a period that was fraught with change and rife with fluid understandings of illness. Rather, their use was determined by multiple mitigating factors. Neither devices alone, nor just the theories behind them were enough in themselves. Understanding devices as the sole catalysts for change would be deterministic; however, the emphasis on theory alone is problematic.

Emphasising theory misses the nuance and incongruencies, which I commented on at the beginning of the chapter. Importantly, it obfuscates some of the experiential details in this shifting and fluid landscape of medical practice, and historians of medicine need to be mindful of this. As I have highlighted, one of the necessities the use of these devices was subject to was a referential body of knowledge, a thought style, which physicians could refer to in order to understand these devices and what they were looking at. Many articles of this nature were published in Danish and Swedish medical journals. The microscope fulfilled an important role here, both as a means of clinical analysis and as an object of reference in building this thought style.

However, this was still not enough. Physicians needed to use these devices with some skill. Medical journals offered help in this area as well, publishing instructional articles with practical suggestions and detailing examinations. These articles were particularly important in helping motivate the use of these devices. This chapter opened with a quote from Camillus Nyrop's trade catalogue *Bandager og Instrumenter* about these devices and "driving away the darkness".[236] Even if Nyrop was speaking figuratively, this was a very real challenge for physicians in these two countries, with long, dark winters and dreary weather. The requisite thought styles and tacit knowledge were not enough. By looking at how the use of these instruments was described in medical journals and moving to the level of practice, it is clear that they encountered other problems involved with device use as well. For instance, in order to properly drive away the darkness, physicians had to literally do

---

[236] Nyrop, *Bandager og Instrumenter*, 149.

just that, which introduced a number of other apparatuses that they had to manage. All this whilst managing a patient and trying to make a diagnosis.

3. Bracing for Impact:
Devices and the Fluid Landscape of Danish Orthopaedics

In 1870, Danish orthopaedists A. G. Drachmann and Immanuel Schøidte noted in an article in *Ugeskrift for Læger* that Denmark employed a method of treatment for scoliosis, a disorder involving the sideways curvature of the spine, which was unique. The authors noted that Denmark relied on the mechanical treatment of the disorder, using braces, to a much higher degree than the other Scandinavian countries.[237] Denmark's distinctive development could be traced back to physicians' early experiments in the use of plaster casts to treat the disorder and their positive results. But more significantly, they claimed that the country's "talented mechanicians and bandagists [...] have thrown themselves over this specialisation, either exclusively or with a certain predilection, and [...] in some sense, taken dominion over this area that most physicians have regarded as outside their realm of expertise".[238]

The practice of orthopaedics concerns itself with musculoskeletal disorders and illnesses, which include trauma, injury, degenerative, and congenital issues. Through much of the nineteenth century, this involved bone-setting and correcting musculoskeletal disorders through mechanical means, e.g., braces, trusses, splints, gymnastics, and prosthetics. At this time, orthopaedic practice was not under the control of physicians. This left room for unlicensed practitioners of varying degrees of training, seriousness and itinerancy, like Danish bandagists. The services provided by bandagists included the application, and sometimes construction, of braces, trusses, and other devices to cure musculoskeletal ailments. Some bandagists were itinerant practitioners, travelling between towns and never staying in one place for very long, with questionable training. All bandagists were not ambulatory, nor were they all untrained. Furthermore, their work was tolerated as long as it did not intrude on the domain of the physician. However, the prevalence of itinerant bandagists of a less-serious nature was attracting the ire of both serious bandagists and physicians.

---

[237] A. G. Drachmann and Immanuel Schøidte, "Beretning om Institutet for medicinsk og ortopædisk Gymnastik fra 1ste Maj 1868 til 30te April 1869". *Ugeskrift for Læger*, Series 3, Vol. 9, No. 14–15, 19 March 1870, 209–225, 210.

[238] Drachmann and Schøidte, "Beretning", 211. [talentfulde Mekanikere og Bandagister, der enten udelukkende eller med en vis Forkjærlighed have kastet sig over denne Specialitet... og I en vis Forstand bemægtiget sig Herredømmet over dette Terræn, der af de fleste Læger betragtes som liggende udenfor deres Omraade.]

At present, the profession is similar to that of orthotists. I will use the Danish term "bandagist" throughout the chapter to avoid hinting at a linear development toward the modern profession and to keep the profession's geographic specificity.[239] Bandagists, in this context, were a Danish phenomenon, who also travelled to Sweden to sell their services and wares. Other countries had unlicensed practitioners of a similar character, for example bonesetters and truss-makers in England and *bandagistes* in France. Applying an English-language term such as bonesetter or truss-maker would not capture the full range of work Danish bandagists engaged in. Furthermore, Denmark already had practitioners equivalent to bonesetters, *benbrudslæger*, who received their authorisation through apprenticeship.[240] Previous research has not done the role of bandagists in nineteenth-century orthopaedics justice. In many cases, patients falling in the above categories were of little interest to physicians in the earlier part of the nineteenth century, where bandagists and other, similar practitioners filled an important role.[241]

This chapter will take a closer look at nineteenth-century Danish orthopaedics and the relationships between medicine, devices and their makers in the 1860s, 1870s, and 1880s. I will begin with a short overview of Danish orthopaedics around the 1860s and 1870s and introduce bandagists, a profession that made and applied bandages and other orthopaedic devices in order to treat physical ailments in particular. This includes a brief contextualisation of the profession in Denmark and its varying degree of seriousness. The individual that provides the most interesting historical example is Camillus Nyrop, and his work in orthopaedics will figure throughout this chapter. Nyrop was a well-known and respected figure in the nineteenth-century Danish medical landscape, and outside of his work as a surgical instrument maker, he was also a proficient truss-maker and undertook some work as a bandagist.[242] His frequent contributions to Danish medical serials illustrate

---

[239] *Bandagist* is still the professional title used in Denmark; whilst in Sweden, *ortopedingenjör* (ortho-pedic engineer) or *ortodpedtekniker* (orthopedic technician) are used.

[240] Birgitte Rørbye. *Mellem sundhed og sygdom. Om fortid, fremskridt og virkelige læger: en narrative kulturanalyse.* Copenhagen: Museum Tusculanmus forlag, 2002, 206.

[241] David LeVay. *The History of Orthopaedics: An Account of the Study and Practice of Orthopaedics from the Earliest Times to the Modern Era.* Lancashire: The Parthenon Publishing Group, 1990, 79. See also John Pickstone, "Bones in Lancashire: Towards Long-term Contextual Analysis of Medical Technology", in *Devices and Designs: Medical Technologies in Historical Perspective*, Carsten Timmermann and Julie Anderson (eds.), 17–36. Basingstoke: Palgrave Macmillan, 2006; Anders Ottosson, "The Manipulated History of Manipulations of Spines and Joints? Rethinking Orthopaedic Medicine Through the 19th Century Discourse of European Mechanical Medicine". *Medicine Studies.* Vol. 3, No. 2 December 2011, 83–116.

[242] I have discussed this in the section "Characteristics of Medical Journals and Surgical Instrument Makers" in the introductory chapter. See pg. 33ff.

that he took his work seriously, was knowledgeable in the treatment of disorders like scoliosis, and maintained a deep interest in medicine more broadly. Nyrop occupied a unique position in that he worked in a liminal space between physicians on the one hand, and itinerant bandagists on the other. He used *Ugeskrift for Læger* as a forum for assessing the orthopaedic work of others and was the initiator behind a call in the 1880s to regulate the work of itinerant bandagists. Drachmann and Schøidte even called him one of the "pillars" of early Danish orthopaedic treatments.[243] Yet he has attracted little historical attention. For these reasons, he serves as a favourable object of study for a closer look at the shifting landscape of Danish orthopaedics and professional orientation.

Nyrop models what Annemarie Mol highlights in her book *The Body Multiple* as a coexistence of difference. The coexistence of difference implies that, on the level of practice, sharp, contested divides between blatantly distinct entities do not exist.[244] Rather than contend with one another, differences might overlap, interact, or exist side-by-side. In practice, the primary stake of practitioners is to treat a given illness. For instance, in doing orthopaedic work, divergent practices could be used simultaneously if the case called for it. More generally, previous research on the status of medicine and the position of physicians in nineteenth-century Denmark highlights terms of coexistence between unlicensed practitioners and physicians [*læger*] of varying backgrounds.[245]

However, general coexistence also includes discrepancy. Mol notes that because the ontology of medical practice contains many different practices, incompatibility will occur and friction between different practices will exist.[246] She further notes that the way friction is expressed differs between venues.[247] In a medical serial, like *Ugeskrift for Læger*, difference might be overstated as conflict or controversy, for example, when it might not be expressed in the same way in practice. Historians have also pointed out the importance of journals in building professional status, in which case friction could help win over allies.[248] Mindful of venue, in this chapter, I will focus on

---

[243] Drachmann and Schøidte, "Beretning", 211.

[244] Annemarie Mol. *The Body Multiple: Ontology in Medical Practice.* Durham, NC: Duke University Press, 2003, 143.

[245] See Rørbye, *Mellem sundhed og sygdom*; Nick Nyland. *De praktiserande læger I Danmark, 1800–1910: Træk af det historiske grundlag for almen medicin.* Odense: Audit Projekt Odense, 2000.

[246] Mol, *The Body Multiple*, 87–88.

[247] Ibid., 116.

[248] See Ana Carneiro, et. al., "Shaping Doctors and Society: The Portuguese Medical Press (1880–1926)". *Media History.* Vol. 25, No. 1, 2019, 23–50.

three cases involving Nyrop in *Ugeskrift for Læger* where frictions came to a head. The following cases may call to mind Thomas Gieryn's term "boundary work", where actors assert epistemic authority to deny the claims of an adversary.[249] However, boundary work is not a suitable way of framing these cases. Because journals are forums where conflict might be overstated, reading the following articles as boundary work misses the nuance present on the practical level. Furthermore, boundary work risks presenting an anachronistic image of nineteenth-century Danish orthopaedics. As such, coexistence of difference according to Mol serves as a more functional way of analysing the following cases because it attends to both medium and practice.

Frictions involving Nyrop were exacerbated for two reasons: forum, and status. They took place in medical journals where conflict could be overstated, and Nyrop was decidedly not a physician, which might have played a role in the exacerbation of difference. The three cases will highlight different aspects of orthopaedic practice–the therapeutical, the technological, and the professional. The first case exemplifies the therapeutic. It examines a conflict that played out between Nyrop and surgeon A. G. Drachmann over Nyrop's orthopaedic work. This discussion illustrates the enactment of difference and divergent approaches to the treatment of patients with musculoskeletal disorders in general, and scoliosis in particular. Following this, I will study the technological. This case centres a discussion between Nyrop and physician Sigfred Levy over a hernia truss. The hernia truss was assessed in *Ugeskrift* by both Levy and Nyrop, and Nyrop's commentary provides a closer look at his expertise as a truss-maker and bandagist. Finally, I will analyse a series of articles in *Ugeskrift for Læger* from the early 1880s that examine the question of profession. This discussion began over a letter penned by Nyrop and several instrument makers and bandagist colleagues over the growing problem with itinerant bandagists. However, it led to physicians positioning themselves against the signatories and attempting to enact their authority over the then-unregulated domain of bandagists.

Bandagists and Nineteenth-Century Danish Orthopaedics

The term *bandagist* in both Danish and Swedish stems from the French word *bandagiste*, which has roots in the eighteenth century.[250] In *The History of*

---

[249] See Thomas Gieryn. *Cultural Boundaries of Science: Credibility on the Line.* Chicago: The University of Chicago Press, 1999.

[250] *Svenska Akademiens ordlista.* [n.a.]. Bandagist. https://svenska.se/saol/?sok=bandagist (Accessed November 5, 2021); *Ordbog over det danske Sprog.* [n.a.]. Bandagist. https://ordnet.dk/ods/ordbog?

Orthopaedics by David LeVay, he describes French *bandagistes* as "appliance-makers" and important figures in the landscape of eighteenth- and nine-teenth-century French medicine. He notes that French orthopaedists typic-ally had long-standing relationships with specific *bandagistes* and that *bandagistes* assisted in bringing new, mechanical treatment methods into practice.[251] In Denmark, the professional situation for some bandagists seems to have been similar. Camillus Nyrop is the most prominent example. Like other Danish bandagists, he constructed and sold orthopaedic appliances, and his extensive work in orthopaedics was clearly important to him. As much is said in his biography, written by his son Camillus, which states that a visit to an orthopaedic institute in Paris had sparked his interest in a more portable way to treat patients than was typical in Denmark at the time, indicating that there was a French connection here as well.[252] He worked together with at least three physicians, in particular, C. Jessen, to treat patients at an orthopaedic clinic, even advertising this in newspapers (see figure 11).[253] Additionally, the most substantial descriptions in *Bandager og Instrumenter*, first published in 1864, were reserved for orthopaedic devices, and they occupied significantly more space in the book than instruments of other varieties. Of the 260-page book, with an additional 88-page supple-ment, over one hundred and fifty pages are descriptions and images of ortho-paedic devices and apparatuses. This includes an extensive guide to measur-ing protheses, hernia trusses, and other devices in order to ensure an optimal fit for the patient. He additionally noted in an article in *Ugeskrift for Læger* from 1872 that orthopaedics had become his primary area of focus, in spite of still making surgical instruments.[254] His work in orthopaedics encom-passed more than just device-making. He was interested in orthopaedic treatment and was also well-acquainted with medical scientific work in orthopaedics.

query=bandagist (Accessed November 5, 2021); *La langue française.* [n.a.]. Bandagiste. https://www.lalanguefrancaise.com/dictionnaire/definition/bandagiste (Accessed November 5, 2021).

[251] LeVay, *The History of Orthopaedics*, 237.

[252] C. Nyrop. *Camillus Nyrop og det kirurgiske Instrumentmageri i Danmark.* Copenhagen: Nielsen & Lydiche, 1884, 105–106.

[253] Camillus Nyrop. [Advertisement]. *Göteborgs Handels- och sjöfartstidning*, 4 April 1866.

[254] See Camillus Nyrop. *Bandager og Instrumenter afbildede og beskrevne med en tilføi et Prisfortegnelse.* Copenhagen: G.E.C. Gad, 1864; Camillus Nyrop, "En Indsigelse". *Ugeskrift for Læger.* Vol. 14, No. 18–19, 26 October 1872, 306–307.

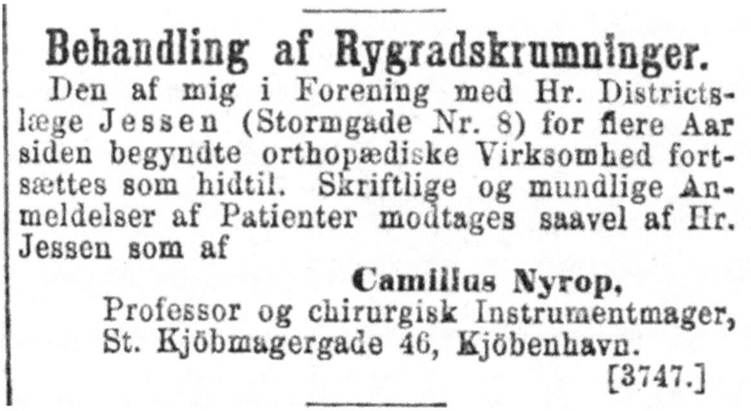

Behandling af Rygradskrumninger.

Den af mig i Forening med Hr. Districts-læge Jessen (Stormgade Nr. 8) for flere Aar siden begyndte orthopædiske Virksomhed fortsættes som hidtil. Skriftlige og mundlige Anmeldelser af Patienter modtages saavel af Hr. Jessen som af

Camillus Nyrop,
Professor og chirurgisk Instrumentmager,
St. Kjöbmagergade 46, Kjöbenhavn.
[3747.]

Fig. 11. An advertisement in a Swedish newspaper for Camillus Nyrop's orthopaedic clinic in Copenhagen. He titled himself "professor and surgical instrument maker". Camillus Nyrop. [Advertisement]. *Göteborgs Handels- och sjöfartstidning*, 4 April 1866.

The relationships between Swedish physicians and bandagists are less clear in medical serials. However, itinerant practitioners, often from Denmark, advertised frequently in Swedish newspapers.[255] Early advertisements from Albert Stille from 1845 also made note of his profession being "surgical instrument maker and bandagist" and he advertised the sale of orthopaedic trusses and bandages as well.[256] Although this chapter focuses on Danish bandagists, the mechanical treatment of orthopaedic disorders through bandages and braces seems to have been more controversial at an earlier stage in Sweden. Anders Ottosson details the work of Pehr Henrik Ling, his gymnastic system, and its subsequent acceptance by the Swedish medical status quo at the time.[257] Ling founded the Royal Central Institute for Gymnastics [*Kungliga Gymnastiska Centralinstitutet*] in Stockholm in 1813 that trained gymnastic instructors, and was eventually elected a member of the

[255] Using the keyword "bandagist" and searching between January 1, 1850 and December 31, 1890 gives 3520 results in the Swedish Royal Library's newspaper archive. There is a significant upswing in the number of results from 1877 onward. I have not systematically looked at the results and a deeper analysis falls outside of the aims of this chapter; however, it is worth mentioning that in 1876 "bandagist" gives 18 results and a year later, in 1877, 328. Most of these results are advertisements about the work of bandagists Niels Peter Heskier and Heinrich Saabye.

[256] In the Swedish Royal Library's newspaper archive, there are at least nine advertisements available referering to Stille as a surgical instrument maker and bandagist, all from 1845 in Stockholm-based newspapers. See Albert Stille. [Advertisement]. *Aftonbladet*, 20 October 1845; 6 November 1845; 21 November 1845; 29 November 1845; Albert Stille. [Advertisement], *Stockholms Dagblad*, 30 October 1845; 6 November 1845; 13 November 1845; 20 November 1845; 27 November 1845.

[257] Ottosson, "The Manipulated History of Manipulations of Spines and Joints?", 90–91.

Swedish Society of Medicine in 1831 but was not trained in medicine. One of the distinctions between Sweden and Denmark in this regard might have to do with educational facilities for gymnastics. Sweden had a qualification in gymnastics/physical education as early as 1813 with the founding of the Royal Central Institute for Gymnastics, whilst Denmark did not have a similar school until 1898 when the Danish Institute of Gymnastics was founded [*Statens etårige Gymnastikkursus*].[258]

In an article series in *Hygiea* from 1862, Swedish orthopaedist Herman Sätherberg provides an additional clue that supports this hunch. Sätherberg himself was a teacher at Ling's institute. In this article series, he discussed the growth of Swedish gymnastics and physiotherapy and its relationship with scientific developments in physiology and illness. His articles are polemic and discuss medical orthopaedics and the so-called "quackery" of unlicensed practitioners.[259] This could have been why subsequent advertisements or other references to Stille's work omitted the title "bandagist" as a means of distancing himself from unlicensed practitioners. I will discuss some of the Danish controversies later on in this chapter; however, discussion of, and serious calls for, professional regulation did not come until the early 1880s in Denmark, whereas regulation had already been established and endorsed in Sweden.[260] But most importantly, this chapter looks at bandagists as a Danish phenomenon in particular, not a Scandinavian one.

---

[258] Else Trangbæk. *Kvindernes idræt: Fra rødder til top.* Copenhagen: Gyldendal, 2005, 106.

[259] See Herman Sätherberg, "Gymnastik och Ortopedi. Belysningar och meddelanden". *Hygiea.* Vol. 24, No. 1, January 1862, 3–27; Herman Sätherberg, "Gymnastik och Ortopedi. Belysningar och meddelanden". *Hygiea.* Vol. 24, No. 3, March 1862, 65–85. Sätherberg wrote several articles about gymnastics in *Hygiea* through the 1850s and 1860s and discussed gymnastics and the problem of offering treatment to patients outside of Stockholm. In one article, he argued briefly for more training in gymnastics for physicians, physical therapists [*sjukgymnaster*] in larger communities in the countryside and for better regulation. See Herman Sätherberg, "Årsberättelse från Gymnastiskt Ortopediska Institutet för år 1859". *Hygiea.* Vol. 23, No. 5, May 1861, 257–262. There were also articles in newspapers discussing the legitimacy of orthopaedics that discussed the problems of itinerant bandagists, and even the legal troubles they encountered in Sweden. See for example [Anon.], "Om senaste försöket att vanställa ortopedien och hos allmänheten inplanta fördomar mot ortopediska institutet". *Aftonbladet.* 30 December 1857; [Anon.], "Om senaste försöket att vanställa ortopedien och hos allmänheten inplanta fördomar mot ortopediska institutet". *Aftonbladet.* 5 January 1858; [Anon.], "Lagskipning". *Öresundsposten.* 1 April 1874; [Anon.], "Elektricitet är lif". *Sölvesborgsposten.* 15 April 1874. Swedish physicians also took out advertisements to warn readers about bandagists. Leif Runefelt mentions this in relation to itinerant bandagist Niels Peter Heskier, who I will discuss later in the chapter. See Leif Runefelt. *Den magiska spegeln: Kvinnan och varan i pressens annonser 1870–1914.* Lund: Nordic Academic Press, 2019 165.

[260] Trangbæk, *Kvindernes idræt*, 106; Ottosson, "The Manipulated History of Manipulations of Spines and Joints?", 89.

Itinerant bandagists typically advertised about their short visits in towns throughout the two countries. Advertisements included addresses where patients could locate them and the times that they were available. For instance, Danish bandagist Julius Schiønning advertised frequently in Swedish newspapers, listing dates and times he would be in cities and towns, particularly in Sweden's southern regions, and his advertisements often included an image of a scoliotic back and the same back with a brace. Schiønning often included testimonials from physicians in his advertisements and medals from industrial exhibitions (see figure 12).[261] Bandagists in these two countries, itinerant and otherwise, constructed, sold and sometimes applied trusses, braces, prostheses, and other devices to treat or manage musculoskeletal disorders, or their physical symptoms. Some of them, like Camillus Nyrop, had close connections with physicians and worked together with them.[262] As such, the profession straddled medicine and mechanics.

---

[261] Julius Schiønning. [Advertisement]. *Nya Kristinehamnposten.* 25 September 1891.

[262] Bandagist Anton Rasmussen also contributed to *Ugeskrift* on occasion. See for example Anton Rasmussen, "Patteflasker med Metalsugerør". *Ugeskrift for Læger.* Series 2, Vol. 41, No. 17, 8 October 1864, 70–71; "Simplifikation af Wintrichs Pandespeil". *Ugeskrift for Læger.* Series 3, Vol. 2, No. 25, 24 November 1866, 390; "Dr. Richardsons anæsthesiske Doucheapparat". *Ugeskrift for Læger.* Series 3, Vol. 3, No. 11, 23 February 1867, 175; "Bekjendtgjørelse." *Ugeskrift for Læger.* Series 3, Vol. 3, No. 12, 2 March 1867, 183. Other studies, like Sabrina Minuzzi's on dealers in medicinal secrets in eighteenth-century Venice, look at similar dynamics. Minuzzi calls these craftspeople "artisans" in her article 'Quick to say Quack'. Rather, networks of social relationships between practitioners of various formal training helped change the pharmacopoeia, and their position in relation to apothecaries was tolerated. Articles like Minuzzi's serve to expand, or at least reevaluate, the role of medical knowledge from sources outside of professional (and licensed) medicine. Sabrina Minuzzi, "'Quick to say Quack': Medicinal Secrets from the Household to the Apothecary's Shop in Eighteenth-Century Venice". *Social History of Medicine.* Vol. 32, No. 1, February 2019, 1–33.

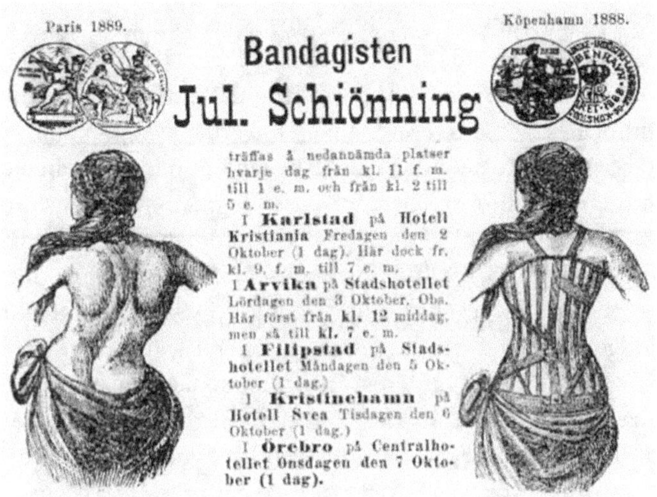

Fig. 12. An advertisement for Julius Schiønning's services. He spent one day in each town and was available between 11am and 1pm and again between 2pm until 5pm. Note the medals from industrial exhibitions in the top corners. Julius Schiønning. [Advertisement]. *Nya Kristinehamnposten*. 25 September 1891.

One issue here is the historiographical difficulty characterising the roles of medical intervention performed by non-physicians. Many bandagists were likely involved in some measure of unsanctioned medical treatment; however, this seems to have been tolerated in Denmark, at least up until the late 1870s and early 1880s. Part of this reason is likely due to the fabric of Danish medical practice at that time. Birgitte Rørbye notes that the sole association of the term physician [*læge*] with university-trained physicians [*universitetslæge*] is problematic in the Danish case, even moving through the nineteenth century. For instance, the Danish equivalent to bonesetters were trained through apprenticeship and called *benbrutslæger*, literally, "fracture physicians".[263] Rørbye also highlights that physicians, especially in the countryside, tried to avoid conflict with or even actively worked together with folk healers [*kloge folk*] throughout the nineteenth century.[264]

Furthermore, even when physicians did not tolerate unlicensed practitioners, quackery laws were of little help. For instance, it was unclear through much of the nineteenth century if the work performed by itinerant bandagists

---

[263] Rørbye, *Mellem sundhed og sygdom*, 205–206.
[264] Ibid., 225–226.

could be legally sanctioned under the Danish quackery law.[265] The authorities were not always on the side of physicians, either. Nick Nyland notes in his study of Danish general practitioners during the nineteenth century that the Danish authorities had a tolerant stance towards "quacks", and were often encouraged by the patients of quacks to be lenient on them when cases were brought to their attention.[266] There were also segments of Danish society that argued for the abolishment of quackery laws altogether, with a bill drafted in 1860 to repeal a quackery law from 1794.[267] The presence and work of bandagists of a more serious calibre complicated the matter and made outright judgement over the profession's general legitimacy more difficult. Physicians' general lack of interest in orthopaedics and the small, professional cadre of physicians in the country were likely some contributing factors to the fluid tapestry of nineteenth-century Danish orthopaedic practice.[268] In other words, a variety of medical practices, licensed and not, coexisted together in the Danish medical landscape, and bandagists were not necessarily on a different playing field than physicians were.

Bandagists were a clear part of nineteenth-century medicine in Denmark and Sweden. However, LeVay gives little mention to their work in the histories of orthopaedics in these countries in his book. More specifically, none of the actors discussed in this chapter are even mentioned. Though his book provides comprehensive overviews of developments and histories elsewhere, the addition of Scandinavia merits only twelve pages including a list of references, few of them in a Scandinavian language. While my intention is not to provide a comprehensive history of nineteenth-century Danish orthopaedics, it is important to underline the value of more locally oriented scholarship in this regard. Unlike the wealth of orthopaedic practitioners that LeVay describes in his chapters on Germany, France, and Britain, the Danish orthopaedists he describes are primarily connected to surgical interventions.[269] The focus on orthopaedics within the realm of surgery follows a

---

[265] T. M. Trautner, "Om Bandagistvirksomheden". *Ugeskrift for Læger*. Series 4, Vol. 5, No. 22, 13 May 1882, 343–344. For more about quackery in the Swedish context, see Sofia Ling. *Kärringmedicin och vetenskap: Läkrare och kvacksalverianklagade I Sverige omkring 1770–1870*. Diss. Uppsala: Uppsala University, 2004. Nick Nyland discusses the relationships between quacks and physicians in his doctoral thesis. See Nyland, *De praktiserende læger*.

[266] Ibid., 221.

[267] Ibid., 306.

[268] On the employment situations and numbers of Danish physicians in the nineteenth century, see Signild Vallgårda, et. al. *Sundhedsvæsen og sundhedspolitik*. Copenhagen: Munksgaard, 2010; Nyland. *De praktiserande læger*.

[269] LeVay, *The History of Orthopaedics*, 329–331. He does briefly discuss Swedish gymnastics and the work of Pehr Henrik Ling and Jonas Zander.

teleological frame of professionalisation, where only practitioners that fit within the profession's current point of reference are worth discussing. This also paints the developments of Danish orthopaedics in a different light than the German, French, and British developments that he details so well, especially regarding the presence, work, and importance of unlicensed practitioners. The work of bandagists in Denmark is wholly absent despite their clearly prevalent position in Danish orthopaedic practice and the contentions with the medical status quo. This flattens the textured landscape of nineteenth-century orthopaedic practice, the professional nuance between practitioners with varying degrees of training and seriousness, and the moves made to amalgamate this field into the larger domain of physician control.

In the Danish context, following LeVay's historiography of orthopaedics in the country would be a mischaracterisation. In this respect, Camillus Nyrop provides an interesting case and a closer look at the legitimacy of at least some Danish bandagists. The profession is, after all, still a common part of Danish healthcare.[270] Nyrop considered his work as more than just constructing instruments. He understood the mechanical principles of devices and how they worked. He worked with physicians as well as reflected over developments in his trade. He also defended his work and assessed the work of others, from his knowledge of orthopaedics and about orthopaedic devices and how they worked. The first two cases will show this. In addition to his interest in medicine, he sent his son, Johan Ernst Nyrop, abroad to study with instrument makers, but also to study anatomy. Nyrop wanted the Danish *Sundhetskollegiet*, the public authority that was in charge of the oversight of healthcare and medical practice, to allow Johan Ernst to take a test in hernial surgery; however, this request that was denied.[271] One of Nyrop's sons, most likely also Johan Ernst, was additionally present with his father during an ovariotomy performed in 1864.[272] Making devices required knowledge and interest in medicine and the body of scientific knowledge being developed in the field. There was no clear-cut and sharp division between licensed and unlicensed practitioners, as Nyrop's work illustrates. Reading all practitioners of this trade as quacks dabbling in the illegitimate treatment of patients mischaracterises the texture of the nineteenth-century medical

---

[270] Vej nr 123 of 20/07/1995, *Vejledning om uddannelse af bandagister (Til sygehusforvaltninger, social- og sundhedsforvaltninger m.fl.)*; Lov nr 431 of 10/06/2003, *Lov om bandagister*. The proposal to the 2003 law notes that bandagists "are an orderly and well-known party for consumers [of health care]". [er en velordnet og for brugerne en velkendt gruppe]
[271] C. Nyrop, *Camillus Nyrop*, 115–116.
[272] F. Howitz, "Et Tilfælde af Ovariotomi". *Hospitals-Tidende*. Vol. 7, No. 12, 23 March 1864, 45–47.

landscape in Scandinavia, as well as the characteristics of the work of bandagists and the trade more specifically.

Therapeutics and Scoliosis Treatments

Even if professional boundaries in orthopaedics might have been relatively fluid, practitioners could take exception. Nyrop's son Camillus eloquently described the situation as follows: "his orthopaedic work changed the prevailing and absolutely idyllic relationship between himself and the medical profession. The crystal-clear skies [he had experienced] thus far had darkened somewhat".[273] Nyrop and Danish surgeon and orthopaedist A. G. Drachmann exchanged words in *Ugeskrift* several times throughout the period, but I will look at two incidents in particular. These two incidents, both from the 1870s, relate to therapeutic matters that called Nyrop's orthopaedic work into question. Drachmann's exception to Nyrop's orthopaedic interventions was primarily because of incongruency between the men's approaches to orthopaedics and treatment. They represented different professions; however, the fact that they were competitors and representatives of different orthopaedic approaches was more pertinent.

Drachmann's career in medicine began as a barber-surgeon apprentice. He later trained as a surgeon and physician. He worked with the Danish navy, including during the First Schleswig War between Germany and Denmark over the Duchies of Schleswig and Holstein. Drachmann was employed as a physician at the Institute for Langgaardian Orthopaedics until 1851. This institute was founded by Danish mechanician Johannes Peter Langgaard in 1836. Langgaard's institute was the first orthopaedic institute opened in Denmark, and Langgaard was inititally granted exclusive rights [*eneret*] for its operation.[274] Langgaard's brother, Otto, trained in Germany and opened a similar institute in Hamburg, where he also worked as a bandagist.[275] Drachmann was interested in gymnastic methods and the physical education of young girls and women.[276] He also visited different gymnastic institutes in Europe, including the Royal Central Institute for Gymnastics [*Kungliga Gymnastiska Centralinstitutet*] in Stockholm, Sweden.[277] He worked extens-

---

[273] C. Nyrop, *Camillus Nyrop*, 106. [Med denne hans ortopædiske Virksomhed forsvand timidlertid det hidtil bestaaende, absolut idylliske Forhold mellem ham og Lægestanden. Den hidtil fuldstændig klare Himmel blev noget formørket.]

[274] Ibid., 103.

[275] Drachmann and Schøidte, "Beretning", 214.

[276] Trangbæk, *Kvindernes idræt*, 63.

[277] Ibid., 60–67.

ively with physician Immanuel Schiødte and they founded an institute for orthopaedics and gymnastics together, Institute for Medical and Orthopaedic Gymnastics [*Institutet for medicinsk og ortopædisk Gymnastik*], in 1865.

In two articles in *Ugeskrift for Læger*, published in March 1870, Drachmann and Schiødte accounted for patient cases at their institute.[278] These two articles mostly highlight the number of patients treated for specific illnesses at the institute–from dyspepsia to paralysis–however, the second article contains a statement that would animate Camillus Nyrop, namely that they called into question the mechanical treatment of scoliosis, i.e., with scoliosis braces, with undertext directed toward bandagists. Drachmann and Schiødte argued that:

> If the mechanical treatment for scoliosis is truly effective and something more than a mere remedy used for the sake of looks, forcing the practitioner to do something that, at least for the layperson's eyes, looks as though it could help, then I believe that the Langgaardian method of treatment can be relied on, with all its consistency, seriousness, and competency. It cannot be restricted to applying any bandage or machine, regardless of what name is attached to it, to a scoliotic back and then leaving it to anyone's ignorant hands to treat this deformity, as is the situation for the majority of cases.[279]

According to Drachmann and Schøidte, treatment was a process that required supervision and assistance, especially if it included a brace. They were proponents of the curative potential of exercises for scoliotic backs rather than the mere application and use of braces. Braces might have given the illusion of being helpful, but knowledgeable practitioners would be able to discern otherwise. The article by Drachmann and Schøidte offers some insight into the differences between the Nordic countries during this period,

---

[278] The first article is primarily a statistical account about what disorders were treated at the institute and how many; whereas, the second discusses scoliosis treatments more specifically. Thus, the first article will not be discussed in great detail, but the second will be. A. G. Drachmann and Immanuel Schøidte. "Beretning om Institutet for medicinsk og ortopædisk Gymnastik fra 1ste Maj 1868 til 30te April 1869". *Ugeskrift for Læger*, Series 3, Vol. 9, No. 13, 12 March 1870, 193–198; Drachmann and Schøidte, "Beretning", No. 14–15.

[279] Drachmann and Schøidte, "Beretning", No. 14–15, 219. [Skal den mekaniske Behandling virkelig udrette Noget mod Skoliosen og være noget Mere end et Middel, som man anvender for et Syns Skyld, fordi man er nødsaget til at gjøre Noget, der idetmindste for Lægmands Øjne ser ud, som om det kunde hjælpe, saa tror jeg, at den maa anvendes med hele Konsekvens, den Alvor og den Dygtighed, som udmærker den Langgaardske Behandlingsmaade, og ikke kan indskrænke til at anbringe en eller anden Bandage eller Maskine, ligegyldig hvilket Navn der er knyttet til denne, paa en skoliotisk Ryg og derefter overlade denne til sig selv eller til hvilkesomhelst ukyndige Hænder,–den almindelige Behandling af denne Deformitet I det store Flertal af Tilfælde.]

namely that while Sweden had adopted gymnastics through Swedish pioneer of physical education Pehr Henrik Ling rather early, and because of this had not relied significantly on mechanical braces, the opposite was true in Denmark.[280]

In Denmark, they noted that the influence of bandagists had led developments in a different direction, where the mechanical treatment of musculoskeletal disorders with braces, trusses, etc., was much more common.[281] At any rate, Drachmann and Schiødte encouraged physicians to test different methods of orthopaedic treatment, including gymnastics. They used a combination themselves, as they did not believe that one method was necessarily more advantageous, rather that the method should always be integrated with anatomical and pathological knowledge.[282] Due to their institute's focus on gymnastics, they would have had interest in contrasting their method of treatment for scoliosis, which combined the use of braces and gymnastics, against the work of bandagists who primarily used mechanical means for treating the disorder. However, they also pointed out that the requisite treatment method depended on what kind of scoliosis the patient had.[283]

Nyrop took exception to Drachmann and Schøidte's declaration that the treatment of scoliosis with braces was becoming an obsolete practice and offered a rebuttal a few months later in *Ugeskrift*. He addressed Drachmann specifically and did not mention Schøidte at all in the article. Given his extensive experience, Nyrop stated that the opposite of what Drachmann was recommending was the case and that the positive results seen by both him and Drachmann using braces for treating scoliosis was proof of this.[284] In this article, he took care to detail the developments in orthopaedics and noted in particular Drachmann's interest in gymnastic physical therapy, rather than the primary use of braces and trusses, which Nyrop constructed and had been commonly used to treat musculoskeletal maladies. In his response, Nyrop focused some of Drachmann's earlier publications. For instance, Drachmann had published articles in *Ugeskrift* in the 1840s and 1850s that illustrated that treating scoliosis with braces worked out favourably and that he had ques-

---

[280] Ibid., 210.
[281] Ibid., 211.
[282] Ibid., 223.
[283] Ibid., 212–214.
[284] Camillus Nyrop, "I Anledning af Hr. Professor Drachmanns Udtalelser i Nr. 13 og 14. 15 af «Ugeskr. F. Læger» d. A.". *Ugeskrift for Læger*. Series 3, Vol. 9, No. 29, 18 June 1870, 449–461, 451.

tioned the usefulness of gymnastics in treating scoliosis earlier.[285] Nyrop chose his words carefully: while he did not dismiss gymnastics as a legitimate method of treatment–he sold some gymnastic apparatuses and stated that it was an "excellent preventative measure"–he also underlined that, based on of the positive results with braces, he did not understand that "now in 1870, [gymnastics] could be declared as the only useful [means of treatment]".[286]

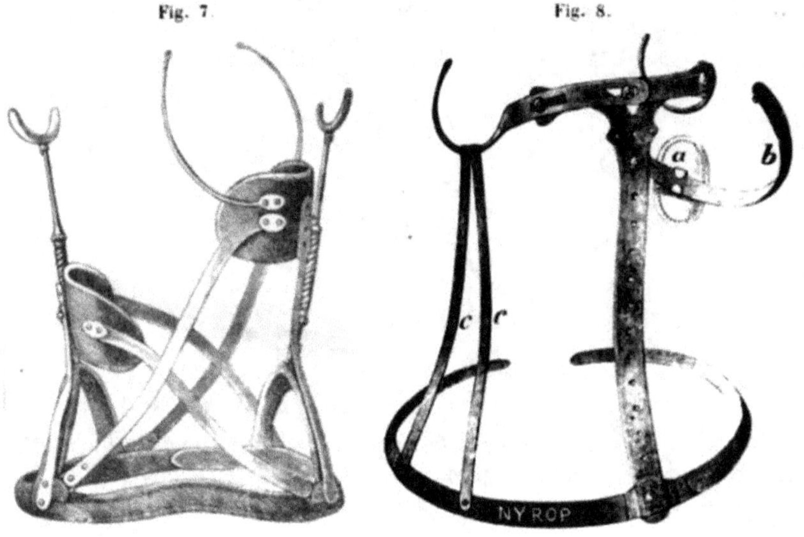

Fig. 13. A side-by-side comparison of the brace Drachmann and Schøidte mention (left) and a similar truss made by Nyrop (right). Camillus Nyrop, "I Anledning af Hr. Professor Drachmanns Udtalelser i Nr. 13 og 14. 15 af «Ugeskr. F. Læger» d. A.". *Ugeskrift for Læger.* Series 3, Vol. 9, No. 29, 18 June 1870, 449–461, 461.

[285] Nyrop, "I Anledning af Hr. Professor Drachmanns Udtalelser", 460. See A. G. Drachmann, "Om den Langgaardske orthopædiske Anstalt". *Ugeskrift for Læger*, Series 2, Vol. 6, No. 26, 29 May 1847, 405–416; A. G. Drachmann. [untitled]. *Ugeskrift for Læger.* Series 2, Vol. 15, No. 6–8, 16 August 1851, 127–128; and, A. G. Drachmann. *Om Rygradens Sidekrumning med særligt Hensyn til dens Diagnose, Ætilologi og Behandling.* Copenhagen: C. A. Reitzel, 1852.

[286] Nyrop, "I Anledning af Hr. Professor Drachmanns Udtalelser", 460. [Gymnastik er et udmærket Forebyggelsesmiddel, ligeom den ogsaa overfor Skoliosen maa kunne være et godt Middle til att styrke Patients Mod; men det forekommer mig ikke, at Hr. Professoren ligeoverfor sine tidligere stærke Udtalelser har givet tilstrækkelig Grund for, at Gymnastiken, som han i 1847 og meget senere kun kunde tilraade en meget ringe Anvendlese af ved Behandlingen af Skoliosen, nu i 1870 skal være det eneste Anvendelige]

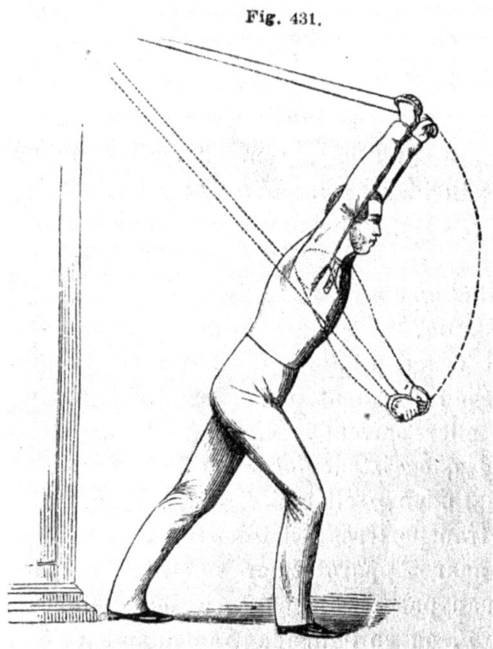

Fig. 14. An illustration from *Bandager og Instrumenter* of an exercise that patients could do on physical therapy apparatus designed by James Chiossos. Camillus Nyrop. *Bandager og Instrumenter afbildede og beskrevne med en tilføi et Prisfortegnelse.* Copenhagen: G.E.C. Gad, 1864, 80.

Nyrop had a long-standing scepticism towards gymnastic apparatuses being used as the sole treatment of orthopaedic ailments; a scepsis that he developed during a trip to Brussels and Paris in 1847. During this trip, he visited an orthopaedist that used trusses and braces as the foremost treatment for orthopaedic disorders like scoliosis, rather than gymnastic apparatuses, which were more common in Denmark at the time.[287] Here, he saw a future in a more portable way to treat patients, outside of an institution. In Nyrop's article, the statements he referred to made by Drachmann on the questionable effects of gymnastics on patients with scoliosis were made in articles from the late 1840s and 1850s, and a book on scoliosis he published in 1852.[288] These statements echoed Nyrop's stance but were not necessarily entirely contrary to the later position of Drachmann, either. Drachmann's position is

---

[287] C. Nyrop, *Camillus Nyrop*, 104–105.

[288] Although the article Nyrop replied to is credited to Drachmann and Immanuel Schøidte, Nyrop refers to Drachmann directly in his article.

worth developing as well. Having been employed at Johannes Peter Langgaard's orthopaedic institute until it closed in the 1850s, he was likely associated with Langgaard's orthopaedist brother, Otto. Both brothers constructed and sold orthopaedic devices, much like Nyrop. However, Otto Langgaard recommended another type of treatment using "machines", so-called *Maskinbehandling*, requiring the patient to stay in a horizontal position for an extended period.[289] Nyrop argued that this was unideal for patients: it required them to remove themselves from daily life, it could delay development in younger patients, and the course of treatment could take several years for some patients.[290] Portable braces, on the other hand, perhaps complimented with gymnastic exercises "to give the patient fortitude", would allow the patient to continue with their life whilst undergoing treatment.[291]

The first article Nyrop referred to was from 1847. It was a report written by Drachmann about the Institute for Langgaardian Orthopaedics and was published in *Ugeskrift*. In this article, Drachmann reported that a combination of gymnastics and mechanics were used at the institute, particularly to strengthen muscles equally on both sides of the body but also to stretch them out with the help of different apparatuses. The apparatuses Drachmann referred to in the article were extension beds that would treat scoliosis through traction, and "machines" [*Maskiner*], that referred to portable braces with springs.[292] Drachmann highlighted that, according to the Langgaardian method, these "machines", i.e., braces, were the primary means of treatment.[293] He further noted the limitations of gymnastics as a sole method of treatment, stating that "[it] strengthens the body, but does not eliminate the deformity".[294] Nyrop interpreted Drachmann's 1870 article as a change in opinion, which no longer emphasised the importance of braces in the treatment of scoliosis.

---

[289] Nyrop, "I Anledning af Hr. Professor Drachmanns Udtalelser", 457.

[290] Ibid., 457.

[291] Ibid., 460. [til at styrke Patientens Mod]

[292] Drachmann, Om den Langgaardske orthopædiske Anstalt", 407. Drachmann did not attribute the devices to Langgaard specifically; however, Langgaard constructed and exhibited an orthopaedic device [*Maskine*] for scoliosis, which may have been the one Drachmann is referring to. He received ten-year exclusive privileges (*eneret*) to construct and sell the device. See C. Nyrop, *Camillus Nyrop*, 135; [Anon.], "Særskilte Bekjendtgjørelser". *Tillæg til den Berlingske politiske og Avertissements-Tidende*. 11 May 1849.

[293] Drachmann, "Om den Langgaardske orthopædiske Anstalt", 406–7.

[294] Ibid., 406. [Gymnastiken, anvendt i dens hele Udstrækning, gjör derfor Legemet i det Hele stærkere, med lader Deformiteten bestaae] For Nyrop's commentary see Nyrop, "I Anledning af Hr. Professor Drachmanns Udtalelser", 450.

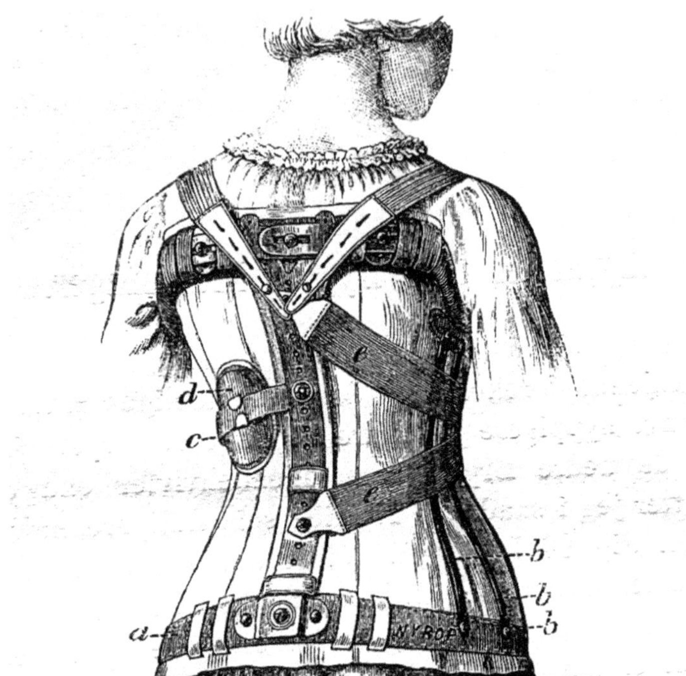

Fig. 15. A scoliosis brace of Nyrop's construction. *Bandager og Instrumenter*. Camillus Nyrop. *Bandager og Instrumenter afbildede og beskrevne med en tilføi et Prisfortegnelse.* Copenhagen: G.E.C. Gad, 1864, 40.

The noteworthy difference in Drachmann's stance from the 1840s and 1850s was that his emphasis on "machines" had changed slightly, from being the primary means of treatment to becoming secondary to gymnastics, and that the braces he used in the 1870s were of a simpler construction.[295] The brace Drachmann referred to here was even claimed to be a modification by Nyrop. However, Nyrop contested this claim, and stated that it was not a modification but a design of his own construction.[296] In his older articles, Drachmann

---

[295] Drachmann and Schøidte, "Beretning", No. 14–15, 224.
[296] Nyrop, "I Anledning af Hr. Professor Drachmanns Udtalelser", 461.

highlighted that braces used at home without performing regular gymnastic exercises could make some conditions worse.[297] In all the articles, he underlined that the combination of the two methods, alongside the attention of a physician, could mitigate eventual problems. Perhaps this was the crux: if patients were merely left on their own, with a portable brace, physicians had less control over the eventual course of treatment. The primary difference between the stances of the two men was around the mechanics of the trusses used. Drachmann, on the one hand, favoured trusses that operated on stretching. Nyrop, on the other hand, designed trusses with springs that applied varying pressure to eventually adjust the spine's problematic curvature.[298] But the other significant difference between the two men was that one was a licensed practitioner, and one was not. This issue would be emphasised directly two years later, along with their stances on braces once again.

In April 1872, a notice in *Ugeskrift* mentioned that a new edition of Nyrop's trade catalogue *Bandager og Instrumenter* had been published; the following month, a review by Drachmann appeared in the same periodical, lambasting Nyrop's book. Drachmann began by pointing out a piece he wrote twenty years prior, in 1852, on scoliosis, how the science behind the condition had developed, and how through medical investigations, the condition and its potential treatment were better understood.[299] Alluding to previous conflicts, Drachmann took issue with Nyrop criticising a treatment method for scoliosis that Drachmann was a proponent of by calling it dangerous, and accused Nyrop of misunderstanding results.[300] He also insisted that one of Nyrop's devices for scoliosis and explanation of how it worked were "contrary to all principles of mechanics".[301]

After dedicating three pages to questioning some of Nyrop's statements about scoliosis, his treatment methods and results, he noted that, with regards to confusing two different conditions synonymously, "that a tilted pelvis and a tilted, fixed pelvis are synonyms for Mr. N, are small things, that are hardly worth mentioning".[302] Drachmann's exasperation over Nyrop's self-confidence

---

[297] Drachmann, "Om den Langgaardske orthopædiske Anstalt", 408.

[298] See Nyrop, *Bandager og Instrumenter*, 76–86.

[299] A. G. Drachmann, "Om Skoliosens Behandling: Nogle Bemærkninger i Anledning af Prof.Nyrops Udtalelser i «Bandager og Instrumenter» 3die Bd. 1ste Hefte. 1872". *Ugeskrift for Læger*. Vol. 13, No. 22, 11 May 1872, 337–345, 337. A note on sources, I have unfortunately not had this edition of *Bandager* at my disposal so that corroborating Drachmann's statements with the correct edition of Nyrop's book has not been possible.

[300] Drachmann, "Om Skoliosens Behandling", 338.

[301] Ibid., 340. [der er modsat alle Mekanikens Grundsætninger]

[302] Ibid., 340. [At «et skævt Bækken» og et skævt stillet Bækken ere Synonymer for Hr. N., ere Smaating, som næppe ere Omtale værd.]

in his orthopaedic work spilled over in stating that Nyrop, "a self-proclaimed representative and spokesman of science behaves as though he is a docent and critic".[303] Along these lines, Drachmann played with Nyrop's statement about the two different conditions of the pelvis used synonymously, and rhetorically asked whether orthopaedist and orthopaedic instrument maker were synonyms as well.[304] Drachmann played off of Nyrop's position as an unlicensed practitioner, without formal medical training.

Nyrop responded to Drachmann's article two weeks later, with a short reply in *Ugeskrift*. He expressed surprise over Drachmann's critique and stated that his reflections in *Bandager og Instrumenter* were not intending to criticise Drachmann. Instead, they were to be read as "generally presenting some results based on experience, and nothing more".[305] He highlighted that some of his examples were misunderstood and that he had perhaps elaborated on his experiences in an unclear fashion. Regarding the synonymous pelvic conditions, he pointed out that the problem was an unfortunate mistake and something that "every understanding reader would quickly move on from".[306] In addition to this, he responded to Drachmann's judgement of his statistics, pointing out that Drachmann's own statistical results had been called into question; by whom, he did not divulge.[307]

When set in relation to the development of orthopaedics and orthopaedic treatments, Drachmann's and Nyrop's surface-level differences were not that stark. They both recommended braces and trusses to some degree; however, their braces operated on different mechanical principles and led to different recommendations, as the discussion from 1870 shows. Annemarie Mol underlines that tensions can be framed as controversy in specific sites of medical practice. She highlights journals as forums for controversy, in particular as a means of establishing scientific consensus.[308] These tensions might have remained unresolved and allowed to coexist in other settings. For Nyrop and Drachmann, the ways that their practices varied were likely overemphasised in *Ugeskrift*, but the reality at the time was that they were two practitioners on a similar professional playing field with competing notions of the best way to treat scoliosis.

---

[303] Ibid., 344. [Hr. N., der som Videnskabens selvskrevne Repræsentant og Talsmand optræder som Docent og Kritiker.]
[304] Ibid., 345.
[305] Camillus Nyrop, "En Replik". *Ugeskrift for Læger*. Series 3, Vol. 13, No. 25, 25 May 1872, 405–407, 406. [hvad jeg vilde, var Ganske I Almindelighed at fremsætte nogle Erfaringsresultater, og Intet videre.]
[306] Nyrop, "En Replik", 406. [en Fejl, som sikkert enhver velvillig Læser let vil komme over.]
[307] Ibid., 407.
[308] Mol, *The Body Multiple*, 114–115.

On the one hand, Drachmann was involved with an orthopaedic institute in Copenhagen that premiered methods involving gymnastics as well as braces and trusses.[309] Patients were required to visit the institution, under the watchful eyes of a physician. Nyrop, on the other hand, made and sold mechanical orthopaedic devices that were portable, in line with other bandagists. Patients could purchase the devices themselves, cutting out the middleman (or physician) so to speak, even if the devices could have been prescribed by a physician and constructed according to the patient's specific needs and measurements.[310] In addition to this, Nyrop was granted privileges in 1852 that allowed glovers to sell his instruments and devices throughout the country. Though this was a welcome development for provincial doctors, who would have been able to procure Nyrop's devices more readily, it opened up for other practitioners to obtain his devices easily as well. Drachmann might have taken exception to this development. According to him, the sole use of braces could harm patients with scoliosis or exacerbate the disorder.[311] But perhaps more acute, cutting out the middleman in Drachmann's case could make visits to his institution superfluous; an operation that was allegedly both profitable and helpful for his career.[312]

More so than the previous controversy, the one in 1872 emphasised the two men's divergent backgrounds, with Drachmann underlining Nyrop's position from the mistakes in *Bandager og Instrumenter*. Nyrop and Drachmann represented two different professional positions: that of the unlicensed practitioner and that of the physician. Within the larger history of orthopaedics, Anders Ottosson notes that narratives involving best practice and quackery could be used by nineteenth-century physicians as a means of securing hegemony over orthopaedic practices. He uses the case of English bonesetters and orthopaedists as an example of how physicians looked toward ancillary professions and amalgamated their collective knowledge as professional strategy.[313] Also regarding bonesetters, John Pickstone highlights how physicians initially worked with this crafts-based, family-oriented profession, built up a body of practical evidence, and eventually formalising and organising the roles of doctors and technicians and their divergent responsibilities.[314] Birgitte Rørbye emphasises that the conflicts between uni-

---

[309] See Jul. Petersen, "Anders Georg Drachmann". *Dansk biografisk Lexikon*, IV Bind Clemens–Eynden. Copenhagen: Gyldendalske Boghandels Forlag, 1890, 319.
[310] C. Nyrop, *Camillus Nyrop*, 107; Nyrop, *Bandager og Instrumenter*, 77, 110–113.
[311] Drachmann, "Om den Langgaardske orthopædiske Anstalt", 408.
[312] Trangbæk, *Kvindernes idræt*, 62.
[313] Ottosson, "The Manipulated History of Manipulations of Spines and Joints?", 86.
[314] Pickstone, "Bones in Lancashire", 26.

versity-trained physicians and other practitioners in Denmark increased toward the turn of the twentieth century when their territories began to overlap to a greater extent.[315] Drachmann's position toward Nyrop's work falls in line with the points made by Ottosson, Pickstone, and Rørbye. But roles were not yet organised, nor was training formalised.

In his study of the British nineteenth-century medical marketplace, Takahiro Ueyama stresses the importance of looking beyond rhetorical demarcations underlining so-called legitimate medical practice. Rather, he highlights the multiplicity and the "substantial divergences within the practice of medicine".[316] This is corroborated in the Danish context by Birgitte Rørbye, who underlines that even the term physician [*læge*] during the nineteenth century did not always indicate what one might associate as a university-trained physician.[317] Unlicensed practitioners aside, Nyrop worked with physicians as well, so even amongst licensed practitioners, there were divergent understandings of the merit of certain orthopaedic treatments, and professional relationships were fluid. Drachmann's comments can be understood in the larger presence of divergent orthopaedic treatments and multiple approaches to treatment, rather than simply as mere slights toward a layperson overstepping some kind of professional boundary. Read in the context of the history of orthopaedics more generally, Drachmann's critique was twofold. His emphasis on Nyrop's standing as a layperson was probably overstated for rhetorical purposes and he may have been attempting to assert control over the still-unlicensed domain of bandagists. However, both men were on a similar playing field and their divergent understandings in orthopaedics would have to continue to coexist.

Technology and the Hernia Truss

A few years later, another orthopaedic device–a hernia truss this time–attracted the attention of Danish physician Sigfred Levy and merited some discussion in *Ugeskrift* in December 1878. While I have not been able to uncover many biographical details about Levy, he was interested in gymnastics and physical activity and their curative potential for certain disorders.[318] Levy wrote an article about a specific hernia truss, which was

---

[315] Rørbye, *Mellem sundhed og sygdom*, 228.

[316] Takahiro Ueyama. *Health in the Marketplace: Professionalism, Therapeutic Desires, and Medical Commodification in Late-Victorian London*. Palo Alto: Society for the Promotion of Science and Scholarship, 2010, 231.

[317] Rørbye, *Mellem sundhed og sygdom*, 205–206.

[318] Trangbæk, *Kvindernes idræt*, 105–106.

designed and patented by Prussian Emil Edel. This truss, according to Levy, appeared to offer possibilities for hernia patients, or "hernia truss patients" [*Brokbaandspatienter*], referencing a comment from the inventor of the truss. Edel's truss allegedly allowed the patient to move more freely without being more expensive.[319] The mention of "patients of hernia trusses" was an indication of Levy's stance regarding the use of trusses, braces, and other, similar devices; Levy was a proponent of the curative potential gymnastics over the use of "machines", much like Drachmann above.[320] Certain kinds of trusses applied or otherwise used incorrectly could be injurious. A less expensive and less cumbersome device used under the guidance of a doctor could be a positive development.

However, according to Levy there was one problem: Edel had patented the truss in "every country" that hindered physicians from free use of the device to help their patients.[321] This also made it difficult to test whether or not the truss functioned as intended, as the patent was perceived to restrict the reconstruction of the device.[322] The issue with the device's patent was thus framed against the possibilities the device offered to hernia patients. The truss' American patent claimed improvement, both from a patient per-spective in that it was less likely to injure the wearer, and in terms of quality.[323] The patent made it seem like a suffering public was missing out on a useful tool to ease their ailment without the problems created by other devices, and the article lamenting the patent corroborated this view.

Looking at the American patent for Edel's hernia truss, Edel made several positive claims, which could make the device sound like a promising alternative. The patent stated that "this invention relates to certain improve-ments in trusses for hernia and other complaints of a similar nature; and it is specifically designed to overcome the objectionable and injurious qualities of the rigid spring body-band".[324] Furthermore, this truss would:

---

[319] Sigfred Levy, "Om Kjæderbrokbaand (Efter Emil Edel. Arch. f. klin. Chir. XXII. 3)". *Ugeskrift for Læger*. Series 3, Vol. 26, No. 28, 14 December 1878, 433–435, 433.

[320] Trangbæk, *Kvindernes idræt*, 105.

[321] Levy, "Om Kjæderbrokbaand", 435. [Forf. har ladet dem patentere i alle Lande.]

[322] Ibid., 435. "Every country" that Levy refers to included neither Sweden nor Denmark. The first multilateral treaty on the protection of intellectual property–the Paris Convention for the Protection of Industrial Property–was not signed until 1883 and did not come into effect until July 1, 1884. Denmark did not have patent laws until 1894.

[323] Emil Edel, "Improvement in Trusses". 1877. United States Patent US198586A, filed 14 July 1876, issued 25 December 1877.

[324] Ibid.

> not exert the undue pressure of the ordinary spring-band [and that] it is a
> well-known fact, demonstrated by experience, that the ordinary truss-spring
> or body-band is, in a number of cases, absolutely injurious to the wearer of
> the truss, for its pressure is so great and unremitting that it will injure the
> person and produce an enlargement of the rupture. Another disadvantage of
> the ordinary spring is, that it is very apt to break, even if it be of excellent
> workmanship.[325]

In other words, Edel positioned his truss in contrast to older models, which
caused, or at least risked causing injury, and claimed that his invention was
sturdier than other models. Based on the information given in the patent, it
may be tempting to believe that this truss would have been a safer and more
durable alternative by setting it against older trusses, showing them to be
injurious and less sturdy.

This was surely Nyrop's domain to offer insight, given his knowledge of
mechanics and experience with similar devices. And indeed, he replied
shortly after Levy's article was published, where he called the truss' benefits
into question. He began his article critically by stating that "as commendable
as it may be to, as soon as possible, make such new inventions available to the
public to serve suffering human beings [and] offer them relief, it is equally
important and necessary to attempt to examine the purported merits of the
new agent in relation to the old before it is praised".[326] And thoroughly
examined, it was. After weighing the supposed benefits against older hernia
technologies, Nyrop concluded that "with the best will, I cannot uncover any
advantage [...] for some simple cases, it can certainly be used, but in these
cases, you have both better and more easily available devices [...] for the
practitioner they are simple trivialities that raise suspicion".[327]

---

[325] Ibid.

[326] Camillus Nyrop, "Kjæderbrokbaand". *Ugeskrift for Læger.* Series 3, Vol. 26, No. 30, 28 December 1878, 469–472, 469, 469. [Ligesaa rosværdigt, som det er hurtigst muligt at overlevere til Offentligheden saadanne nye Opfindelser, der kunne tjene lidende Medmennesker til Lindring, ligesaa vigtigt og nødvendit er det at prøve og undersøge det nye Middels foregivne Fortrin fremfor det gamles–forinden det anbefales.]

[327] Nyrop, "Kjæderbrokbaand", 471–472. [Med bedste Villie kan jeg ikke opdage nogensomhelst Fordel ved denne af en Mængde Led sammensatte Kjædefjeder… og for enkelt lette Tilfælde kan den jo nok benyttes, men man har i disse Tilfælde baade bedre og lettere tilgængelige Apparater, som af den daglige Praktik stadig ville blive foretrukne… men ogsaa disse Oplysninger tage sig godt ud i en Reklame–for Fagmanden ere de rene Trivialiteter, og de opvække hans Mistænksomhed.]

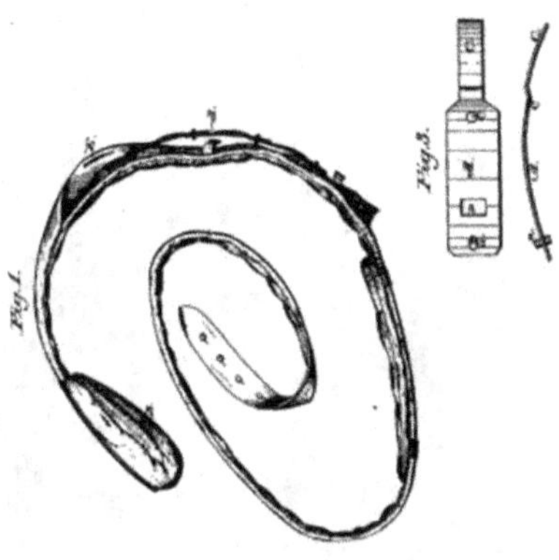

Fig. 16. Emil Edel's patented hernia truss. A series of plates are connected to the belt, which Edel argued in the patent made the device more flexible and able to withstand movement. This design, he stated, could be used in a number of different hernia trusses. Emil Edel, "Improvement in Trusses". 1877. United States Patent US198586A, filed 14 July 1876, issued 25 December 1877.

Nyrop's mechanical expertise was well-known in Denmark and internationally, and his expertise would have made him qualified to offer commentary on the construction of the truss.[328] His skill in metalwork and orthopaedics was acknowledged multiple times in Danish newspapers.[329] His orthopaedic work was also praised in the Swedish newspaper *Aftonbladet* over the attention it had received at the 1873 World's Fair in Vienna. For example, according to the article, the springs used in his orthopaedic devices "are

[328] See for example his account of praise from German physicians in Nyrop, "I Anledning af Hr. Professor Drachmanns Udtalelser", 460–461. See also the introduction to *Bandager og Instrumenter*, where he cites French praise for his work. Nyrop, *Bandager og Instrumenter*, [not paginated].

[329] See for example [Anon.], *Fædrelandet*. 15 January 1856; [Anon.], "Industriudstillingen i Malmø". *Lolland-Falsters Stifts-Tidende*. 17 September 1861; [Anon.], *Fædrelandet*. 2 June 1862; [Anon.], "Den danske Afdeling af Udstillingen i London". *Fyens Stiftstidende*. 22 August 1862; [Anon.], "A. Den industrielle Afdeling af Udstillingen". *Lolland-Falsters Stifts-Tidende*. 31 May 1863.

immensely yielding [but] strong [...] Mr. Nyrop has, by perfecting the springs, even attempted to minimise injury and injurious qualities often caused by cumbersome orthopaedic apparatuses".[330] Nyrop's review should not be understood merely as a maker examining whether or not the device itself would work, but rather as an individual with knowledge of both orthopaedic treatments *and* orthopaedic devices, assessing the device of a potential competitor with this complex knowledge in mind.

Fig. 44.

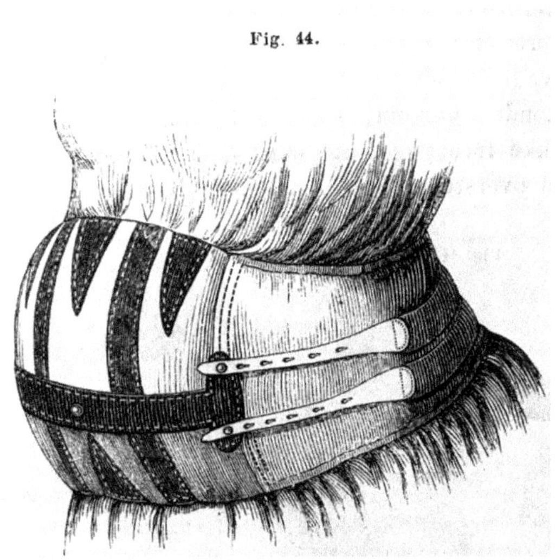

Fig. 17. A hernia truss designed by Camillus Nyrop for an umbilical hernia. The small screw in the middle of the wide band running lengthwise across the front would be where a pad with a spring would be attached on the backside to apply pressure on the hernia. Nyrop designed this larger almost corset-like apparatus to apply consistent pressure and keep the pad from moving. Camillus Nyrop. *Bandager og Instrumenter afbildede og beskrevne med en tilføi et Prisfortegnelse.* Copenhagen: G.E.C. Gad, 1864, 40.

In his review of the truss, Nyrop did not directly criticise patents as Levy did. He did, however, indicate that patents were not necessarily formulae for success and that they could be a form of advertisement. According to Nyrop, the hernia truss may not have been as useful as Levy's article makes it seem, which calls into question whether or not patents could be read as a mark of actual quality. According to Levy's article, the patent illustrated a system

---

[330] [Anon.], "Werldsutställning i Wien". *Aftonbladet.* 28 May 1873. [Fastän dessa stålfjedrar ege en ofantlig mjukhet… de äro dessutom starka… Hr Nyrop har dessutom genom fjedrarnes fullkomnande sökt minska de skador och farligheter, som ortopedien ofta gifvit upphof till, när klumpiga apparater af den begagnas.]

where a suffering public was missing out on a useful tool to ease their ailments. If patents are understood as claim-making texts, the claims made in patents of medical devices must imply some kind of new technology or improvement to older ones.[331] Edel's patent makes several beneficial claims, for example, that "forming the truss spring or band of a series of plates, which are connected to each other by means of studs or rivets and interlocking tongues [...] that will yield to all muscular movements of the body", but the integrity of these claims was implicit.[332]

Instead, Nyrop's reservations over the truss itself raises further questions about it: did it actually work and was it really as innovative and beneficial as the author states? Nyrop himself encouraged examination of the merits of these claims and explained why it might not work according to description. He stated that many of the descriptions accompanying the truss would raise suspicions for anyone well-versed in truss mechanics and their function and he had indeed examined the truss himself.[333] For instance, in his examination of the truss, he attempted to work with it according to instructions and some of the rivets fell out. This led to costly repairs, contrary to Edel's claims.[334] From Nyrop's perspective, this would have hardly been an improvement to other models and spoke poorly of the craftsmanship and construction of the device.

[331] Eva Hemmungs Wirtén notes that patents are claim-making in similar ways that academic papers are claim-making. They have authors, imply readership, rely on collection, storage and archiving and relate to the construction of public knowledge. See Eva Hemmungs Wirtén, "The Patent and the Paper: A Few Thoughts on Late Modern Science and Intellectual Property". *Culture Unbound: Journal of Current Cultural Research.* Vol. 7, 2015, 600–609. See also Mario Biagioli, "Rights or Rewards?: Changing Frameworks of Scientific Authorship", in *Scientific Authorship: Credit and Intellectual Property in Science,* Mario Biagioli and Peter Galison (eds.), 253–279. New York: Routledge, 2003.

[332] Edel, "Improvement in Trusses", US198586A.

[333] Nyrop, "Kjæderbrokbaand", 472.

[334] Ibid., 471.

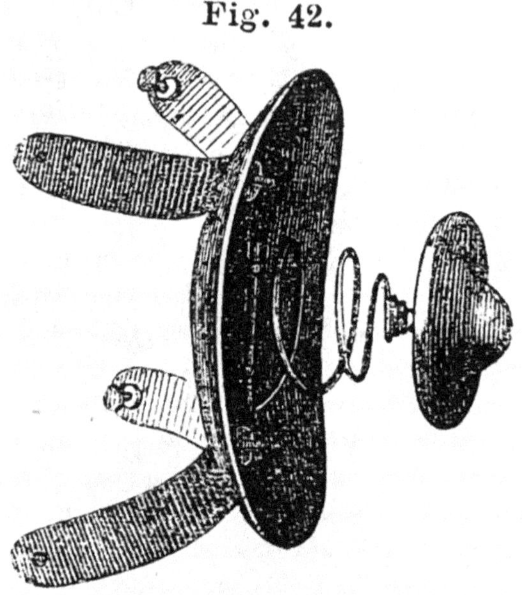

Fig. 18. An illustration of a pad attached to a hernia truss designed for umbilical hernias. The spring apparatus is enclosed in the pad, which would sit around the hernia and apply pressure to it. Camillus Nyrop. *Bandager og Instrumenter afbildede og beskrevne med en tilføi et Prisfortegnelse*. Copenhagen: G.E.C. Gad, 1864, 39.

Nyrop's article examining the mechanical merits of Edel's truss was not the final interjection on Edel's truss. Levy responded to Nyrop a few weeks later, having misunderstood a point that Nyrop made about advertisement. He misread Nyrop to such a degree that the editor had to interject with comment in a footnote.[335] Levy had presumed that Nyrop was accusing him of advertising Edel's truss and stated that "advertisement is a form of expression that is completely disharmonious and foreign for a scientific debate".[336] Nyrop's original article was no critique against Levy or Levy's query, but rather a

[335] Sigfred Levy, "Om Kjædebrokbaand". *Ugeksrift for Læger*. Series 3, Vol. 27, No. 2, 11 January 1879, 21–22.

[336] Levy, "Om Kjædebrokbaand", 22.[Reklame er overhovedet et Udtryk, der klinger lidt disharmonisk og fremmed i videnskabelig Debat.] This was not the final contribution to this "scientific debate" (using Levy's words), however. See Camillus Nyrop, "Om Kjædebrokbaand". *Ugeksrift for Læger*. Series 3, Vol. 27, No. 3 & 4, 18 January 1879, 52–53; Sigfred Levy, "Om Kjædebrokbaand". *Ugeksrift for Læger*. Series 3, Vol. 27, No. 5, 25 January 1878, 62.

thorough review of the truss in question. Nyrop's point about advertising was that "the present day is bustling with advertisements for all kinds of curiosities as cures for all possible human weaknesses and this trend has even reached Denmark".[337] Accordingly, Nyrop remarked that a patent could shine favourable light on the device in an advertisement.[338] These remarks indicate that, according to Nyrop, Edel's truss fit well into the growing culture of commodity in medicine and that despite its pitfalls, obvious to anyone knowledgeable in truss mechanics, it could be made to look favourable in advertisements.

And, indeed, Edel's patented truss was used in an advertisement, albeit for itinerant bandagist Niels Peter Heskier. The advertisement for Heskier's services in figure 19 mentioned Edel's truss as being "patented everywhere in Europe and America".[339] Heskier mentioned Edel's truss in at least one other advertisement during the 1870s, both from 1879.[340] Takahiro Ueyama notes that mentioning patents in advertisements was particularly popular amongst these kinds of practitioners, and was a means of gaining access to the healthcare market.[341] Nyrop, on the other hand, already had access to the healthcare market, in particular in exchange directly with legitimate practitioners, so the necessity of highlighting a device was patented would be less pertinent for him. A patent, or mention of one, would have been a means of legitimisation and a way of building trust, especially by a quasi-legitimate practitioner like Heskier. The connection between Edel's truss and Heskier is interesting in itself, as Heskier was a bandagist of the less serious calibre. In an article in *Ugeskrift* from 1882, physician T. M. Trautner noted that

[337] Nyrop, "Kjæderbrokbaand", 469. [Nutiden er saa fuld af Reklamer for allehaande Kuriositeter, der helbrede for alle mulige menneskelige Svagheder, og Danmark begynder ogsaa godt at komme med denne Retning.]

[338] Nyrop, "Kjædebrokbaand", 471–472 .

[339] P. Heskier, [Advertisement]. *Lolland-Falsters Folketidende.* 22 February 1879. [patenterede overalt i Europa og Amerika.]

[340] Heskier, [Advertisement], 22 February 1879; P. Heskier. [Advertisement]. *Sorø Amtstidende.* 14 February 1879. It is worthwhile to note that Heskier mentioned that he was from Copenhagen in many of his advertisements, and that both the above newspapers are from smaller locales. While outside the scope of this chapter, the relationship between city and countryside and the legitimacy given from using a title under false pretences and mentioning the capitol were likely ways of trying to boost his reputation for potential clients. He also travelled and advertised his visits frequently in newspapers. See for example P. Heskier, [Advertisement]. *Horsens Folkeblad.* 12 January 1877; [Advertisement]. *Horsens Folkebland.* 19 January 1877; [Advertisement]. *Bornholms Tidende.* 14 Feburary 1878; [Advertisement]. Aarhus Amstidende. 5 November 1881; [Advertisement]. *Stubbekøbing Avis.* 21 February 1882; [Advertisement]. *Svendborg Amtstidende.* 6 September 1882; [Advertisement]. *Kolding Folkeblad.* 11 December 1883.

[341] Ueyama, *Health in the Marketplace*, 152.

attempts to have Heskier indicted under the quackery law were unsuccessful, despite Heskier's endeavours in treating patients.

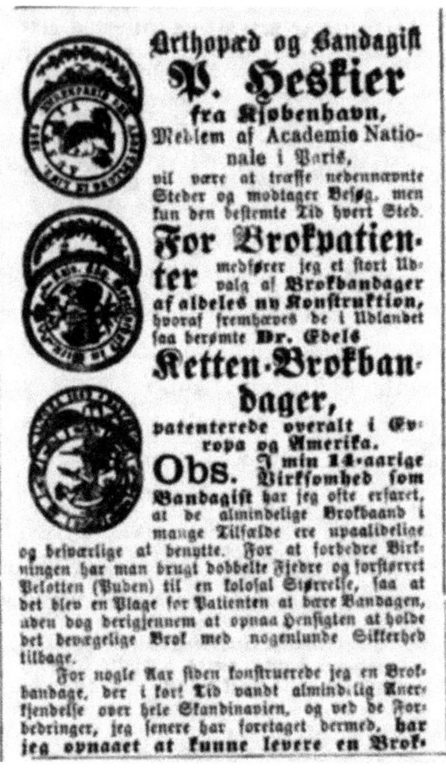

Fig. 19. An advertisement for bandagist P. Heskier, where he mentioned Edel's patented hernia trusses, noting they were patented in the United States and Europe. P. Heskier. [Advertisement]. *Lolland-Falsters Folketidende*. 22 February 1879.

Heskier also advertised under the moniker "Professor Heskier". According to Trautner, a physician had inquired about Heskier's title, and it was apparently an honorary title bestowed upon Heskier by "Dante's Institute" in Naples in 1881. Trautner queried if it was possible to sanction Heskier for the illegitimate use of a title somehow.[342] Heskier's later use of "professor" after 1881, whether the title was acquired through legitimate means or not, plays off Nyrop's use of the same–he frequently used his, albeit legitimate, title in

---

[342] Trautner, "Om Bandagistvirksomheden", 343–344.

advertisement as well as authorship (see figure 11 for example).[343] While the Heskier-connection to Edel's truss appeared after the above discussions in *Ugeskrift*, the timing is convenient: Heskier may have also been familiar with the discussion between Nyrop and Levy. His advertisements also serve as a testament to Nyrop's point about patents and promotion: they look convincing in advertisements but are not necessarily a stamp of legitimacy.

Professional Regulation and Orthopaedics

As a response to the problem of itinerant bandagists like Heskier, moves were made to try to give bandagists official professional status in Denmark in the 1880s. This set out to define the requisite forms of knowledge and training required, and formally organise the profession. The following case will look at some of the strategies used by practitioners, both physicians and non-physicians, in establishing and organising orthopaedic practice. The three men, Nyrop, Drachmann and Levy, were central figures in discussions about this matter in *Ugeskrift* as well.[344] The background to this move was the presence of itinerant bandagists specialised in selling and applying orthopaedic treatments with bands and braces, without any particular training or knowledge in orthopaedics or medicine. Heskier and Schøinning were two examples of the problematic bandagist. One of the issues raised about ambulatory bandagists was that some were untrained, prone to do more harm than good and could potentially harm patients.[345] It was difficult to sanction quacks in nineteenth-century Denmark and it was unclear if they could be penalised as quacks or if their work even qualified as quackery under contemporary law. But the issue of itinerant and unlicensed practitioners, who were only available in a given locale under a brief period, would have been detrimental if a patient encountered problems after he had left town and would allocate the burden of treatment on a local physician. [346]

---

[343] His colleagues referred to him as "Hr. Prof." as well. See for example Drachmann, "Om Skoliosens Behandling"; C. R. Struckmann, "Et Instrument for Ikke-Kirurger". *Ugeskrift for Læger*. Series 4, Vol. 5, No. 1–2, January 7, 1882, 1–5.

[344] Immanuel Schiødte, who authored the first articles mentioned in this chapter with Drachmann, died in 1873.

[345] See for example C. Nyrop, *Camillus Nyrop*, 116; Camillus Nyrop, "Om Virksomheden som kirurgisk Instrumentmager og Bandagist". *Ugeskrift for Læger*. Series 4, Vol. 5, No. 21, 6 May 1882, 313–326, 314.

[346] His ads included an image of a scoliotic back and an image of the same back with a corset-like brace over. See fig. 91 in Nyrop, *Bandager og Instrumeter*, 75. I have not been able to uncover any direct relationship between the Nyrops and Schiønning, which makes his use of this image all the more interesting.

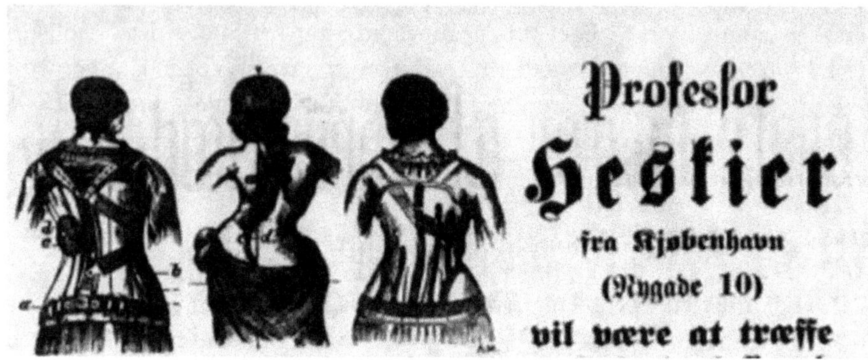

Fig. 20. "Professor Heskier from Copenhagen". Note the image in the middle, which is the same as the one on the left in Schøinning's advertisement in fig. 12. P. Heskier. [Advertisement]. *Aarhus Amstidende.* 5 November 1881.

However, it was not a physician who presented a motion to alter this situation: it was Camillus Nyrop, along with eight other bandagists and instrument makers, including one of Nyrop's sons, Johan Ernst. In the spring of 1882, Nyrop and the other signatories presented a formal request to the Ministry of Ecclesiastics and Education as well as the Ministry of Internal Affairs, which was republished in *Ugeskrift*. The letter highlighted the problem of "so-called [...] bandagists" who "travel around the country and peddle various apparatuses, bandages and machines trumpeted as miracle cures, with previously arranged promotion in the form of fantastical advertisements", much like Heskier and Schøinning.[347] The letter argued that surgical instrument makers and bandagists were complimentary trades. Legitimate bandagists who were not also instrument makers and trained in metal work would not be able to construct proper devices due to the metal frame in most devices they worked with.[348] The letter also argued for formal recognition of the knowledge required to work as instrument maker or bandagist. It noted the need for some kind of regulatory system for medical devices, including suggestions for formalised training opportunities for the construction, sale, and modification of these devices. One of its key arguments was the potential danger for patients if instrument makers and

[347] Nyrop, "Om Virksomheden som kirurgisk Instrumentmager og Bandagist", 313. [at saakaldte Elektrikere, Bandagister, o.s.v. rejse Landet igjennem og falbyde forskjellige Apparater, Bandager og Maskiner, som efter en forud arrangeret Reklame, navnlig storartede Avertissementer, ere udbasunede som næsten mirakelgjørende.]
[348] C. Nyrop, *Camillus Nyrop*, 117.

bandagists were not knowledgeable enough, used false titles or purchased professional certificates without undertaking training and offering braces and trusses under the principle of one size fits all.[349]

The call for regulation made in the letter presented a potentially reasonable solution to a problem experienced by surgical instrument makers and bandagists of less dubious character as well as physicians and offered potential for a united front. This would not be the case, however. An editorial response to Nyrop's letter agreed that itinerant practitioners were a problem, but also pointed out that there were penial measures that could be taken against people who sold goods and services under false pretences.[350] Two weeks later, in the same issue of *Ugeskrift*, responses by both A. G. Drachmann and Sigfred Levy were published. While both welcomed the call for better regulation, they highlighted the differences in expertise between the three professions and argued for the diagnosis and ordinated treatment of an ailment to be the sole responsibility of the physician. One of the tasks both men undertook was analysing the relationship that surgical instrument makers and bandagists had with medical practice. For bandagists, it was technical expertise, but for surgical instrument makers, it was unclear how closely related to medical practice they were at all.

The editorial response also highlighted the difficulties with requiring some kind of examination for instrument makers, as they sold other goods, including kitchen knives and cutlery. The situation was, however, different for bandagists. Bandagists worked, according to the editor, with devices that treated injuries and afflictions that could potentially be life-threatening and, in some cases, "many people turn to bandagists directly [...] The bandagist is, in reality, the patient's physician and in these situations rational treatment can have a significant impact on healing and [the patient's] life".[351] The important difference between the two professions was the therapeutic value of their work and their roles in contact with patients. Bandagists, he argued, were different from surgical instrument makers, as their work had therapeutic value and would benefit from regulation through a knowledge test in order to practice. He stated that "the next logical step would be that the community supports that the bandagist profession is reserved for those with

---

[349] Nyrop, "Om Virksomheden som kirurgisk Instrumentmager og Bandagist", 314.

[350] Ibid., 318.

[351] Ibid., 320. [Det maa nu ikke glemmes, at mangfoldige Mennesker henvende sig direkte til Bandagisten med disse og andre lignende Tilfælde, Bandagisten bliver i Virkeligheden Patientens Læge, og det for Tilfælde, hvor en rationel Behandling kan have den allerstørste Betydning for Helbred og Liv.]

medical training as a specific specialisation".[352] The commentary ended by thanking Nyrop for bringing this issue to light and encouraging further discussion.

In his article, Drachmann underlined the importance of analysing the relationships bandagists had with medicine and medical practice. Bandagists, according to him, could provide "expert technical assistance" and perhaps assist in other ways for patients with incurable physical disabilities where "the help they would require is significantly or exclusively of the technical-mechanical variety", i.e., patients who could not be helped with physical therapy.[353] The bandagists' role, in this case, would not be curative, but take a therapeutic character–assisting those whom medicine could not cure, but who could be assisted in some way by mechanical means. Drachmann also argued that physicians specialised in orthopaedics should "like American orthopaedists and our own [Danish] dentists, acquire the mechanical and technical knowledge and skills necessary [...] and construct apparatuses and bandages required at their own workshops".[354] This would mean that orthopaedists would have more mechanical knowledge and be able to readily construct their own devices. Levy, on the other hand, likened bandagists to pharmacists, who "under no circumstances should be encumbered with any responsibility for the effects of the prescription and would especially not take it upon oneself to prescribe medicines".[355] They could continue to carry out their work, but it should not be their responsibility to diagnose and ordinate devices used to treat patients. Rather, "that which cures the ill must be decided by physicians–and not by anyone else".[356]

Nyrop responded to all three articles a few weeks later. He stated that he was pleased that his letter attracted so much interest; however, he seemed unsatisfied with some of the suggestions offered up by *Ugeskrift*'s editor,

[352] Ibid., 323. [Men ogsaa her fremtræder det da som en logisk Selvfølge, at Samfundet vilde staa sig bedst ved, at Bandagistvirksomheden blev forbeholdt Lægestanden som en særlig Specialitet.]

[353] A. G. Drachmann, "Om Virksomheden som kirurgisk Instrumentmager og Bandagist". *Ugeksrift for Læger*. Series 4, Vol. 5, No. 23, 20 May 1882, 345–349, 346. [Bandagistens sagkyndige tekniske Bistand... da den Hjælp, de trænge til, væsentlig eller udelukkende er en teknisk-mekanisk.]

[354] Drachmann, "Om Virksomheden", 349. [i Lighed med de amerikanske Orthopæder og vore egne Tandlæger, erhverve sig de mekaniske og tekniske Kundskaber og Færdigheder, som ere nødvendige til en saadan Stilling, og paa deres egne Værksteder lade forfærdige de Apparater og Bandager, som de have Brug for.]

[355] Sigfred Levy, "Om Virksomheden som kirurgisk Instrumentmager og Bandagist". *Ugeskrift for Læger*. Series 4, Vol. 5, No. 23, 20 May 1882, 349–353, 351. [men i ingen Henseende bebryder sig med noget Ansvar for Virkningen af det Ordinerede, end mindre paatager sig selvstændig at forordne Medikamenterne]

[356] Levy, "Om Virksomheden", 353. [at hvad der baader Syge, det skal afgjøres af Læger–og ikke af nogensomhelst anden.]

Drachmann, and Levy. "This is a serious issue for me", he stated in the concluding paragraph after reiterating his stance and arguing against several of the suggestions presented by the other commenters.[357] He questioned the suggestion Drachmann presented about orthopaedists-cum-bandagists with workshops. In this case, he noted that while bandagists and surgical instrument makers might seek to study medicine, he thought it unlikely that "the educated physician, who stands in the service of science" would consider studying a mechanical trade.[358] But most importantly, for Nyrop, the entanglements between the work of a bandagist and that of an instrument maker necessitated that bandagists also had training in and knowledge of metalwork to properly construct the springs, frames, and other metalwork in more complicated orthopaedic braces and devices.[359] Furthermore, many surgical instrument makers, including Nyrop, made orthopaedic devices as well. In this sense, he considered the two professions hardly separable, in contrast to the suggestions presented in the editorial.

Although the above discussion illustrates an attempt to, at least rhetorically, draw boundaries between the work of physicians, instrument makers and bandagists, it also highlights fluidity. All four men presented different solutions to the perceived problem. By drawing bandagists closer whilst pushing instrument makers away, physicians would have allocated tasks to bandagists that would have typically fallen under their domain. For instance, although Drachmann's overarching stance argued for orthopaedists taking over the construction of orthopaedic devices, he did acknowledge that bandagists could be of assistance for patients with physical disabilities that were incurable. Bandagists would serve a more supplementary role and acquiesce to the assessment of physicians. Levy suggested that, like pharmacists, the bandagist's professions should follow "a natural order to achieve correct, rational, and therefore less burdensome work", i.e., that diagnostics remain firmly in the physician's domain and bandagists operate according to this system.[360] It was the physician's task to mull over diagnoses.

The reallocation of certain kinds of labour, including that of a more manual character, to ancillary professions, whilst keeping diagnosis as the domain of physicians is a means of power assertion, according to Rosemary

---

[357] Camillus Nyrop, "Om Virksomheden som kirurgisk Instrumentmager og Bandagist". *Ugeksrift for Læger*. Series 4, Vol. 5, No. 28–29, 17 June 1882, 433–437, 437. [For mig er Sagen fuld Alvor.]

[358] Nyrop, "Om Virksomheden", 434. [uddannede Læge, der staar ved et langt videnskabeligt Arbejdes Maal]

[359] Ibid., 434.

[360] Levy, "Om Virksomheden", 351. [Forholderne ogsaa for hans Vedkommende fi ken naturlig Ordning, kunne opnaa en korrekt, fornuftig og derfor mindre byrdefuld Gjerning]

Stevens.[361] The different moves physicians made to attempt to claim aspects of the bandagist's work as their own, distance their profession from that of surgical instrument makers and their proclamation of diagnosis as their domain also illustrate the assertion of power. In John Pickstone's study of bonesetters in nineteenth-century England, he outlines the rationalisational moves that physicians made to organise unlicensed practice. He identifies them as, firstly, a professional medical interest in a small, crafts-based practice, which, secondly, led to the practice's professional promotion, which, thirdly, lead to the collection of evidence and placement within a professional analytical framework, and then lastly, could be organised socially.

Much like Danish bandagists (and indeed, Nyrop as well), the nineteenth-century bonesetter family in Pickstone's study, the Taylors, were seemingly uncontroversial to mainstream medical doctors and their medical cosmology and work was "easily compatible with ordinary medicine".[362] Nyrop was, and at least some other bandagists were, accepted by the medical status quo, and had previously filled a practical gap. But the number of physicians was increasing, and physicians were increasingly undertaking orthopaedic work. By 1880, there were over 500 private practicing physicians in Denmark, and the number had increased significantly since mid-century even when accounting for general population growth.[363] This shift, with a growing number of trained physicians, seen in conjunction with the moves Pickstone identifies, may have motivated the likes of Drachmann and Levy to assert their control over an area once covered by bandagists. An example of this is Levy's insistence on the "natural order" where the work of bandagists was limited to that of fulfilling what a physician ordinated. He also underlined that future association between the two professions was dependent on maintaining and understanding this hierarchy, stating that "the continual and intimate cooperation between the physician and the bandagist in this form is conditional on their different areas of responsibility".[364]

This issue was not easily resolved, and bandagists, surgical instrument makers, and physicians would have to continue to find ways to coexist with one another without reform. A year after the articles above, in 1882, the editor of *Ugeskrift* left a comment to another article on the problem of

---

[361] Rosemary Stevens. *In Sickness and in Wealth: American Hospitals in the Twentieth Century.* Baltimore: Johns Hopkins University Press, 1999, 12.

[362] Pickstone, "Bones in Lancashire", 21.

[363] Vallgårda, et. al.. *Sundhedsvæsen og sundhedspolitik,* 142.

[364] Levy, "Om Virksomheden", 352. [der i sidste Instans forudsætter et stadigt og intimt Samarbejde mellem Lægen og Bandagisten i den Form, som betinges ved disse Tvendes forskjellige Art af Ansvar.]

itinerant bandagists and stated that "this question was discussed extensively one year ago [...] and has not seemed to reach fruitful results in practice".[365] He was open for further discussion about how to conclusively deal with the situation but reminded practitioners that itinerant bandagists engaged in illegitimate practice could technically be punished by law. However, he acknowledged that the problem was exacerbated by lack of physicians in the countryside. The best way to resolve this problem and regulate the influx of illegitimate bandagists was to "see to it that there is a physician who specialises in orthopaedics and the adjacent field of the practical healing arts as a bandagist, in every larger town in the country."[366]

Concluding Remarks

In this chapter, I have used the work of Camillus Nyrop as a guide to examine three cases where friction arose regarding orthopaedic practice. Bandagists were generally tolerated, and generally sanctioned, practitioners in nineteenth-century Danish orthopaedics. Nyrop was no exception. However, the work of bandagists and physicians began to overlap all the more, causing friction between different actors. The three cases highlight examples of this in different spheres: the therapeutic, the technological, and the professional. The differences in opinion on therapeutics between Nyrop and Drachmann prevailed; neither Levy nor Nyrop found resolution over Edel's hernia truss; itinerant bandagists remained unregulated following the letter to the Ministry of Ecclesiastics and Education and the Ministry of Internal Affairs, and its subsequent responses. If anything, tensions quickly evaporated again. Because the frictions ebbed out, differences were left to coexist. Thus, these cases illustrate what Annemarie Mol calls the coexistence of difference. This means that, on the level of practice, differences coexisted alongside one another, and even overlapped, but that tensions could arise under certain circumstances. Even if physicians may have tried to mobilise and enact authority in their favour, they were unsuccessful in doing so. There were no clear losers in any of these cases, nor were any of the actors directly excluded from engaging in this chapter's specific forum for discussion, *Ugeskrift for Læger*.

---

[365] V. Budde. [unititled]. *Ugeskrift for Læger*. Series 4, Vol. 8, No. 6, 4 August 1883, 80–81, 80.
[366] Budde, [untitled], 81. [at der i enhver større By her i Landet fandtes en Læge, som med Virksomheden som Specialist i Orthopedi og nærstaaende Gren af den praktiske Lægekunst tillige forbandt Virksomheden som Bandagist]

I have chosen not to frame this chapter around quacks or quackery for a few reasons. When licensed practice still had little control over some areas of the healing arts, such as orthopaedics, conflating all forms of unlicensed practice as quackery would misrepresent the work, skill, and training of some practitioners. Actors like Nyrop operated on a similar playing field as physicians in orthopaedics during the period examined. While I acknowledge that some bandagists engaged in quackish practices, orthopaedics was still yet to be put under the explicit control of physicians, and as I have stated, patients with musculoskeletal disorders at this time, especially those with disorders deemed untreatable, were often left in the care of unlicensed prac-titioners like bandagists anyway. All bandagists were not lacking in requisite knowledge or skill, either. Labelling them largely or solely as quacks does not acknowledge the formal and informal channels of training that they partook in and would misrepresent the skill and competency of some practitioners. Their general position seems to have been relatively uncontroversial, at least as far as *Ugeskrift for Læger* is concerned. Further research will hopefully be able to look more closely at other sources and perhaps engage with the question of quackery more directly by, for example, looking at the authorit-ies' unwillingness to sanction quacks in some cases. Perhaps difference was also forced to coexist here.

Finally, as Anders Ottosson has highlighted in his research on the history of orthopaedics, physicians were active in rewriting the history of ortho-paedics as a more physician-centred discipline than it actually was in the nineteenth century.[367] Ottosson does not, however, examine the Danish case, which needs to be studied further. Indeed, Nyrop as a figure in Danish orthopaedics stands in contrast to the image David LeVay presents in his book *The History of Orthopaedics*. The first significant figures he mentions, Niels Stensen and Jakob Benignus Winslow, were born in the seventeenth century. The next one he presents is Poul Guildal. Guildal was born in 1882 and did not sit his final medical examinations until 1906.[368] To be sure, Guildal was a significant figure in Danish orthopaedics; however, the absence of the nineteenth century in LeVay's book works from a narrative that Ottosson attempts to nuance in his article, as I have also done in this chapter. Hopefully, it will inspire further consideration and a closer look at the work of bandagists in this regard. Though it is unclear what specific training Nyrop had in orthopaedic remedies, his work with physicians and his position in

---

[367] Ottosson, "The Manipulated History of Manipulations of Spines and Joints?", 86–87.
[368] LeVay, *History of Orthopaedics*, 329; Harald Nilsonne, "Poul Guildal: In Memoriam". *Acta Orthopaedic Scandinavica*. Vol. 20, No. 3, 1951, 181–183.

Danish medicine serves to sanction his practice and skill in truss making and as a bandagist, at least until this chapter's final case, a little over a year before his death on Christmas Eve 1883.

4. Faithful Followers:
Listerism, Surgical Practice, and Antiseptic Enactment

In an article on antisepsis in *Hygiea* from 1878, Swedish surgeon Carl Rossander remarked that "as we can see now, and a number of further examples could be presented, the cases in this question cannot be considered closed, regarding theory. But in practice, the matter is definitive thus far. Antiseptic injections present a much greater effect than other methods of treatment for cystitis, regardless of how it [the illness] developed".[369] Cystitis is an inflammatory condition of the bladder. What Rossander suggested was that the positive, clinical results of antiseptic injections were more important than the illness' unclear aetiology. Theory and aetiology were debatable, but practice was clear and definitive.

Antisepsis is a method of wound care based on the destruction of germs through the use of chemicals in order to prevent infections. There were multiple understandings of infection and inflammation during this time, and much like in the second chapter, interest in cellular pathology and chemical changes in the body varied. As Michael Worboys highlights in his book *Spreading Germs*, inflammation was primarily associated with trauma around mid-century, and while practitioners could identify wounds that were liable to cause problems such as mortification and sepsis, the aetiology was not well understood, and theories behind disease processes were diverse. Furthermore, he points out that surgeons in particular were, at this time, largely empirically inclined clinicians, not theorists.[370] Both statements are reflective of Rossander's statement above, and of the general attitudes Swedish and Danish physicians and surgeons had towards antisepsis. Even if they were unsure of the theory behind the practice, its empirical results were clear.

The method most associated with antiseptic wound care in the nineteenth century is Listerism, pioneered by surgeon Joseph Lister and described first in the *British Medical Journal* in 1867. This is the type of antisepsis that I will discuss in this chapter. Listerism employed the use of strong chemicals,

---

[369] Carl Rossander, "Nya området för den antiseptiska sårbehandlingen". *Hygiea*. Vol. 40, No. 10, October 1878, 529–541, 530. [Som man ser, och exempel skulle kunna i än större mängd framdragas, äro akterna i denna fråga ej att betrakta såsom afslutade, hvad teorien beträffar. Men i praxi synes saken så till vida afgjord, att de antiseptiska insprutningarna visa en långt större verksamhet än andra, när det gäller att behandla en blåskatarr, den må nu hafva uppkommit huru som helst.]

[370] Michael Worboys. *Spreading Germs: Disease Theories and Medical Practice in Britain, 1865–1900.* Cambridge: Cambridge University Press, 2000, 33.

carbolic acid solutions in particular, according to explicit methods. Lister altered the method several times during his lifetime, and introduced a toolkit in the 1870s that included the use of carbolic acid spray and bandages and ligatures prepared with the chemical solution. There were, however, multiple, simultaneous antiseptic systems of wound care circulating at the time, and practitioners used antiseptic terminology to delineate other methods. Thus, the term antisepsis should be read fluidly, in that what it entailed varied based on factors like subdiscipline, training, and other factors.[371]

This chapter will examine antisepsis in Sweden and Denmark and its relationship to medical practice by looking at articles commenting on Joseph Lister's method of antiseptic wound management. In Denmark and Sweden, the method was often described as "the Listerist dressing" [*forbinding/förband*]. This language emphasises that it was understood by contemporaries as method of wound care and management, rather than a strictly invasive surgical technology. This is an important distinction for the method, and in discussing surgery around mid-century. Few surgeries at this time were elective. For example, Seraphim Hospital in Stockholm accounted for 153 "larger" operations during 1850; whereby, the majority were cataract extractions and amputations, and many of the disorders treated by surgeons here were the result of accidents.[372] Even more than two decades later, operations requiring opening the abdominal cavity were rarities.[373] While some of the procedures discussed below are invasive, Listerist wound care

---

[371] Antisepsis and antiseptics were also used to describe methods of and recommendations for food hygiene, meaning it was used outside of medical practice as well and connected to other, more general conceptions of disinfection. Additionally, while disinfection was used occasionally in relation to antisepsis, the term, through the 1860s, 1870s and 1880s was typically used in reference to the cleaning of rooms and wards due to communicable diseases, e.g., dysentery, cholera and typhoid fever or questions of hygiene. See for example Edward Edholm, "Lehrbuch der Militär-Hygiene, bearbeitet von Dr C. Kirchner, mit 75 Holzschnitten und 6 lithografirten Tafeln. 445 sid. Erlangen 1869". *Hygiea*. Vol. 31, No. 8, August 1869, 359–366; A. A. Langell, "Om Ileo-typhus och Typhus exanthematicus å Allmänna och Sahlgrenska sjukhuset i Göteborg". *Hygiea*. Vol. 32, No. 9, September 1870, 441–451; A. Kullberg, "Den tredje internationella medicinska kongressen i Wien 1873. Om karantäner mot kolera". *Hygiea*. Vol. 35, No. 11, November 1873, 658–673; Andreas Brünniche, "Til Belysning af den I Efteraaret 1875 her I Byen forekomme Epidemi af Dysenteri". *Hospitals-Tidende*. Vol. 19, No. 23, 7 June 1876, 354–357; Frederik Trier, "Nogle Tilfælde af Blodgang som Hospitalssygdom". *Hospitals-Tidende*. Vol. 19, No. 31, 2 August 1876, 481–489; R. Wawrinsky, "Om desinfektion efter smittosamma sjukdomar. Föreläsning å Karolinska Insitutet den 4 oktober 1890. Af dr R. Wawrinsky". *Hygiea*. Vol. 52, No. 11, November 1890, 798–828.

[372] Wolfram Kock. *Kungl. Serafimerlasarettet, 1752–1952: En studie i svensk sjukvårdshistoria.* Jönköping: H. Halls Boktr. A.-B., 1952, 182–183 & 186. Michael Worboys also points this out in his contextualization of Listerism. See Worboys, *Spreading Germs*, 74.

[373] Kock, *Kungl. Serafimerlasarettet*, 186.

was also highlighted as a method of managing infection more generally, outside of surgical practice.

In this chapter, I will examine how practitioners motivated and used the method. I argue that this was done on the basis of practice rather than theory. Its theoretical foundations seem to have been of little importance here. To illustrate this, I begin by framing the introduction of Listerism in Sweden and Denmark within an ongoing discussion about the problems and challenges of amputation. Here, I will tie the spread of Listerist antiseptic wound care in these two countries together with discussions about amputation, its problems and challenges. At the time, this surgical intervention would have severely impacted the patient's quality of life and introduced a substantial wound that was at a great risk for infection, which could be fatal. Listerism was initially framed by Lister himself, as well as followers in these two countries, as a means of assisting surgical interventions that could save limbs and mitigating sepsis. This section will also include a brief historical overview of Listerism.

The next section studies how Listerism was enacted in practice and relates training in the method to apprenticeship. By enacted I mean Annemarie Mol's term that highlights how objects and phenomena unfold in practice.[374] I will do this by focusing on practical descriptions of Listerism in journal articles that describe the method and its performance. The focus on developing physical skill and craft tradition involved in apprenticeships aligns with surgery as a discipline, even if Listerist antisepsis could be applied as a method of wound care outside of surgical intervention. I argue here that Listerism was a locally situated practice; something that Lister's own writings support. Because his articles were detailed, complex, and often practically inclined, the knowledge he was communicating was not always self-evident, in particular in translation and for non-native English speakers. Articles were communicating how to perform Listerism and the method's clinical results were more interesting for practitioners, even if they were unsure of its theoretical basis.

Because surgery can be understood as a technology in itself, the role devices play in practice is important. For Listerism, practice was often discussed in relation to different kinds of medical devices, in particular chemicals, soft articles, and instruments. The final section studies some of the tools that were used in and assisted with Listerist antisepsis, and the problems that practitioners encountered with them. This method of wound manage-

---

[374] Annemarie Mol. *The Body Multiple: Ontology in Medical Practice*. Durham, NC: Duke University Press, 2003, 99.

ment was chemical-heavy, which caused problems in its application. However, Lister also introduced new devices, including bandages and ligature recommendations. This challenged the ways physicians and surgeons were used to working, but also led to practical problems that were detailed in the local medical presses. This section also includes a brief look at local discussions about carbolic acid and Lister's carbolic acid sprayer and its use. The, albeit sparse, information that exists about these tools suggests that they were adapted locally, with surgeons making some things, such as ligatures and bandages, themselves and working together with instrument makers to procure others.

Surgery, Change, and the Advent of Listerism in Sweden and Denmark

Amputation had long been a method of treating complex limb injuries, like compound fractures.[375] However, it was not an ideal method of treatment. It entailed a significant reduction in the patient's quality of life and introduced a new, open wound that could put the patient at risk of infection and death. The underlying prospects for the nineteenth-century amputee were well-understood by practitioners and presented somewhat of a dilemma. On the one hand, removing the limb could save the patient. On the other hand, it was both a risk in itself and could put patients in the crosshairs of social stigma around disability.[376] For instance, in 1850, Swedish physician H. J. Carlsson pointed out the "questionable value" of amputation in an article in *Hygiea*, noting that "generally amputation implies a tragic admission to the

---

[375] See E. J. Chaloner, et. al., "Amputations at the London Hospital, 1852–1857". *Journal of the Royal Society of Medicine*. Vol. 94, No. 8, August 2001, 409–412; Faith Wallis, "Pre-Modern Surgery: Wounds, Words and the Paradox of Tradition", in *The Palgrave Handbook of the History of Surgery*, Thomas Schlich (ed.), 49–70. London: Palgrave Macmillan, 2018. *Hygiea*'s index for volumes 11–22 covering the years 1849–1860 lists a total of seven articles with the subject "amputation" (*amputation*). See "amputation" in *Hygiea: Register öfver banden elfva (1849)–Tjugutvå (1860)*. P.A. Norstedt & Söner, 1863, 3. Articles in *Ugeskrift*'s index covering the years 1839–1860 indexes articles after their title, which includes five articles. There are eighteen articles on fractures, some of which may have discussed amputation depending on the injury's complexity. See *Ugeskrift for Læger: Sag- og Navneregister til Ugeskrift for Læger. Förste Række I–X Bind og anden Række I–XXXI Bind (1839–1860)*. Copenhagen: C. A. Reitzels Forlag, 1860, 2, 6.

[376] See David Turner, "Disability and Prosthetics in Eighteenth- and Early Nineteenth-Century England", in *The Routledge History of Disease*, Mark Jackson (ed.), 301–319. New York: Routledge, 2017; Stephen Milm, "'A Limb Which Shall Be Presentable in Polite Society': Prosthetic Technologies in the Nineteenth Century", in *Artificial Parts, Practice Lives: Modern Histories of Prosthetics*, Katherine Ott, et. al. (eds.), 282–299. New York: NYU Press, 2002.

art's [medicine's] inability to help".[377] Carlsson further highlighted that amputation was risky business. According to him, physicians should carefully reflect over the necessity of the procedure, because it did not eliminate wounds, but introduced new ones.[378] Carlsson encouraged physicians to consider other options and not make hasty decisions in cases where amputation was an option, and noted that limbs could have been saved if a better method of treatment was developed and used.[379]

One alternative to full amputation was partial resection, i.e., the surgical removal of part of a tissue, structure or organ.[380] In *Ugeskrift* in 1858, a long, translated summary of a British article on resection as an alternative to amputation appeared in several parts, highlighting the challenges, successes, and failures of this surgical technique, and how to make use of it on injured joints. Joint resection, as described in this series of articles, focused on trying to save a limb or body part, in contrast to amputation. The author and/or translator highlighted that there were factors where amputation might be preferable, but that resection techniques allowed surgeons to potentially save limbs by removing damaged structures in and around joints, for instance.[381] According to Swedish physician G. A. Landgren, amputation and resection techniques needed to be improved because they were "much too complicated: difficult for the operator and unnecessarily agonising for the ill".[382] The nature of surgery at the time is worthwhile to keep in mind. Anaesthesia, though used to some degree by the 1850s with the introduction of chloroform, was still unreliable and potentially deadly.[383] Surgical procedures were

---

[377] H. J. Carlsson, "Utdrag ur en till Kgl. Sundhets-Collegium afgifven berättelse om en, med understöd af statsmedel företagen vetenskaplig resa". *Hygiea.* Vol. 12, No. 7, July 1850, 393–410, 407. [Amputation är i och för sig en operation af ofta rätt tvetydligt värde… I allmänhet innebär amputation ett sorgeligt erkännande af konstens oförmåga att hjelpa.]

[378] Carlsson, "Utdrag ur en till Kgl. Sundhets-Collegium afgifven berättelse", 408.

[379] Ibid., 407–408.

[380] Tissues, structures and organs can be fully resected as well.

[381] [Anon.], "Om Resektion af de större Led (The brit. and for. med. chir. review. October 1857)". *Ugeskrift for Læger.* Series 2, Vol 28, No. 1–2, 2 January 1858, 1–23; [Anon.], "Om Resektion af de större Led (The brit. and for. med. chir. review. October 1857)". *Ugeskrift for Læger.* Series 2, Vol 28, No. 3, 9 January 1858, 25–33; and, [Anon.], "Om Resektion af de större Led (The brit. and for. med. chir. review. October 1857)". *Ugeskrift for Læger.* Series 2, Vol 28, No. 4, 16 January 1858, 41–53.

[382] G. A. Landgren, "Om amputation med tibio-tarsalleden och förenkling af operationssätt dervid". *Hygiea.* Vol. 13, No. 5, May 1851, 285–288, 286. [syntes den mig vara alltför invecklad: besvärlig för operatören och onödigt plågsam för den sjuke.]

[383] See Carl Santesson, "Ett fall af död efter Chloroform; jemte en öfversigt af alla hittills kända likartade olyckshändelser". *Hygiea.* Vol. 12, No. 10, October 1850, 599–624; G. Böttiger, "Om Etherisationen. Tal, hållet vid franska Wetenskaps-Academiens Årssammankomst d. å., af VELPEAU. Medd. Af D:r G. Böttiger". *Hygiea.* Vol. 12, No. 6, June 1850, 350–364; G. Böttiger, "Om Etherisationen. Tal, hållet vid

often not elective and conducted as quickly as possible. However, as Thomas Schlich points out, surgeons have had a long-standing relationship with and interest in technological developments that interest their practice.[384] For example, in an article in *Hygiea* from 1850, G. Böttinger summarised a speech at the French Academy of Sciences that underlined the importance of opening up for new technical developments in medicine. The article highlighted that the surgeon's goal has always been to reduce pain and make operations less dangerous: "to stop the actual occurrence of pain shall always be of benefaction".[385]

Amputation introduced a significant lifestyle change for patients, and the subsequent loss of a limb in the nineteenth century affected the patient's sense of self and means of supporting oneself. In her article "Fractions of Men", Erin O'Connor highlights that nineteenth-century sensibilities involving amputation changed in the British and American contexts. She notes that the visibility of amputees in the United States grew throughout the century due to a rise in industrial accidents and the American Civil War, and that methods of wound management made survival more viable.[386] Denmark fought two wars over the region Schleswig-Holstein, the first from 1848 to 1851 against German separatists supported by Prussia, and the second in 1864 against Prussia and the Austrian Empire. Although the Swedish state was not directly involved in any wars at this time, Swedish military volunteers, including physicians, joined the Danes in both wars.[387] In any case, physicians would have been well-attuned to foreign publications from and about battlefields and war wounds. This might have underscored the prevailing problems with amputation and resection in the minds of physicians in both countries, not in the least in relation to the

franska Wetenskaps-Academiens Årssammankomst d. å., af VELPEAU. Medd. Af D:r G. Böttiger". *Hygiea*. Vol. 12, No. 7, July 1850, 411–415; [Anon.], "Et Tilfælde af Chloroformdød: Klinisk Foredrag, af Prof. Billroth (Wien. med. Wchschrift 1868, Nr. 46, 47, 48 og 49)". *Ugeskrift for Læger*. Vol. 6, No. 5, 25 July 1868, 65–77. Some later examples involing the use of ether and other anaesthetics are: E. Engdahl, "Om eteriseringen". *Hygiea*. Vol. 39, No. 9, September 1877, 489–505; E. Engdahl, "Om eteriseringen". *Hygiea*. Vol. 41, No. 4, April 1879, 227–232; [Anon.], "Nordisk kirurgisk förenings samforskning angående kirurgisk narkos". *Hygiea*. Vol. 59, No. 2, February 1897, 291–292.

[384] Thomas Schlich, "Introduction: What Is Special About the History of Surgery", in *The Palgrave Handbook of the History of Surgery*, Thomas Schlich (ed.), 1–24. London: Palgrave Macmillan, 2018.

[385] Böttiger, "Om Etherisationen", 361. [Att hindra sjelfva uppkomsten af smärta, skall väl alltid vara en välgerning.]

[386] Erin O'Connor, "'Fractions of Men': Engendering Amputation in Victorian Culture". *Comparative Studies in Society and History*. Vol. 39, No. 4, October 1997, 742–777.

[387] Swedish surgeon Carl Santesson volunteered in the second war in 1864, for example. At the time he was chief of surgery at Seraphim Hospital and Professor of Surgery at Karolinska Institute, both in Stockholm. See Mikael Boox, "Svenska frivilliga till Danmark: Krigen 1848–1850 och 1864". *Militärhistorisk tidskrift*. 2004, 13–68.

effects on patients and the possibilities for wound management in unsanitary conditions.[388] For instance, Danish instrument maker Camillus Nyrop was acutely aware of this dilemma as well, as he served as a volunteer in the first war and noted the difficulties facing amputees upon return in *Bandager og Instrumenter*, like the poor quality of some prosthetic devices and his attempts at improving them.[389]

By the 1870s, a Danish article from 1870 on resection used the term "conservative surgery" to distinguish this so-called triumph of operative surgery, which stood in contrast to what the author called "radical surgery".[390] The term "conservative" distinguished the retention of a bodily structure, while "radical surgery" involved the complete excision of a structure, e.g., the amputation of a limb. But, the procedure gave unsatisfactory results, according to the author. The anonymous author drew on earlier literature and the difficulties resection patients had faced after their surgeries, with poor outcomes, and surgeons who had previously praised the method recanting their support after it had been performed extensively by German military surgeons during the war.[391] Part of the problem with joint resection was the procedure's deep, penetrating wound. Probably even riskier in poor hygienic conditions, like during war, the wound could lead to deep infection that could require amputation of the limb anyway, or even death.[392] Despite these significant problems and concerns, the development had helped in reassessing surgery and wound care. In 1881, Swedish surgeon Ivar Svensson underlined that surgeons were increasingly willing to intervene at an earlier stage of illness, undertake riskier procedures, and that "modern surgery has little in common with the older, more apprehensive".[393] This context, as it relates to nine-

---

[388] Michael Worboys, "The History of Surgical Wound Infection: Revolution or Evolution", in *The Palgrave Handbook of the History of Surgery*, Thomas Schlich (ed.), 215–233. London: Palgrave Macmillan, 2018. For a broader discussion of the relationships between surgery, innovation and war see Leo van Bergen, "Surgery and War: The Discussions About the Usefulness of War for Medical Progress", in *The Palgrave Handbook of the History of Surgery*, Thomas Schlich (ed.), 389–407. London: Palgrave Macmillan, 2018.

[389] Camillus Nyrop. *Bandager og Instrumenter afbildede og beskrevne med en tilføi et Prisfortegnelse.* Copenhagen: G.E.C. Gad, 1864, 1–4.

[390] [Anon.], "Resektionsspørgsmaalet". *Ugeskrift for Læger.* Series 3 Vol. 9, No. 3, 8 January 1870, 35–37, 35.

[391] See [Anon.], "Resektionsspørgsmaalet", 36–37; Adolph Hannover, "Resektioner fra Krigen 1864 i den danske Armes Underklasser". *Ugeskrift for Læger.* Series 3, Vol. 7, No. 12–13, 6 March 1869, 169–195, 171.

[392] Carl Rossander, "Nya områden för den antiseptiska sårbehandlingen IV fortsättning". *Hygiea.* Vol. 41, No. 2, February 1879, 85–98, 87.

[393] Ivar Svensson, "Från kirurgiska afdelningen af Sabbatsbergs sjukhus". *Hygiea.* Vol. 43, No. 7, July 1881, 321–381, 330. [är den moderna kirurgi en ej i likhet med den gamla hufvudsakligen exspekterande].

teenth-century medicine's ethical premises and the consequences of modern warfare, plays into the introduction of Lister's antiseptic system in these two Nordic countries after 1867.

While "conservative surgery" was not directly connected to Listerism in 1870, the case was different just seven years later. In a summary of a German article about complex fractures, "conservative" surgery rather referred to techniques other than amputation, which worked to save rather than remove the limb. This article underlined the importance of Listerist antisepsis in achieving positive results with conservative techniques.[394] These procedures, including amputation and resection, exposed patients to at least two risks–from the operation as well as the wound. However, this article on conservative surgery highlighted the importance of wound care in surgical practice and the development of "conservative" methods, like joint resection. Carl Rossander remarked in 1879 that while resection was "a procedure that had been praised long before anyone had thought about [Listerist] antisepsis", it was "self-evident that resection had become more valuable through its union with antiseptic treatment".[395] In 1881, Ivar Svensson remarked about his own surgical ward's implementation of Listerism, that "in treating illnesses of the joints, the surgeon goes now under the aegis of antiseptics, with valour motivated by success".[396] In other words, antiseptic wound care seemed to improve the outcome of joint resections, tying them in to the development and proliferation of antisepsis in these two countries as a whole.

The method of antisepsis discussed in the articles mentioned above was Listerism. Surgeon Joseph Lister presented the following at the annual meeting of the British Medical Association in Dublin on August 9, 1867:

---

[394] [Anon.], "Behandlingen af komplicerede Benbrud. Efter Richard Volkmann (klin. Vorträge 117–118)". *Ugeskrift for Læger*. Series 3, Vol. 24, No. 17, 6 October 1877, 249–256, 253–4. An overview of this article appears in *Hygiea* as well. See Carl Rossander, "R. Volkmann: Die Behandlung der complicirten Fracturen. Klinische Vorträge N:o 117 och 118". *Hygiea*. Vol. 40, No. 4, April 1878, 200–205.

[395] Rossander, "Nya områden", 87. [Resektionen är äfven ett medel, som var kommet till heders, långt innan någon menniska tänkte på antisepsis. Det är dock sjelfklart, att resektionen vunnit betydligt värde genom föreningen med den antiseptiska behandlingen.]

[396] Svensson, "Från kirurgiska afdelningen", 331. [Vid behandling af ledgångssjukdomar går kirurgen under antiseptikens egid nu tillväga med en djerfhet, som berättigas af framgångar.]

> All local inflammatory mischief and general febrile disturbance which follow severe injuries are due to the irritating and poisoning influence of decomposing blood or sloughs. For these evils are entirely avoided by the antiseptic treatment, so that limbs which otherwise would be unhesitatingly condemned to amputation may be retained, with confidence of the best results.[397]

Lister's proposed method of wound care through systematic procedures and the use of harsh chemicals would later prompt historians and physicians to regard him as the "father" of antiseptic surgery.[398] Listerism attracted admirers, detractors, and nonchalance, and like with many new technologies, it was met with practical resistance and challenges.[399] As the quotation illustrates, the method hoped to change the outcomes of certain injuries. Lister's address detailed the serious injury of a young boy, which included a compound fracture. Lister noted that "without the assistance of antiseptic treatment, I should certainly have thought of nothing else but amputation at the shoulder-joint; but [...] I did not hesitate to try to save the limb".[400] This did not go unnoticed in Sweden and Denmark, for, outside of amputation, the prognosis for compound fractures around mid-century was not particularly good. One translation of a German article published in *Hygiea* in 1878 noted that mortality rates were between 40–68% before the introduction of Listerist principles.[401]

Physicians in these two countries were naturally interested in this method, like many international developments in their profession, and the method was rather quickly employed in both countries. Denmark's *Ugeskrift for Læger* even translated Lister's presentation into Danish and printed it the

---

[397] Joseph Lister, "On the Antiseptic Principle in the Practice of Surgery". *British Medical Journal*. Vol. 2, No. 246, 21 September 1867, 246–248, 246.

[398] See Jacques Borelius, "Joseph Lister, An address on a new antiseptic dressing' Brit. Med. Journal 1889, nov 9, 1890, jan. 4. Referat af Jacques Borelius". *Hygiea*. Vol. 52, No. 6, June 1890, 589–591. Historians, Michael Worboys in particular, have later challenged this label, arguing that Lister championed *one* method of antiseptic wound care, whilst many had been in circulation during the same period. Additionally, Lister's method was not universally accepted by physicians and frequently criticised; a narrative that Worboys argued shifted after Lister's death. Worboys, "The History of Surgical Wound Infection", 228. See also Nancy J. Tomes and John Harley Warner, "Introduction to the Special Issue on Rethinking the Reception of Germ Theory of Disease: Comparative Perspectives". *Journal of the History of Medicine and Allied Sciences*. Vol. 52, No. 1, January 1997, 7–16.

[399] Worboys, *Spreading Germs*; and Thomas Schlich, "Farmer to Industrialist: Lister's Antisepsis and the Making of Modern Surgery in Germany". *Notes and Records of the Royal Society of London*. Vol. 67, No. 3, 20 September 2013, 245–260.

[400] Lister, "On the Antiseptic Principle", 247.

[401] Rossander, "R. Volkmann", 201.

same year, 1867.[402] In Sweden, though nothing related to Lister or Listerism was published in 1867, interest started to grow amongst surgeons the following year, with the surgical ward at Seraphim Hospital implementing the practice in 1868.[403] The method was introduced at this hospital by Swedish surgeon Alrik Törnblom, who had travelled to learn the method from Lister and was one of the country's foremost advocates of it.[404] Lister had a follower in Copenhagen-based physician Mathias Saxthorph as well, who, like Törnblom, spent time in Glasgow with Lister to study the method.[405] One Swedish source names Saxthorph as "perhaps the first faithful follower of Lister", suggesting Listerism was particularly prevalent in Denmark.[406] The Danish surgeon responsible for translating Lister's *Lancet* address, Harald Philipsen, had also spent time studying under an earlier follower of Lister's in Edinburgh where he witnessed operations "of a very invasive and dangerous character [with] not one example of an infection disease amongst these patients, let alone a death".[407]

Managing risk from the wounds inflicted by the aforementioned procedures was on the minds of many practitioners throughout the century and European medical journals are rife with recommendations, accounts over methods and tips about chemicals that could be helpful in wound care. Michael Worboys stresses in his book *Spreading Germs* that other antiseptic chemicals and methods besides Listerism were widely used by practitioners, so antiseptic wound care in itself was not "new".[408] This is no different in Denmark and Sweden. Other articles on surgical procedures from the 1850s mentioned aftercare in the form of applying oatmeal porridge and beeswax

---

[402] Harald Philipsen, "Om antiseptisk Forbinding. Efter Prof. Joseph Lister i Glasgow («The Lancet», 21de Septbr. 1867)". *Ugeskrift for Læger.* Series 3, Vol. 4, No. 25, 23 November 1867, 381–390.

[403] Kock, *Kungl. Serafimerlasarettet,* 185.

[404] See *Förhandlingar vid Svenska läkarsällskapets sammankomster.* 26 March 1872.

[405] *Förhandlingar vid Svenska läkarsällskapets sammankomster.* 26 March 1872; see also Alrik Törnblom, "Notiser ur den kirurgiska journallitteraturen". *Hygiea.* Vol. 34, No. 3, March 1872, 144–159; Ole Hart Hansen, "Saxtorph, Holmer og Listers antiseptic". *Ugeskrift for Læger.* Vol. 169, No. 35, 24 August 2007, 2863.

[406] Per Söderbaum. *Listers antiseptiska method.* Diss. Uppsala University, 1877, 75. [Den, som kanske först blef en trogen efterföljare af Lister]. The physician Söderbaum refers to in Copenhagen is Matthias Hieronymus Saxtorph, who, at the time was chief of surgery at Fredriks Hospital in Copenhagen and professor of surgery at the University of Copenhagen. He travelled to Glasgow to observe Lister directly, and in 1868 began employing and teaching the method.

[407] Philipsen, "Om antiseptisk Forbinding", 390. [Uagtet der blev foretraget en stor Mængde Operationer, tildels af meget indgribende og farlig Beskaffenhed, saa indtraf der iblandt disse Syge ikke et eneste Tilfælde af Infektionssygdomme, endsige Dødsfald.]

[408] Worboys, *Spreading Germs.* See in particular his first chapter, *Medical Practice and Disease Theories, c. 1865.*

or baths with cold or warm water.[409] Despite this, one article on amputation aftercare noted that "the frequent reapplication of the dressing is tormenting for the patient and the physician, and it is often, regardless of the best caution, impossible to prevent the wound from developing infection".[410] As I have shown in the second chapter, many articles like these detail how physicians tried to improve their techniques and methods. They did much of the same here, in both surgical procedures and in aftercare.[411]

Hygiea frequently published correspondence from Swedish physicians on educational visits abroad, with descriptions of other disinfection technologies. These accounts illustrate the multitude of disinfection methods circulating at the time and highlight the importance of personal preference depending on what methods were favoured by whom.[412] Moreover, some of the articles discussing the application of other disinfection technologies noted the importance of the constitution of the room the patient was treated in. As early as 1854, a Danish article accounted for a variety of different "antiseptica" in the context of clearing rooms of miasma, noxious bad air, which would have been in correlation with its constitution.[413] In one of the Swedish Society of Medicine's meetings in 1873, a physician detailed a method of open-wound healing, i.e., without a dressing, used in Austria, which led him to conclude that as long as the hospital had a good constitution, the choice of wound care method perhaps did not matter.[414] This method built on the principle of following a healthy, natural healing process

[409] [Anon.], "Tracheotomi for et fremmed Legeme I Luftröret". *Ugeskrift for Læger.* Series 2, Vol. 21, No. 15, 14 October 1854 235–238; [Anon.], "Lagenbech: Det permanente varme Vandbad (Prager Vierteljahrschr. 1856. 3 Bd.)". *Ugeskrift for Læger.* Series 2, Vol. 25, No. 6, 26 July 1856, 73–85.

[410][Anon.], "Lagenbech", 73. [Ved Behandlingen af större Saar, navnlig efter Amputation og Resektion, saavelsom ved komplicerede Frakturer er den hyppige Fornyelse af Forbindningen en sand Plage baade for Patienten og for Lægen, og det er ofte, uagtet den störste Omhyggelighed, ikke muligt at forebygge, at Saaret antager en ondartet Charakter.]

[411] See [Anon.], "Om nogle Desinfektionsmidler (Wilson: Pharmacol. Journ. Decbr. 1852, Schmidts Jahrb. 1853, Nr. 6)". *Ugeskrift for Læger.* Series 2, Vol. 20, No. 3–4, 28 January 1854, 62–63; [Anon.], "Tracheotomi for et fremmed Legeme I Luftröret", 235–238; N. E. Ravn, "Et Tilfælde af Strubehoste helbredet ved Tracheotomi". *Ugeskrift for Læger.* Series 2, Vol. 21, No. 16, 21 October 1854, 241–253; [Anon.], "Lagenbech", 73–85; [Anon.]. "Om operative Behandling af Kroup". *Ugeskrift for Læger.* Series 2, Vol. 30, No. 6, 29 January 1859, 73–85. See also Chapter 2 for further discussion on the relationships between technique and improvement journal articles.

[412] See for example disinfection power, cotton boiled in caustic soda, cotton treated in iron chloride and "chloralum wool". *Förhandlingar vid Svenska läkarsällskapets sammankomster.* 17 September 1872, 26 November 1872, 17 December 1872; [Anon.], "Vatforbinding. Efter Hervey (Arch. gén. de méd. Dcbr. 1871–Juni 1872)". *Ugeskrift for Læger.* Series 3, Vol. 15, No. 11, 1 March 1873, 161–172; John Berg, "Resebref från Dr John Berg. Uppläst i Medicinska Föreningen den 28 Februari 1880". *Hygiea.* Vol. 42, No. 5, May 1880, 286–291, 286.

[413] [Anon.], "Om nogle Desinfektionsmidler", 62–63.

[414] *Förhandlingar vid Svenska läkarsällskapets sammankomster*, 15 June 1873.

as closely as possible, where oxygen assisted in promoting the growth of new tissue.[415]

While Listerism is an antiseptic practice, all antiseptic practices in circulation during the period are not Listerism, even if they were often used synonymously.[416] The challenge here for the historian is to pick apart the conflation of Listerist practice as *the* antiseptic treatment, and other means of antisepsis, which were described using the same or similar terminology. For example, Carl Rossander used Listerism and antisepsis synonymously in his article series "Nya områden för den antiseptiska sårbehandlingen" [New areas for the antiseptic treatment of wounds], which appeared in *Hygiea* in 1878 and 1879. He began by discussing the achievements of antisepsis more generally, to then refer to "this, the Listerist method".[417]

But many of these articles, including those about Listerism, were focused on explaining how to follow a specific method and the method's empirical results rather than detailing its scientific basis. In the early years of Listerism, wound care methods were often framed around less invasive surgical procedures involving fracture care, rather than abdominal surgery, which was associated with significant risk.[418] Rossander's article series from 1878 and 1879 is an example of this: even though the articles did highlight some technical surgical details, their primary focus was antiseptic wound care in correlation with surgical procedures that did not open the abdomen. In the first instalment, he detailed the use of antiseptic gauze, carbolic solutions and spray for different forms of ocular surgery.[419] Subsequent instalments included hernias, bladder stones, and joint illnesses, and their positive, empirical results after the application of Listerist wound care. Even Lister's own publications focused on the treatment of abscesses, compound fractures

---

[415] *Förhandlingar vid Svenska läkarsällskapets sammankomster*, 15 June 1873. See also, Worboys, *Spreading Germs*, 83.

[416] Ibid., 82. See also "The History of Surgical Wound Infection", 222.

[417] Rossander, "Nya områden", 315. [Denna den Listerska metodens]

[418] For a history of abdominal surgery see Sally Frampton, "Opening the Abdomen: The Expansion of Surgery". in *The Palgrave Handbook of the History of Surgery*, Thomas Schlich (ed.), 175–194. London: Palgrave Macmillan, 2018. See also Sally Frampton, "Defining Difference: Competing Forms of Ovarian Surgery in the Nineteenth Century", in *Technological Change in Modern Surgery: Historical Perspectives on Innovation*, Thomas Schlich and Christopher Crenner (eds.), 51–70. Rochester: University of Rochester Press, 2017. In the Swedish context, Ulrika Nilsson includes a chapter that deals in part with the expansion of abdominal surgery from the 1870s in her thesis on the establishment of Swedish gynaecology. See Ulrika Nilsson. *Kampen om Kvinnan: Professionalisering och konstruktioner av kön I svensk gynekologi 1860–1925*. Diss. Uppsala University, 2003, 77–109. See also Torsten Sørensen, "Træk af ovariotomiens historie: Privathospitalet på Jelling Mark", in *Dansk Medicinhistorisk Årbog*, Nils Rosdahl, et. al. (eds.), 40–55, Viborg: Specialtrykkeriet Viborg A/S, 2008.

[419] See Rossander, "Nya områden", 319–324.

and the influence of decomposition in wound health at first.[420] Lister's focus on decomposition, wound secretions, and the treatment of abscesses indicate that some of the wounds that Lister based his method on were already infected. This shows that his method was not just for invasive surgical wounds but wound care and aftercare more broadly.[421] Because of the early emphasis on wound care and management, the interest in the method was equally broad. For example, one Swedish provincial doctor detailed a complicated case from 1873 involving a needle lodged in a woman's thigh; whereby, the method's successful application in the patient's home eventually led to full recovery, in spite of early infection.[422]

Even if Listerism had a broader application outside of surgery, the surgical application of the method was often highlighted in journals as particularly important. In March 1872, at one of the Swedish Society of Medicine's meetings, surgeon Carl Santesson claimed that "antiseptic practice" was "next, after chloroform, perhaps the greatest newer discovery in [this] field of science".[423] Just a few years later, in 1879, Rossander remarked in *Hygiea* that "hardly any area of external medicine has changed in character as this one has", referring to the antiseptic treatment of illnesses of the joint.[424] Indeed, physicians had become emboldened to some degree in treating these kinds of illnesses, with physician John Berg also remarking that surgical procedures to treat *osteomata* (bone tumours) and *genu valgum* (knock-knee) had increased according to German literature, after the associated surgical procedures for these disorders were conducted according to antiseptic principles.[425] "Antiseptic practice" and "antiseptic principles" in this case worked explicitly from Listerist practice. Rossander also stated that "issues, red-hot iron, flies, leeches or cupping have vanished [...] and they have been replaced by, without question, more rational and therefore more

---

[420] For a detailed account of Lister's publications through his career, see Michael Worboys, "Joseph Lister and the Performance of Antiseptic Surgery". *Notes and Records of The Royal Society*. Vol. 67, No. 3, September 2013, 199–209, 207. See also Joseph Lister, "On a New Method of Treating Compound Fracture, Abscess, &c., with Observations on the Conditions of Suppuration. Part I". *The Lancet*. Vol. 89, Issue 2272, 16 March 1867, 326–329; Joseph Lister, "On a New Method of Treating Compound Fracture, Abscess, &c.. Part II". *The Lancet*. Vol. 89, Issue 2274, 30 March 1867, 95–96.

[421] See the first paragraphs of Lister, "On a New Method", 326–7. See also Worboys, *Spreading Germs*, 82.

[422] *Förhandlingar vid Svenska läkarsällskapets sammankomster*, 15 July 1873.

[423] *Förhandlingar vid Svenska läkarsällskapets sammankomster*, 26 March 1872. [näst efter kloroform kanske vara den största nyare upptäckt inom vetenskapsgren.]

[424] Rossander, "Nya områden", 85. [knappt någon enda gren af den utvärtes medicinen så fullständigt ombytt gestalt som den.]

[425] John Berg, "Några ord om subkutana osteomier i allmänhet och behandling af genu valgum i synnerhet". *Hygiea*. Vol. 41, No. 11 & 12, November/December 1879, 721–731, 721.

useful methods of treatment".[426] The comment pitted older treatment methods against newer ones by referring to the development of Listerist antiseptic practice in particular. According to Rossander, the character of medicine was changing. This juxtaposition differs from that highlighted in the second chapter, where the "exacting pathologist" was still reliant on knowledge from "older schools" in order to treat patients.[427]

By 1877, the "dressing" addendum was on the way out of the Swedish nomenclature, at least according to a doctoral thesis by Per Söderbaum on Lister's antiseptic method. Söderbaum criticised the association strictly with simple wound management, the bandage/dressing [*bandage/förband*] terminology many used and its connotations, and provided a detailed description of what had developed into a system of disinfection.[428] The lexical difference here points to a distinct methodology behind the performance of Listerist antisepsis on a broader scale versus just the application of germ-killing wound care, and Söderbaum pointed out that what Listerism offered was more than applying a bandage doused in carbolic acid to a wound; rather, it was an empirically based method of preventing infection in wounds. This points to a shift in understanding antisepsis, its role in surgical practice and systematisation.[429] Söderbaum highlighted that, in addition to this, the method had not yet been thoroughly described in Swedish, and did just this in his thesis, which included details on the method's accoutrements as well as its application during certain surgical procedures.[430]

Communicating Listerist Practice

Part of the challenge with Listerism and its principles of practice was learning how to follow Lister's instructions, and this was not always easy. The performative aspects of antisepsis were of fundamental importance to prac-

---

[426] Rossander, "Nya områden", 85. [Fontanellerna, glödjernen, flugorna, iglarne eller koppningarne hafva försvunnit… och i deras ställe ha trädt helt andra och utan tvifvel mera rationela och derför äfven mera lönande behandlingsmetoder.]

[427] See Chapter 2. See also [Anon.], "Pathologisk Physiologi–Cellularpathologi." *Ugeskrift for Læger.* Series 2, Vol 31, No. 13-14. 12 March 1859, 193–202.

[428] Söderbaum, *Listers antiseptiska metod*, 1.

[429] Michael Worboys details the developments of Listerism after he was appointed Professor of Clinical Surgery at Kings College in London in 1877, at which point surgeons began reconsidering the role of germs in surgery and attempting to find better ways to deal with them practically. This was, according to Worboys, also interconnected with contemporary laboratory research on germs, sepsis and aetiology. See Worboys, *Spreading Germs*, 150–192. See also Worboys, "The History of Surgical Wound Infection".

[430] See Söderbaum, *Listers antiseptiska metod*, 23–40. The third chapter (43–52) discusses general pre-operative procedures including handwashing, disinfecting the operating field and the patient, etc., as well as methods for abscesses, trauma, septic wounds, etc.

titioners. It is perhaps more fruitful to see Listerist practice then, from a similar framework as the training of surgical instrument makers: that between master and apprentice. In both instances, for surgeons as well as surgical instrument makers, training the hand, and the tacit knowledge embodied within, was of paramount importance. Surgical instrument makers also had a vested interest in keeping up with technological developments in medicine. Physicians and surgical instrument makers were part of a network, with local convergence.

Swedish instrument maker Albert Stille and Dane Camillus Nyrop undertook training abroad, much like their physician counterparts and early Listerists Törnblom and Saxthorph. Nyrop and Stille spent time in Paris studying under instrument maker Joseph-Frédéric-Benoît Charrière, and in Nyrop's case, former-Charrière apprentice Amatus Lüer as well, before returning to their home countries.[431] The time spent abroad was likely favourable for Stille and Nyrop, as it acquainted them with a well-known style of instrument making and allowed them to hone their skills. The work of Charrière, and Stille and Nyrop's connections to him in addition to their relationships with physicians in their respective countries, would have meant they were well-read, or at least understood the principles behind antiseptic treatments.[432] It also opens up the sites of knowledge in medicine to instru-

---

[431] See "Characteristics of Medical Journals and Surgical Instrument Makers" in Chapter 1. See [Anon.], "Inrikes". *Najaden*. 31 January 1840. "Student in surgical instrument making Stille has received 500 riksdaler banko in support from the manufacturing fund to work under surgical instrument maker Charrière in Paris, in order to help him further his work during his stay abroad" [Kirurgiske Instrumentmakare-eleven Stille har erhållit 500 Rdr Banko understood, att utgå af Manufaktur-fonden, för att under sitt utrikes vistande äfven kunna komma i tillfälle att i yrket ytterligare fullkomma sig hos Kirurgiske Instrumentmakaren Charrière i Paris.]; Michael Sachs. *Geschichte der operativen Chirurgie*, ii; *Historische Entwicklung des chirurgischen Instrumentariums.* Heidelberg: Kaden Verlag, 2001, 270; C. Nyrop. *Camillus Nyrop og det kirurgiske Instrumentmageri i Danmark.* Copenhagen: Nielsen & Lydiche, 1884, 62; C. Nyrop. *Slægten Nyrop: Nogle biografiske oplysninger.* Copenhagen, Nielsen & Lydiche, 1908, 138.

[432] The first edition of *Bandager og Instrumenter* was published in 1864, three years prior to Lister's first address, and antisepsis or Listerism are not mentioned in subsequent editions. However, given Nyrop's frequent publication in medical journals, and Albert Stille's participation in society meetings in Stockholm, it, although speculative, seems reasonable that they would have been aware of, and followed these developments. Both Stille and Nyrop attended ovariotomies, for instance. One of Nyrop's sons, probably Johan Ernst Nyrop, was also present. At least two of the three records of their attendance predate Listerist antisepsis; however, their attendance indicates that they would have understood at least some of the challenges involved in opening the abdominal cavity, like sepsis. Ulrika Nilsson mentions Stille's presence during ovariotomies in her thesis. See Nilsson, *Kampen om Kvinnan*, 58. One ovariotomy attended by Stille was performed in 1863, and the patient survived. Stille also attended another ovariotomy performed by Sköldberg, this time in 1868. In this case, the patient did not survive. Neither case details the use of antiseptics. The ovariotomy performed in 1868 was attended by this

ment makers and highlights them as actors in the production of medical knowledge.[433] This facilitated their working together with physicians to accommodate technologies like Listerism, but their training also draws parallels to the ideal Listerist tutelage, given the emphasis on performance and the association with knowledge of the hand.

In an article about Listerist practice, Michael Worboys examines Listerism as professional performance that required attention to detail and a sense of improvement. Listerist protocols, he argues, were flexible and allowed the surgeon to craft new solutions; however, close attention to detail in practice was paramount. He further stresses the performance aspect of Listerism, where the written publication of his lectures should be read as retellings of performance and attempts by Lister to detail movement and manipulation, but according to exacting protocol.[434] In these terms, the proximity-based successes of Listerism bore apprenticeship-like qualities and interpersonal instruction, rather that textual, would have facilitated the method's enactment in practice. If we look at Törnblom and Saxtorph, the successes of Listerism in their respective surgical wards seem to be interrelated with their studies in Glasgow with the "master", Lister himself, and the reliance on a network of "apprentices" to further spread the method locally. Lister's written work and lectures were criticised for being difficult to follow and complicated to put into practice, something that may have been exacerbated for non-native English speakers, in which case, seeing Lister or one of his followers perform surgery according to this system might have helped them grasp the method's practical details. Thomas Schlich notes that in the German context, the method's success was dependent on proximity to Lister's home base, which also had bearing on whether or not all the specific details taught by Lister were followed correctly or at all.[435] One Danish physician made a remark about this in 1873, stating that it was difficult to

---

chapter's oft-mentioned Rossander and Törnblom, however. See Sven Sköldberg, "Fall af Ovariotomi, III". *Hygiea*. Vol. 29, No. 11, November 1867, 479–481; Sven Sköldberg, "Fall af Ovariotomi, VIII". *Hygiea*. Vol. 31, No. 7, July 1869, 316–318. For Nyrop and his son's attendance, see F. Howitz, "Et Tilfælde af Ovariotomi". *Hospitals-Tidende*. Vol. 7, No. 12, 23 March 1864, 45–47. Though Howitz does not detail disinfection procedures he does mention that "we made sure that all our hands were fully cleaned and warm". [vi sørgede Alle for at vore Hænder vare fuldkommen rene og varme]

[433] See Lisa Roberts, "Introduction", in *The Mindful Hand: Inquiry and Invention from the Late Renaissance to Early Industrialisation*, Lissa Roberts, et. al. (eds.), 1–7. Amsterdam: Edita KNAW, 2007, 3.

[434] Worboys, "Joseph Lister and the Performance of Antiseptic Surgery", 200.

[435] Schlich, "Farmer to Industrialist", 249.

prove "Lister's disciples" wrong because they always equated problems with the method to improper use.[436]

Many method-descriptions were long-winded because the element of performance was difficult to convey in words, and many of Lister's articles were transcriptions of lectures.[437] The first point is easy to concur with in Swedish and Danish contexts–this was the case with many of the articles in *Hygiea, Ugeskrift,* and *Hospitals-Tidende.* Many offered detailed retellings of procedures performed, instrument tests, and other practical matters, and a number longer of articles were split into several parts and published over the course of several issues.[438] In the Danish translation of Lister's 1867 address, the translator, Harald Philipsen, noted that he had difficulty following all of Lister's pathological digressions, but that they might still be of interest for colleagues.[439] Although physicians might have been used to reading these types of articles, they could still prove to be a challenging read. Worboys' point about the complexity of Lister's own body of work might also have to do with what it was communicating about practice. As Michael Polanyi points out in *The Tacit Dimension,* both conveying and comprehending tacit knowledge in textual forms is difficult. If the knowledge Lister and his followers communicated was mostly performance-based, discerning the essential actions of a performance involved putting together clues about what aspects of the performance were essential to know. [440] This was likely difficult the further afield a practitioner was from Lister or one of his followers.

Conveying performance through text is complicated. In his article on the performance of antiseptic surgery, Worboys uses following recipes when cooking as an example to illustrate this. As a knitter, I think of knitting. I have books about stitch patterns and casting on and binding off; however, follow-

---

[436] [Anon.], "Journalistik". *Hospitals-Tidende.* Vol. 16, No. 40, 1 October 1873, 159–160.

[437] Worboys, "Joseph Lister and the Performance of Antiseptic Surgery", 200.

[438] Carl Rossander's article series on antiseptic dressings, which I refer to several times in this chapter, is one example. Valdemar Holmer additionally published an article series in several parts in *Hospitals-Tidende* in 1872 on resection that included information on antisepsis, as did surgeon Oscar Bloch in 1876. Holmer's article series was a republished lecture he held for the Danish medical society Filiatrien. See Bibliography for detailed references for each article. Valdemar Holmer, "Om Resektion af Knæleddet i kroniske Knæledssygdomme". *Hospitals-Tidende.* Vol. 15, No. 43–47, 23 October 1872, 30 October 1872, 6 November 1872, 13 November 1872, 20 November 1872. Oscar Bloch, "Om den forskellige Saarbehandling i forskellige kirurgiske Services". *Hospitals-Tidende.* Series 2, Vol. 3, No. 18–20, 3 May 1876, 10 May 1876, 17 May 1876. Carl Rossander, "Nya områden för den antiseptiska sårbehandlingen". *Hygiea.* Vol. 40, No. 6–Vol. 41, No. 2, June 1878, July 1878, October 1878, December 1878, February 1879.

[439] Philipsen, "Om antiseptisk Forbinding", 389.

[440] Michael Polanyi. *The Tacit Dimension.* Garden City, New York: Doubleday & Company, 1966, 30–31.

ing written instructions is always more challenging than looking at a video where I can see the knitter's hands communicating where and how to wrap the yarn. But even seeing someone do it does not always translate well in practice: everyone has encountered someone with skill making something inexplicably difficult look easy. The knowledge communicated by Lister is no different. In Worboys' readings of Lister's articles, he concludes that Lister, "as an experienced and effective clinical teacher himself, he [Lister] was only too aware of the problems of communicating surgical methods and that he sought to deal with this by including the performative aspects of antiseptic and other methods in his writings".[441] These practical aspects of antiseptic technology are further illustrated in the training involved in their performance and training relationships with Lister or someone else well-versed in the method and all its components. The importance of these kinds of training relationships is corroborated in a study of the history of total hip replacement by Julie Anderson, Francis Neary, and John Pickstone, although the scope of their study is situated in the twentieth century. They note that while surgeons can work from books in the operating theatre, seeing the procedure done or spending an extended period learning these techniques from the source is also common, and works in accordance with "master-pupil relations".[442]

Given Lister's written descriptions, the tension of putting the hands to work and following instructions could elicit problems. If we turn to tacit knowledge, and Polanyi in particular, Lister's ability to convey the details of his method in words, either verbally or written, would have been difficult. The knowledge conceived in following the method would have been interiorised for him. This process of interiorisation according to Polanyi "relies further on our attending from these unspecifiable particulars to a comprehensive entity connecting them in a way we cannot define".[443] In other words, to understand the performance, the observer is required to coordinate the practical movements as well as the pattern of these movements, and interiorise the movements themselves.[444] The performance of Lister's method accurately seemed to have benefited from this kind of interiorisation, which was helped by studying under Lister, or working with one of his pupils, rather than relying on studying complicated retellings of how to follow Listerist principles. Lister's faithful followers Saxthorph and Törnblom, both of whom

---

[441] Worboys, "Joseph Lister and the Performance of Antiseptic Surgery", 207.
[442] Julie Anderson, et. al. *Surgeons, Manufacturers and Patients: A Transatlantic History of Total Hip Replacement.* Basingstoke: Palgrave Macmillan, 2007, 151.
[443] Polanyi, *The Tacit Dimension*, 24.
[444] Ibid., 30.

travelled to Glasgow to see Lister work directly, could communicate and perform these retellings for their respective local medical communities.

This is akin to another study by Thomas Schlich on the proliferation of osteosynthesis in the twentieth century, where control over the method's use was dependent on the development of a reliable network and building cooperation between practitioners in that network.[445] Though Saxthorph and Törnblom could spread Listerism to their local communities, it likely changed the amount of control over the method Lister could reasonably have, which might have emboldened practitioners to make modifications. Törnblom offered commentary along these lines concerning the work of French surgeons, where he hoped that they "should not neglect the small details, and one could then hope that mortality amongst their patients would become somewhat less horrific".[446] Another Swedish physician, the provincial doctor Axel Gustaf Virgin, remarked in 1873 that critics of Listerism had not applied the method correctly, inferring that correct application predicated success.[447] The "small details" likely made the method less user-friendly and more difficult to adopt without an instructive means of proliferation with intervention from the master and watchful eyes on Lister's application. But, like training more generally, practice makes perfect.

The introduction of new devices and examination technologies was dependent on understanding what information was conveyed to the physician via visual examination as well as knowing how to handle the instruments used for the examination itself, their relationships with specific patient anatomies, and spatial conditions like lighting and weather. These factors also played a role in antiseptic methods and technologies. Worboys highlights that while many historians have focused on the ways that Listerist antisepsis evolved from wound management to a system and later paved the way for aseptic practices, the newness of Listerist performance, the instruments, and the techniques involved were perhaps more important for surgeons practicing at the time.[448] These practical relationships are reflected

---

[445] Thomas Schlich. *Surgery, Science and Industry: A Revolution in Fracture Care, 1950s–1990s*. Basingstoke: Palgrave MacMillan, 2002, 242.

[446] Törnblom, "Notiser ur den kirurgiska journallitteraturen", 158. [en gång lära sig att man icke bör försumma de "minutiösa detaljerna", och då kan man hoppas att dödligheten bland deras patienter blifver något mindre fasaväckande.]

[447] *Förhandlingar vid Svenska läkarsällskapet*, 15 July 1873.

[448] Worboys, "Joseph Lister and the Performance of Antiseptic Surgery", 207.

in my material as well, with many of the early articles about antisepsis focusing on the how-to's, rather than the principles behind them.[449]

Early articles on Listerism from 1868 in the Danish periodical *Hospitals-Tidende* only detailed case studies. The authors highlighted positive results in Lister's ward in contrast to others at the same hospital, and with infections and injuries like complicated fractures. They also mentioned issues with carbolic acid.[450] This is akin to Harald Philipsen's praise of the method in his 1867 translation of Lister's *Lancet* address. Philipsen's uncertainty about the theory behind Listerism did not affect his exuberance over the positive results he observed, witnessing no instances of infection or death during his time in Edinburgh. Another example of this type of article is Rossander's article series, where he positioned antiseptic practice against older methods.[451] Rossander's articles also detailed the use of antisepsis in a variety of different surgical techniques, with summaries and references. Rossander included references, even if he had not read the work in question, so that curious readers could refer to the more detailed, original accounts, often published in *Hygiea*. Though he did mention different theoretical ideas, in particular in the article's third part in the October 1878 edition of *Hygiea*, the articles primarily focus on practical performance of certain varieties of surgery.

Even Per Söderbaum's thesis focused primarily on practical details of Listerism. In summarising the basis of the method, he noted that Lister's principle was that there was a poison [*gift*] present in the air and in everything in the air that affected wound care negatively. The exact form and composition of this "poison" was unclear, but disinfection prevented it from reaching the wound and affecting healing, regardless of how.[452] While he does discuss theoretical objections to Listerism and the theoretical basis of the method, he argued that Lister frequently returned to practical matters in defending his method and that "he, in other words, wanted his practical method judged practically".[453] By shifting focus to practice, as Annemarie Mol suggests in her

---

[449] See for example [Anon.], "Om Anvendelsen af Karbolsyren i Chirurgien". *Hospitals-Tidende*. Vol. 12, No. 21, 26 May 1869, 82–83; [Anon.]. "Vatforbinding"; [Anon.], "Kloral som antisepticum. Efter Dujardin-Beaumetx og Hirne (L'un. méd. 1873. Nr. 62 og Nr. 63)". *Ugeskrift for Læger*. Series 3, Vol. 16, No. 12, 6 September 1873, 177–181; [Anon.], "Behandlingen af komplicerede Benbrud"; Jacques Borelius, "Antiseptiken på Listers afdelning på Kings College Hospital i London". *Hygiea*. Vol. 51, No. 11, November 1889, 665–669.

[450] P. C. Larsen, "Prof. Listers antiseptiske Forbinding". *Hospitals-Tidende*. Vol. 11, No. 32, 5 August 1868, 126–127; [Anon.], "Om Anvendelsen af Karbolsyren i Chirurgien".

[451] Rossander, "Nya områden för den antiseptiska sårbehandlingen", Vol. 40, No. 6–Vol. 41, No. 2. See Bibliography for detailed references to each article.

[452] Söderbaum, *Listers antiseptiska method*, 56–57.

[453] Ibid., 67 [med andra ord sin praktiska method vill han ha praktiskt bedömd]

ontology of practice, in the case of Listerism the enthusiasm over the method's practical effects despite its unclear theoretical basis undermines the notion that practice needed to have solid theoretical foundations in order to be adopted.[454] This is particularly the case in Swedish and Danish practice. The lack of theoretical consensus or unclear aetiologies of certain disorders did not stop Rossander from declaring Listerism to be rational or useful.

Works of these kinds highlight the importance of the practice and performance of Listerism and offer textual retellings for practitioners to work from. They would have served as case studies and as instructional guides. Importantly, they also illustrate that a sound understanding of the theoretical basis for Listerism was not as important for practitioners in its adoption here as positive empirical results were. Rather, the empirical evidence supports Worboys' argument that "germ practices" around mid-century were "deliberately decoupled" from theory and that empirical results were, generally speaking, more important for surgeons even if they would have liked to better understand the nature of infections.[455]

This stands slightly in contrast to the conclusions drawn in the second chapter, where practitioners needed a clear frame of reference to discern the clinical applications of these instruments. With antisepsis, the direct, empirical results seemed to have been clearer for physicians, and the aetiological explanations of infection were of less consequence. In her thesis on the rise of bacteriology in Swedish medicine, Ulrika Graninger introduces the term "theoretical disorientation" [*teoretisk vilsenhet*] regarding the slow establishment of bacteriology in Swedish medicine. This term points to medicine's lack of clarity over what caused infectious diseases in the 1860s up until the 1880s.[456] The term *vilsenhet* is difficult to translate into English without losing some of its character, but the notion of being disoriented compels the opposite, orientation. However, this term is teleological and prioritises the establishment of theory over its clinical implications and therapeutic labour, neither of which have a solid, empirical basis in the historical materials I have studied. It is important to underscore that Listerism was practically deployed in Sweden and Denmark relatively early, still in the 1860s, despite bacteriology's alleged slow establishment according to Graninger.

---

[454] See Annemarie Mol on using the practitioner's hands as the focal point of theorising in Mol, *The Body Multiple*, 152.

[455] Worboys, *Spreading* Germs, 6 & 78.

[456] Ulrika Graninger. *Från osynligt till synligt: Bakteriologins etablering i sekelskiftets svenska medicin.* Diss. Linköping University, 1997, 29.

This problem is in part due to how the development of bacteriology in Sweden is approached in Graninger's thesis. In the chapter "Den teoretiska vilsenheten" [The Theoretical Disorientation] she questions the "theoretical preparedness" [*teoretiskt beredskap*] of Swedish physicians in "accepting, spreading and developing the knowledge that had been developed in the new science of bacteriology".[457] But what if a bacteriological thought style, using Fleckian terms, was not yet well established? The historical actors that I discuss, during the same period Graninger connects to bacteriology, seldom discussed "bacteria" as such. Rather, they most commonly used terms like poison [*gift*], germs [*kim*], contagion [*smitte*/smitta/*farsot*], and substance [*stof*], although some articles do use bacteria [*bakterie*]. At least in the British case, Michael Worboys points to the establishment of bacteriology in the 1880s.[458] Framing discussions from the 1860s, 1870s, and at least the early 1880s in these two countries in terms of bacteriology's theoretical preparedness is anachronistic and implies a theoretical frame that simply did not exist at the time, even outside of Sweden and Denmark. Rather, this thought style was under establishment and reading early Listerism as indicative of unprepared-ness or disorientation ignores the variation and work involved in the establishment of a bacteriological thought style.[459] Reframed with Worboys' periodisation in mind, with a closer relationship with the terminology practitioners actually used, and a closer focus on practice, bacteriology's development in Sweden did not occur particularly late. In fact, practitioners seemed to be interested in one practical method, Listerism, which would later fall under the bacteriological umbrella, relatively early, even if they were not acutely in tune with its theoretical background.

Listerist Practice and Devices

Surgeons were interested in technological developments that assisted their practice, which the above discussions highlight. Furthermore, because of the very hands-on nature of surgery, surgical practice itself can be understood as

---

[457] Graninger, *Från osynligt till synligt*, 69. [Frågan är om det i Sverige fanns teoretisk beredskap att ta emot, sprida och vidareutveckla de kunskaper som utvecklades inom den nya vetenskapen bakteriologi.]
[458] Worboys, *Spreading Germs*, 18.
[459] Ludwik Fleck, "To Look, To See, To Know", in *Cognition and Fact: Materials on Ludwik Fleck*. Robert S. Cohen and Thomas Schnelle (eds.), 129–151. Dordrecht: D. Reidel Publishing Company, 1986, 140. Fleck even uses bacteriology as an example. Observers needed to know what they were looking at and distinguish features of what they were observing in the establishment of this thought style.

a technology.[460] This relationship between technology and surgery is significant, because technology has direct bearing on the tools used in surgical work, which is illustrative of many of the practical discussions involving Listerism. Thus far, I have framed the introduction of Listerism in Sweden and Denmark alongside problems with amputation. I have also shown that, for practitioners, clinical results were more important than the method's theoretical basis. A number of the discussions involving practice at the time implicated the construction and use of devices; problems with them; subsequent modifications; and, occasionally, exasperation. Devices were not just tools with a solely instrumental function, they were implements of assisting with, or even hindering, the implementation of Listerist aims in wound care. This method introduced a different way of thinking of and relating to devices used in practice. This involved cleaning them in particular ways, changing their construction, and the delegation of task. Listerism eventually developed into a method that encompassed other aspects of surgical practice than wound management, and into a more all-encompassing surgical technology, as Per Söderbaum suggested.[461] This increasingly required not only techniques, but also a specific set of tools.

By the 1870s, the Listerist system included a potential toolkit, and Lister himself worked with instrument makers to produce devices specific to the method. For example, in the 1870s, Lister introduced a carbolic acid sprayer to eliminate airborne pathogens. Lister first experimented with using a sprayer in 1871 and his sprayer was adapted from a Richardson's spray that was typically used for etherisation (figure 21).[462] The introduction of a Listerist toolkit might have entailed that practitioners in Sweden and Denmark introduced local adaptations themselves and/or with the help of trusted instrument makers, like the Stilles and Nyrop; however, medical journals provide little indication of this specifically. Lister himself had described ways to prepare bandages and ligatures, which surgeons would have done themselves or delegated to an assistant, if available.[463] As such,

---

[460] Schlich, "Introduction", 7. See also Thomas Schlich and Christopher Crenner, "Technological Change in Surgery: An Introduction Essay", in *Technological Change in Modern Surgery: Historical Perspectives on Innovation*, Thomas Schlich and Christopher Crenner (eds.), 1–20. Rochester: University of Rochester Press, 2017, 1.

[461] Söderbaum, *Listers antiseptiska metod*, 1.

[462] Joseph Lister, "Address in Surgery Delivered at the Thirty-Ninth Annual Meeting of the British Medical Association, Held in Plymouth, August 8th, 9th, 10th and 11th, 1871. 26 August 1871". *British Medical Journal*. Vol.2, No. 556, 26 August 1871, 225–233, 227. Lister's address was republished in translation in *Hospitals-Tidende* in several parts. For the part on Richardson's spray see Joseph Lister, "Den antiseptiske Metode". *Hospitals-Tidende*. Vol. 14, No. 47, 22 November 1871, 186–188, 187.

[463] Söderbaum, *Listers antiseptiska method*, 31.

Listerism, followed according to Lister's instructions and including the purchase of the necessary devices, offered a packaged alternative for the practitioner with recommended tools and other articles, but with room for further development and/or modification based on well-founded knowledge and practical experience.[464]

An example of this was the growing prevalence of ready-prepared "Listerist" ligatures, as well as soft articles, like dressings, for sale. Lister had given instructions on the preparation of dressings according to his method.[465] For example, by 1872, specific "Listerist" dressings could be purchased at pharmacies in Sweden.[466] These dressings were soaked or otherwise treated with carbolic acid or another antiseptic chemical, and the sale by apothecaries indicates broader use than just by surgeons or even the medical profession itself.[467] Despite their direct availability, however, physicians continued to prepare dressings themselves due to cost.[468] Two methods were detailed in *Hygiea* in 1878. One involved soaking curtain cloth in aseptin, a type of boric acid produced by Swedish chemical company Henrik Gahns AB; while the other method involved carbolic cotton. Both dressings could be reused under certain conditions, i.e., that the wound was not gangrenous, and with appropriate chemical treatment afterwards.[469]

Lister also had recommendations for the preparation of ligatures. He began experimenting with catgut ligatures, which were made from the intestines of animals, in the late 1860s, and published his recommendations in 1869 and 1881.[470] In contrast to other ligature materials at the time, ligatures of catgut were absorbable. This would mitigate irritation and inflammation, which would be particularly hazardous for more invasive surgical procedures. In operations involving internal structures of the body or other subcutaneous procedures, irritation and inflammation would require reopening the patient to remove sutures, whilst absorbable ligatures would be

---

[464] Worboys connects this "package" as an example of Lister's attempts to professionalise surgery. See "Jospeh Lister and the Performance of Antiseptic Surgery", 207.

[465] Lister, "On a New Method of Treating Compound Fracture", 95. Worboys also notes that one of Lister's students, William Watson Cheyne's book *Antiseptic Surgery*, which details Lister's system, provided illustrations of both dressings and instruments. See Worboys, "Joseph Lister and the Performance of Antiseptic Surgery", 204.

[466] *Förhandlingar vid Svenska läkarsällskapets sammankomster.* 26 March 1872.

[467] Worboys, *Spreading Germs*, 184.

[468] *Förhandlingar vid Svenska läkarsällskapets sammankomster.* 26 March 1872.

[469] A. Wiborgh, "Om antiseptiskt förbandstyg". *Hygiea*. Vol. 40, No. 8, August 1878, 413–416; *Förhandlingar vid Svenska läkarsällskapets sammankomster* 15 June 1873.

[470] Joseph Lister, "Observations on the Ligature of Arteries under the Antiseptic System". *Lancet*. Vol. 93, No. 2379, April 1869, 451–455; "An Address on the Catgut Ligature". *British Medical Journal*. Vol. 1, No. 1055, 5 February 1881, 183–185.

absorbed by the body, or at least remain inert. In July 1881, just a few months after Lister delivered an address on his new method of ligature preparation, surgeon Ivar Svensson described this method in *Hygiea*, which he hoped to begin using at Sabbatsberg Hospital in Stockholm. The method involved soaking catgut in a solution of chromic acid, water and carbolic acid for forty-eight hours, and after drying them thoroughly, storing them in a solution of carbolic acid and oil. [471] The compromised preparation time was also a Listerist innovation, with other preparation methods taking several months or years.[472] This would have hindered probable supply issues and made stocking ligatures less time-sensitive, meaning restocking could be done in a more time-sensitive manner.

The Listerist system included protocols for disinfection more broadly, with Lister underlining two primary sources for infection: contact and atmospheric.[473] This had broader implications for the use of surgical instruments and conventions for their correct and thorough disinfection. A translated article in *Hospitals-Tidende* from 1885 looked at the effects of different methods of disinfection on these two means of infection. In the case of infectious air, the author concluded that it was impossible to create a room completely free of germs and that surgeons should rather focus more intently on hindering contact infections.[474] This could be done in several different ways, depending on the material in question. For sponges, gauze, and bandages, the author recommended thorough rinsing with water and disinfectant soap with a rinse in a chemical solution such as carbolic, sublimate or choral water. Hands were trickier, but thorough hand washing with warm water, soap, and a brush was recommended, including under the nails. The author noted that it was difficult to make them completely germ-free and recommended carbol or choral water in addition to hand washing.[475]

Instruments offered further challenges. Other strategies were required to clean and keep them disinfected, with awareness for their material composition and form. The author of the translated article in *Hospitals-Tidende* recommended thoroughly cleaning instruments with warm water and disinfectant soap and soaking them in a disinfectant solution. Polished instruments could be thoroughly disinfected after soaking ten minutes in a carbolic

---

[471] Svensson, "Från kirurgiska afdelningen", 342.

[472] Lister, "An Address on the Catgut Ligature", 184.

[473] Lister, "Address in Surgery", 226.

[474] [Anon.], "Kontakt- og Luft-Infektion i den praktiske Kirurgi; Kümmel (Hamborg) (Beil. zum Centrabl. für Chirurgie 1885. Nr. 24. Meddelt paa den 14de tyske Kirurg-Kongres)". *Hospitals-Tidende.* Vol. 28, No. 29, 22 July 1885, 691–698, 697.

[475] [Anon.], "Kontakt- og Luft-infektion", 693–694.

acid solution, but disinfection after shorter soaks was not always guaranteed, even after brushing them with carbolic solution. Unpolished instruments were difficult to clean thoroughly per Listerist principles. Even after longer soaks in a disinfectant solution, they still developed "germs" [*Kim*] and "mould" [*Skimmelsvampe*], and the author underlined that thoroughly disinfecting unpolished instruments was dependent on their construction: "ribbed tweezers, serrated hooks were, for example, much more difficult to rid of germs than the smooth blade of a knife".[476]

Plating mitigated some of the problems encountered with disinfecting instruments properly. For instance, nickel plating was initially used because it made instruments easier to clean and offered some resistance to rust.[477] But even this was not a perfect solution. Some nickel-plated instruments were still prone to rust and difficult to resharpen, according to a report from Albert Stille at a Swedish Society of Medicine meeting in 1877.[478] Stille recommended it only for instruments that were not used for incisions and those that could be cleaned thoroughly before plating, as uneven plating would leave the instrument prone to rust. In cases where plating could not be done adequately, he recommended unplated, but polished steel.[479] Rust and issues with the plating's integrity would likely make them more difficult to disinfect. As Stille's expertise indicates, the chemical-laden disinfection processes used for some instruments merited a change in their composition. A translated article from 1878 also discussed an alternative to carbolic acid, thymol, which was said to be less caustic for instruments.[480] Sabbatsberg Hospital in Stockholm noted in their annual report from 1884 that instruments utilised in intraperitoneal operations, i.e., involving the abdominal organs were thoroughly disinfected. Also, in cases where instruments that had "shafts of bone [ivory] or wood are used, [they were] replaced over time with ones of iron".[481] Lavish designs and the use of materials other than metal for handles were not uncommon features of surgical instruments in nineteenth-century medicine; however, as the statement indicates, they were difficult to clean in

---

[476] Ibid., 692. [Riflede Pincetter, 4-takkede Hager kunne f. Ex. langt vanskeligere befries med Kim end glatte Knivsblade.]

[477] *Förhandlingar vid Svenska läkarsällskapets sammankomster*, 6 November 1877; see also James M. Edmonson. *American Surgical Instruments: An Illustrated History of Their Manufacture and a Directory of Instrument Makers to 1900*. San Francisco: Norman Publishing, 1997, 114.

[478] *Förhandlingar vid Svenska läkarsällskapets sammankomster*, 6 November 1877.

[479] Ibid.

[480] Carl Rossander, "Hans Ranke: Ueber das Thymol und seine Benutzung bei der antiseptischen Behandlung der Wunden". *Hygiea*. Vol. 40, No. 4, April 1878, 205–208, 206.

[481] F. W. Warfvinge. *Årsberättelse från Sabbatsbergs sjukhus i Stockholm för 1884*. Stockholm, 1885, 116. [i allmänhet användas skaft af trä eller ben, men dessa ersättas efter hand med sådana af järn.]

accordance with new disinfection protocols, in particular after invasive surgical procedures.[482] The archive for the Stockholm nurse's college, Sophiahemmet, registers costs for tin plating, sharpening, and repair, in particular in 1885 and 1886, and additional, unspecified invoices from instrument makers Stille and Werner could have included these services.[483]

Outside of affecting instruments, carbolic acid itself began to illustrate some of the downsides of this chemical-heavy system. Physicians remarked on its toxicity, irritability, and potential to cause burns. In *Ugeskrift,* a physician retold a case first published in *British Medical Journal* in 1868, where three women being treated with carbolic acid were poisoned by mistake, whereby two died. "When he [the physician] entered the room, he noticed the air was strong with the fumes from carbolic acid and the three women had collapsed".[484] Other articles highlighted the problems with the chemicals and either detailed personal experiences or translated articles from abroad to caution colleagues.[485] Simultaneously, experiments with other chemicals came up short, as, despite finding carbolic acid to be toxic, there had been disappointing results with substances that were less so.[486] Practitioners continued looking for other solutions, using local alternatives and experimenting with other chemicals. For larger wounds, boric acid or thymol were suggested initially as alternatives: thymol had a strong antiseptic effect and "boric acid does not possess the same injurious qualities of carbolic acid [toxic and irritating]".[487] There were cons in practice. Boric acid was a weaker antiseptic than carbolic acid, and thymol "promotes epidermis regeneration to a lesser degree than boric acid and, on more sensitive areas like the fingers, etc., causes significant pain".[488] Furthermore, thymol was found to attract flies, due to its sweet smell: a quality perhaps not particularly

---

[482] Edmonson, *American Surgical Instruments,* 119.

[483] SE/SSA/0252/A Riksarkivet, Sabbatsbergs sjukhus administrativa arkiv, G 1 B: Inventariehuvudböcker.

[484] [Anon.], "Forgiftning med Karbolsyre: Efter Dr. Machin (Brit. med. journ. Marts 1868.–L'un. méd. 1868. Nr. 108)". *Ugeskrift for Læger.* Series 3, Vol. 6, No. 20, 17 October 1868, 295–296, 295. [Da han kom ind i Stuen, fandt han Luften stærkt opfyldt af Karbosyredampe, og de tre Kvinder laa i en dyp Prostration.]

[485] [Anon.], "Karbolsyreforgiftning". *Ugeskrift for Læger.* Series 3, Vol. 13, No. 25, 25 May 1872, 403–404.

[486] Carl Rossander, "Sonnenburg: Zur Diagnose und Therapie der Carbolintoxicationen. Deutsche Zeitschrift für Chirurgie. Band. 9, sid. 356". *Hygiea.* Vol. 40, No. 9, September 1878, 499–501, 499–500.

[487] G. Naumann, "Om antiseptisk behandling af brännsår". *Hygiea.* Vol. 40, No. 6, June 1878, 282–286, 282. [Borsyran besitter deremot ej dessa karbolsyrans skadliga egenskaper.]

[488] Naumann, "Om antiseptisk behandling af brännsår", 282. [att tymolen långt mindre än borsyran gynnar epidermisbildningen och å mer känsliga ställen såsom fingrarne etc., förorsakar en ej obetydlig sveda.]

advantageous for a practice involving the chemical elimination of germs.[489] Correct storage was also necessary, with one practitioner commenting that dressings would be essentially useless if they were not stored in liquid-filled containers with tight-fitting lids.[490]

William Bynum points out that the growing reliance on technology in medicine more generally during the nineteenth century increased the financial investment required, which shifted the responsibilities to institutions rather than individuals.[491] This was no different for Listerism, with sources showing that following Listerist developments in wound care led to increased operating costs. Sabbatsberg Hospital detailed in a report on their economic situation in 1879 that their surgical ward had higher daily operational costs than other wards.[492] Expenses for preparations were more expensive as well. Reporting in *Hygiea*, the hospital director, F. W. Warfvinge, indicated that this was attributed to "the strict antiseptic treatment... [that] has made the utilisation of large quantities of carbolic acid necessary".[493] Medicines, which included carbolic acid, contributed to 44% of the ward's total yearly expenditures.[494] Aside from carbolic acid, bandages, drainage tubes, etc. were also required, of which the surgical ward's expenditures were four times higher than the medical ward's.[495] The dressings and wear and tear on instruments would have burdened individual practitioners without institutional support, which not all physicians had at this time. Still, responsibility to the patient was priority: one physician implored that physicians should avoid worrying about the cost of antiseptic methods, and instead focus on the safest and best method of treatment.[496]

---

[489] M. Sondén, "Diskussion om antiseptica, Berliner kiln. Wochenschr. N:o 17. 1878". *Hygiea*. Vol. 40, No. 5, May 1878, 254–255, 254.

[490] *Förhandlingar vid Svenska läkarsällskapets sammankomster*, 25 November 1873.

[491] William Bynum. *Science and the Practice of Medicine in the Nineteenth Century*. Cambridge: Cambridge University Press, 1994, 99.

[492] F. W. Warfvinge, "Redogörelse för sjukvården och ekonomien inom Sabbatsbergs sjukhus under år 1879". *Hygiea*. Vol. 42, No. 4, April 1880, 241–255, 244.

[493] Warfvinge, "Redogörelse för sjukvården", 245. [Till hufvudsakliga del härleder sig detta förhållande från den stränga antiseptiska behandling... gjort förbrukning af stora qvantiteter karbolsyra nödig.]

[494] Ibid., 245.

[495] Ibid., 246.

[496] Söderbaum, *Listers antiseptiska method*, 110.

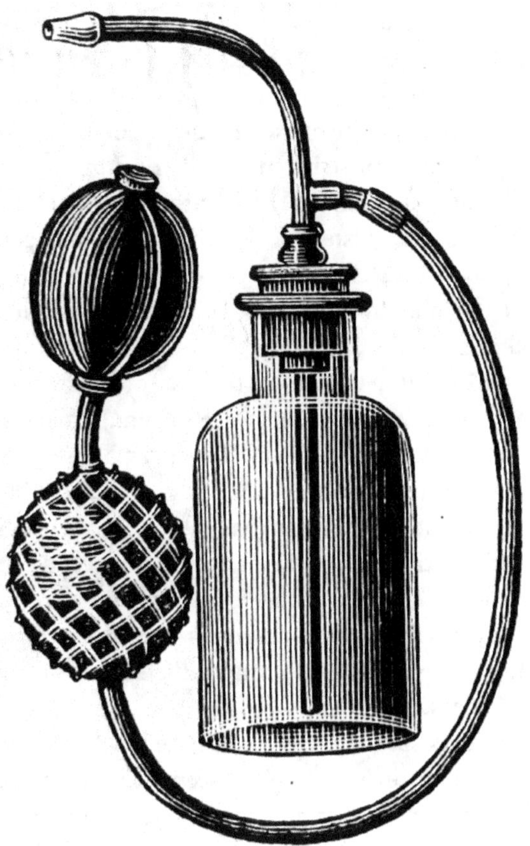

Fig. 21. Though not the sprayer of Lister's design, Lister's first experiment with a carbolic acid spray was with Richardson's spray, pictured above, which he modified. This device was primarily used for etherisation. Camillus Nyrops etablissement. *Illustreret Katalog.* Copenhagen: Nielsen & Lydiche, [n.d.], 34.

But sometimes following Lister's methods was difficult for solely practical, rather than economic, reasons. Perhaps the most controversial piece of Lister's toolkit was the carbolic acid sprayer. The science behind the use of Lister's spray was the notion that the infection of surgical wounds could be introduced through contact, e.g., instruments and/or the surgeon's or assistant's hands, or from germs in the air, or "atmospheric gas" and "particles of dust", as Lister referred to them.[497] The carbolic spray, in this

---

[497] Lister, "Address in Surgery", 226.

sense, would mitigate wound sepsis from these atmospheric influences. Lister would later renounce the spray, referring to it in 1881 as probably the least necessary part of the method.[498] However, in the address that introduces the sprayer, Lister highlights some of the practical problems with it. For example, the sprayer that he had constructed for distributing carbolic vapours over larger surgical fields, like amputations at the hip, was "in a cumbrous and heavy form".[499] Instead, Lister noted that surgeons could use "two of Richardson's spray-producers, worked by two assistants" (see figure 21).[500] In another case, detailed by Swedish surgeon M. Salin, administering the spray and paying attention to the operation proved to be difficult. During a surgery in London in 1879, Salin witnessed the use of the spray "but during the operation, the surgeon and assistants were so engulfed in their work that they did not realise for quite some time that the spray doused one assistant's back instead of the field of operation".[501] The spray could also be contraindicated, because of carbolic acid's toxicity and irritability. In an article in *Hygiea* from 1881, the author mentioned that, in a knee joint resection on a two-year-old, the spray was not used due to the length of time the patient had to be anaesthetised and because of the patient's young age.[502] Carbolic acid was, again, a well-known irritant at this time, which likely prompted the surgeon to forego it in this case.

The carbolic acid sprayer was highlighted at least twice in *Hospitals-Tidende* as a challenge, even though it seemed to have been adopted by at least one Danish surgeon a year after Lister's experiments with the device in 1871. Danish surgeon Valdemar Holmer mentioned the sprayer in 1872, in an article series on resection in *Hospitals-Tidende*. Holmer noted in that the number of assistants required to follow the method correctly during surgery was difficult. He stated that he thought it pertinent to apply the "antiseptic method" as closely as possible during and after the operation in question, but that keeping two sprayers with a carbolic acid solution operating throughout

---

[498] Joseph Lister, "An Address on the Treatment of Wounds". *The Lancet*. Vol. 118, No. 3038, 19 November 1881, 863–866. Michael Worboys notes in addition to this that the spray was the most commonly forsaken. See Worboys, *Spreading Germs*, 169.

[499] Lister, "Address in Surgery", 228.

[500] Ibid., 228.

[501] W. Netzel, "Utdrag ur bref från Dr M. Salin". *Hygiea*. Vol. 41, No. 2, February 1879, 98–104, 100. [Äfven här användes spray, men under operationens gång blef såväl operatörens som assistenternas uppmärksamhet tagen i så starkt anspråk, att de ej märkte, att spray'n längsta tiden bearbetade den ena assistentens rygg i stället för operationsfältet.]

[502] O. F. Hallin, "Om lasarettsväsendet i Sverige 1880". *Hygiea*. Vol. 43, No. 11, November 1881, 601–632, 619.

the procedure required "several assistants".[503] The use of two sprayers likely indicates that he did not use the heavy and cumbersome apparatus Lister mentioned, but used two smaller sprayers instead. In two countries where physicians and surgeons were, at the time, not plentiful resources, the delegation required of exacting Listerist principles would likely have been a difficult task. This problem would have been exacerbated outside of the respective capitols, particularly at smaller hospitals and clinics. It also placed control over the space outside of the hands of the surgeon, requiring one or more assistants to control the sprayer and the room.

Using the sprayers was not necessarily a simple task either. Another article in *Hospitals-Tidende* noted that the assistants using them had to ensure that they were positioned correctly over the operating field; that they sprayed steady streams of solution consistently; that the spray did not change direction; that all windows and doors were closed; that no one could leave or enter the room during the procedure; and, perhaps most importantly, that the sprayers actually contained the carbolic acid solution and not just water.[504] This ties into the scene witnessed by Salin in London, where even with a few assistants on hand, the surgeon would have to delegate as well as ensure the right field was being doused with carbolic acid spray, and errors risked diverting the surgeon's focus from the task at hand. Attention, economy, and preparation were all implicated in the method's practice, illustrated by devices, introducing new ways of working, and different ways of relating to surgery's tools.

Concluding Remarks

The focus on antiseptic theory over antiseptic practice has misrepresented the goals of surgeons during this period. They were clinically inclined, and the importance of clinical results is highlighted in journal articles discussing the method. Rather than mulling over theoretical implications or foundations, practitioners in Sweden and Denmark in the 1860s and 1870s were more concerned with the positive, practical results of Listerist antisepsis. This chapter began by framing the introduction of Listerism in these two countries around a prevailing problem: amputation. By looking at the introduction of Listerims vis-à-vis amputation, subsequent discussions could be better centred around practice, which figures most significantly in medical journals from these two countries. This does not negate an interest in germ theory or

---

[503] Holmer, "Om Resektion af Knæleddet" No. 45, 177. [den fordrer flere Assistenter]
[504] Bloch, "Om den forskellige Saarbehandling", No. 18, 276–277.

Listerism's theoretical foundation; however, theory was less important for practitioners than the method's empirical results were. The dissemination of Listerism in Sweden and Denmark can be better understood in similar terms as an apprenticeship. Communicating Listerist practice and its tacit knowledge was difficult through text. Listerist practice should be understood as locally situated, as it was disseminated through local retellings by practitioners who had visited Lister or one of his students, or through translation. As such, the details communicated in medical serials may appear convoluted; however, the details of practice are notoriously difficult to communicate through text, in particular knowledge that has been internalised by the practitioner. Furthermore, many articles about Listerism appeared in translation, which adds a further layer to their complexity. Fundamentally though, articles in Swedish and Danish medical serials were highly focused on the method's clinical applications over its theoretical foundations, suggesting that they were published to communicate just that: practice.

Many details of Listerist practice often focused on the use of chemicals and devices, the issues physicians encountered with them, and, in some instances, potential solutions. Listerism introduced different ways of relating to devices and their use in practice. Practitioners were given distinct methods of preparing dressings and ligatures, which included new materials. This also introduced issues that practitioners resolved to overcome. Some of these challenges related to the local adaptation and development of antisepsis, where devices and chemicals had to be procured, used, and paid for. Other practical challenges included the use of harsh chemicals on patients as well as instruments and the significant cost of these chemicals. In the case of the carbolic acid sprayer that Lister introduced, it was difficult to motivate its use practically due to manpower during operations and raised questions involving the surgeon's capability to manage the suite and focus on the task at hand. It is questions like these, of a practical character, that seemed to matter most to Swedish and Danish physicians concerning Listerism, not necessarily explanations of the method's theoretical underpinnings. Given the surgeon's relationship with device technologies, many of the practical discussions about Listerism implicated these technologies in particular and bore important meaning for the proliferation of Listerist practice and its enactment.

5. Asepsis, Surgery, and a System of Cleanliness: Two Cases in Stockholm

In February 1894, the Swedish newspaper *Smålandsposten* commented that "[Max] Stille's well-known operating table, which has already spread around the whole of Europe, has also found its way over the Atlantic. Dr. Edebohls, the director of the grand Rosewell Hospital in New York, has spoken with the most laudatory words about the elegant and solid workmanship regarding the table, chairs and accompanying accessories".[505] Stille's operating table attracted the attention of the press due to its recognition abroad. But it was not just his operating tables that attracted attention. There were other newspaper articles about a Stille-constructed model surgical suite, designed to conform to new standards of cleanliness, which included examples of "some of the firm's famous, award-winning and patented excellent operating tables".[506] Later that same year, in April, Stille set up another model suite, this time at the Eleventh International Medical Congress in Rome. The newspaper *Stockholms Dagblad* reported on the suite and Stille's impressions, stating that "the Swedish work attracted broad attention of the most flattering kind, in particular because of the care placed in every detail to ensure an entirely antiseptic treatment, ease in cleaning all aspects, as well as comfort for the patient, physician, and assistants. [...] Mr. Stille could also enjoy the practical acknowledgment in the form of orders that have been placed from Italy, England, Germany, Russia, Serbia, and Romania, as well as promises of orders upon returning home have been left by physicians from America, Hungary, and Egypt".[507]

---

[505] [Anon.], "Erkännande från Amerika åt svensk industri". *Smålandsposten*. 9 Feburary 1894. [Alb. Stilles kända operationsbord, som redan spridits kring snart sagdt hela Europa samt också hittat vägen öfver Atlanten. D:r Edebohls, direktör för det storartade Roswell hospital i Newyork (sic), har skriftligen i de mest berömmande ordalag uttalat sig om det eleganta och solida arbete, som utmärker dessa operationsbord, dito stolar och tillhörande utensilier]
Though the article mentiones "Alb. Stille" (Albert Stille), the author presumably means the firm rather than the person. Albert Stille had died several months prior on October 23, 1893 and had already passed on the firm to his son, Max.

[506] [Anon.], "En mönster-operationssal". *Dagens Nyheter*. 28 February 1894. [Der finnas följaktligen några af firmans kända, prisbelönta och patenterade utmärkta operationsbord]

[507] [Anon.], "Stilles operationssal vid läkarkongressen i Rom". *Stockholms Dagblad*. 22 April 1894. [detta svenska arbete ådragit sig en vidsträckt uppmärksamhet af den mest smickrande art, särskildt på grund af den omsorg, som blifvit nedlagd på hvarje detalj för att försäkra såväl fullkomlig antiseptisk behandling, lätthet att rengöra alla delar samt beqvämlighet för patent, läkare och assistenter... Hr Stille

In this chapter, I will use Max Stille's model surgical suite and operating table as cases that highlight the respatialisation of surgical practice that occurred in conjunction with the rise of aseptic surgical practices in the late 1880s and 1890s. Asepsis is a microbe-free state, while antisepsis is the method of destroying microbes. The two operate from different premises. On the one hand, antisepsis principally acknowledges the presence of microbes but uses chemicals to destroy them to prevent infection. Asepsis, on the other hand, anticipates an environment free of microbes. However, a microbe-free state was both difficult to discern and difficult to achieve. Surgeons noted problems with furnishings, rooms, and other objects. Because of this, surgeons did not immediately discard antiseptic practice and used it together with other, aseptic, means of disinfection in order to maintain a sense of control over the process. Additionally, Listerism had been a significant influence on Swedish and Danish surgery, though this chapter will primarily centre Sweden. Some historians have argued that asepsis developed independently to Listerism, which may have been the case in some regions.[508] However, Listerist antisepsis and aseptic practices were used simultaneously in this period in both these two countries. This period, in this geographical context, can be understood as transitional, which called for the fluid use of these two methods, often together.

The requirements of aseptic practice introduced what I will refer to as a system of cleanliness. This system required more of surgical spaces and the cleanliness of rooms, devices, and surgeons. This would eventually give surgeons a sense of control over the process. However, initially it was not always easy for practitioners to discern whether or not spaces, devices, and bodies were microbe-free, so the introduction of the aseptic system of cleanliness should be understood as overlapping with antiseptic practices. From antisepsis, a method that was less bound to a specific space, asepsis was quite specific to institutional space. With the use of asepsis, surgical practice became increasingly dependent on space, the sterility of that space, and its ability to be disinfected. Some historians have examined changes in surgical and hospital spaces in relation to different technological changes like anaesthesia, whilst others have argued that architecture rather than technology

har också haft att glädja sig åt ett praktiskt erkännande i form af beställningar, som ingått från Italien, England, Tyskland, Ryssland, Serbien och Rumänien, hvarjemte löften om beställningar efter hemkomsten lära hafva lemnats af läkare från Amerika, Ungern och Egypten.]

[508] See N. J. Fox, "Scientific Theory Choice and Social Structure: The Case of Joseph Lister's Antisepsis, Humoral Theory and Asepsis". *History of Science.* Vol. 26, No. 4, December 1988, 367–397; T. H. Pennington, "Listerism, its Decline and Persistence: The Introduction of Aseptic Surgical Techniques in Three British Teaching Hospitals, 1890–1899". *Medical History.* Vol. 39, No. 1, January 1995, 35–60.

predicated change.[509] Neither architecture nor surgical technology alone were entirely fundamental in surgery's respatialisaton in Sweden. Rather, Max Stille's work illustrates that the shift in venue also demanded more of the furnishings and interiors of surgical spaces in accordance with aseptic principles of cleanliness, and Stille's surgical tables and model suite are examples of this. As I will show, many of the articles about the suite and the table noted their conformation to new surgical principles. Stille made both his tables and suite to conform with the aseptic system of cleanliness. But outside just conforming to new standards of cleanliness, they also exemplify a practical shift. They could not conceivably be marketed to individual physicians only. One was an entire room dependent on a hospital setting, and the other was an expensive furnishing. The suite and the table serve to illustrate that, unlike Listerist antisepsis, aseptic practice was dependent on institutional support.

Surgical Space, Antisepsis, and Asepsis

The previous chapter ended with a discussion about practical problems with Listerism and some changes made to the method of wound care. By the late 1880s, Lister had renounced the carbolic acid spray and had begun adapting other methods of wound management and disinfection.[510] The foremost challenge Swedish and Danish practitioners had with the method was the chemicals used. Practitioners were particularly troubled with the method's primary chemical, carbolic acid, and had been experimenting with alternatives to it for nearly as long as Lister made his method known.[511] Additionally, surgeons were retooling their practice to accommodate greater control over surgical outcomes and spaces. However, as Ulrika Graninger points out in her study on the establishment of bacteriology in Sweden, the theoretical underpinnings of the move from antisepsis to asepsis were not straightforward. She notes that despite bacteriology being seemingly uncontroversial in the late 1880s and 1890s, many practitioners still discussed it from a frame

---

[509] For space and anaesthesia, see Jeanne Kisacky. *Rise of the Modern Hospital: An Architectural History of Health and Healing, 1870–1940*. Pittsburgh: University of Pittsburgh Press, 2017. For architecture as a catalyst for change see Jeremy Taylor. *The Architect and the Pavilion Plan Hospital: Dialogue and Design Creativity in England, 1850–1914*. London: Leicester University Press, 1997; Katherine Carroll, "Creating the Modern Physician: The Architecture of American Medical Schools in the Era of Medical Education Reform". *Journal of the Society of Architectural Historians*. Vol. 75, 2016, 48–73.

[510] Michael Worboys. *Spreading Germs: Disease Theories and Medical Practice in Britain, 1865–1900*. Cambridge: Cambridge University Press, 2000, 191.

[511] See Chapter 4, pg. 150ff.

of reference founded on miasma theory.[512] In the previous chapter, I highlighted that theory was secondary to a method that worked. This seems to be the case here as well. Based on Graninger's research, bacteriology's theoretical foundation in relation to the evolution and implementation of an aseptic system of cleanliness seems to also have been secondary to its results.[513] Listerism was implemented quickly and with relative ease in Sweden, and it remained important even as surgeons began experimenting with methods of asepsis.

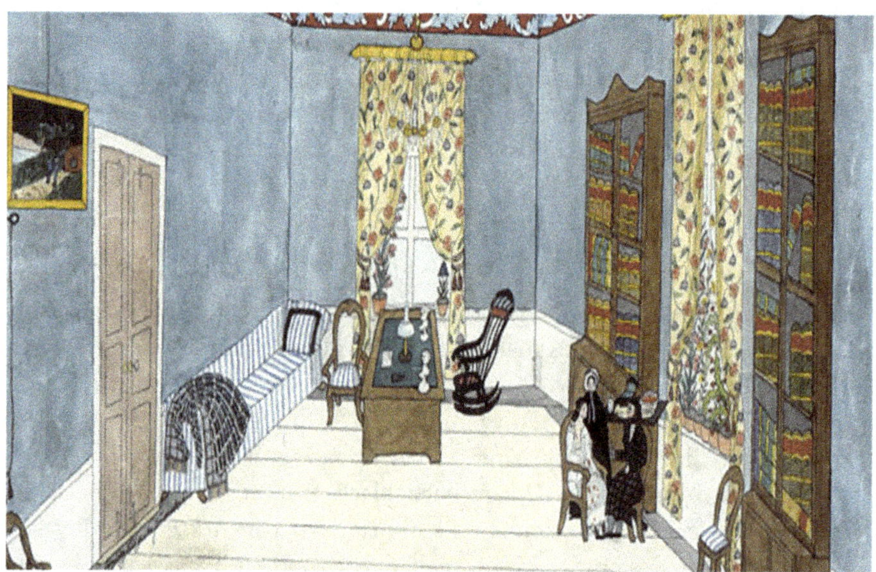

Fig. 22. An example of a space where surgery could have taken place, the patient underwent a smaller operation in the physician's examination room. Josabeth Sjöberg, D.L.'s (Dr. Levin) examination room No. 14 near Götgatan, Block Jupiter Större, one floor up, Operation Wednesday 24 April year 1850. Dr. Levin is the figure in the checkered jacket, with a knife in his hand. The piece is cropped. Stockholms stadsmuseum, Inventarienummer SSM 502493

One of the physicians who will make frequent appearances in this chapter because of his interest in antisepsis, asepsis, and their practical concerns is Swedish surgeon Jacques Borelius. Borelius visited Lister's ward in 1889, now at King's College Hospital in London, and published his observations in an

---

[512] Ulrika Graninger. *Från osynligt till synligt: Bakteriologins etablering i sekelskiftets svenska medicin.* Diss. Linköping University, 1997, 230.
[513] For a thorough account of the establishment of bacteriology in Sweden, see Ibid., 189–230.

article *Hygiea*. While some of the articles mentioned in the previous chapter were less about surgical space, with one even detailing an operation in a patient's home, Borelius' article, and many of the others discussed in this chapter, were tied explicitly to a specific space and the maintenance of that space per the aseptic system of cleanliness. That space was the operating room.

Specific spaces for surgery were not new inventions, but many of the articles discussed in the third chapter did not specify space. In some instances, authors noted that operations were carried out in patients' homes.[514] Thomas Schlich highlights that, historically, surgery could be and was performed in a multitude of different spaces including homes, and surgeons generally had little control over their work environment.[515] Surgery was performed in emergency situations, or it was less invasive, involving disease of the skin.[516] In Denmark, the first successful ovariotomy that did not result in the death of the patient was performed outside a hospital setting, in a house in Jelling, a small town in the western part of the country.[517] Julius Boye, the physician who performed the ovariotomy, even suggested that surgeons should consider keeping the patient close to their family and "find a detached, hygienic space in the countryside" to operate in.[518] On an individual level, antisepsis could be implemented in any space, even if its use in hospital settings activated questions of "hospital airs" or miasma.[519] Boye

---

[514] See for example *Förhandlingar vid Svenska läkarsällskapet*, 15 July 1873 where Axel Gustaf Virgin details the removal of a needle from a patient's thigh and subsequent antiseptic treatment in the patient's home of the infected wound. For a more general discussion about hospital admissions in Denmark and Sweden, see for example Signild Vallgårda, "Who Went to a General Hospital in the Eighteenth and Nineteenth Centuries in Copenhagen?". *European Journal of Public Health*, Vol. 9, No. 2, June 1999, 97–102; Anders Brändström, "The Silent Sick: Life-Histories of 19th Century Swedish Hospital Patients", in *Society, Health and Population During the Demographic Transition*, A. Brändström & L. G. Tedebrand (eds.), 343–368. Umeå: Almqvist and Wiksell, 1988.

[515] Thomas Schlich, "Surgery, Science and Modernity: Operating Rooms and Laboratories as Spaces of Control". *History of Science*. Vol. 45, No. 3, September 2007, 231–256, 236.

[516] Michael Worboys, "The History of Surgical Wound Infection: Revolution or Evolution", in *The Palgrave Handbook of the History of Surgery*, Thomas Schlich (ed.), 215–233. London: Palgrave Macmillan, 2018, 217.

[517] J. Boye, "Et Tilfælde af Ovariotomi med heldigt Udfald". *Hospitals-Tidende*. Vol. 10, No. 12, 16 October 1867, 165–167. Boye was not a surgeon and part of his article lifted the question of whether or not surgical training was important in a positive outcome, or if the constitution of the space was of more significance. See also Klas Larsen, "Her fødtes dansk underlivskirurgi". *Ugeskrift for Læger*. 25 June 2018. https://ugeskriftet.dk/nyhed/her-foedtes-dansk-underlivskirurgi (Accessed 27 November 2021).

[518] Boye, "Et Tilfælde af Ovariotomi", 167. [Kan man derfor skaffe sin Patient et fritliggende, sundt Lokale paa Landet]

[519] Jeanne Kisacky discusses the relationships between environment and disease prevention in a New York City hospital in the nineteenth century. Jeanne Kisacky, "Germs are in the Details: Aseptic Design and General Contractors at the Lying-In Hospital in the City of New York, 1897–1901". *Construction*

noted further that the constitution of the countryside might have provided a better environment than the large, city hospitals.[520] However, in contrast, the aseptic system of cleanliness was closely tied to space and the sterilisation of that space.

Although ovariotomies did not generally move to hygienic, countryside locales, Boye's article highlights that practitioners were thinking about the constitutions of the spaces they were performing surgery in and how they might relate to surgical outcomes even before aseptic practice.[521] They were also performing, successfully, more difficult and invasive surgeries. While the association with space was not new, the shift in space was necessitated in part by the changing nature of surgical procedures. This is highlighted by Michael Worboys. While Worboys considers understanding asepsis as an evolution of Listerian antisepsis, he also underlines the importance of other variables that affected the nature of surgical practice and the outcomes of surgical procedures. The factors he notes include, but are not limited to, different types of procedures, new techniques, societal factors affecting the health of patients, better facilities, and fewer last-resort procedures.[522] However, aseptic practice was also more specific to space and the qualities of that space than Listerism and other antiseptic practices were. Boye's countryside location would have been difficult to conform to the spatial standards of asepsis due to factors involving ventilation, material composition, sterilisation equipment, and control.[523]

Control over space and circumstance are frequent points made in articles on the technologies of disinfection and sterilisation in medical serials during the 1880s and 1890s. This was not always straightforward for practitioners, as new technologies and methods introduced uncertainty, which in turn required further examination.[524] One of the first areas of control that physicians had grappled with was over disinfection practice. Chemicals had

---

History. Vol. 28, No. 1, 2013, 83–106. See also Worboys, *Spreading Germs*, 37–38, on miasma and sanitary conditions. Though not hospital-related, Annelie Drakman discusses shifting perspectives on air and air circulation in relation to health in Sweden in her thesis. See *När kroppen slot sig och blev fast: varför åderlåtning, miasmateori och klimatmedicin övergavs vid 1800-talets mitt.* Diss. Uppsala University, 2018, 99–119.

[520] Boye, "Et Tilfælde af Ovariotomi", 167.

[521] See Kisacky, "Germs are in the Details", 86–87; Kisacky, *Rise of the Modern Hospital*, 13–15, 78–79; Worboys, *Spreading Germs*, 73–107, Worboys, "The History of Surgical Wound Infection", 216–223.

[522] Worboys, "The History of Surgical Wound Infection", 225.

[523] Kisacky, "Germs are in the Details", 89–90.

[524] Sally Frampton, "Defining Difference: Competing Forms of Ovarian Surgery in the Nineteenth Century", in *Technological Change in Modern Surgery: Historical Perspectives on Innovation*, Thomas Schlich and Christopher Crenner (eds.), 51–70. Rochester: University of Rochester Press, 2017, 66.

long been a problem for Listerism but gave results. The use of chemicals was also a means of disinfection that physicians were well-acquainted with by the 1880s.[525] The familiarity with disinfection chemicals, how they worked and in what quantities, were, by this time, part of a collective body of knowledge that gave physicians a sense of control. At this point, physicians worked with different dilutions depending on the material composition of the object in question. For example, Borelius noted in his article about Lister's ward the composition of dilute solutions of the different chemicals, their concentrates, and in what situations different dilutions were used. Weaker dilutions and different chemicals were used for the skin and hands than for instruments, that, given the discussion in the previous chapter, tied into physician's practical experience with chemicals.[526]

However, this began to change. As other historians point out, it was not the presence of airborne germs, but Robert Koch's demonstration in 1878 that diseased organisms were inhabited by germs and could be transferred to other organisms, that had a significant impact on germ theory and wound management.[527] A year after his visit to Lister's ward, in 1890, Borelius published a short overview in *Hygiea* about Lister's work using different chemicals in his wound management system and Lister's recommendations. Despite the changes made to Listerism, and Lister's recommendations, Borelius stated that "this [Lister's] dressing does not and will not have large practical meaning. The majority have now gone over to or are willing to go over to the simplest and safest of all dressings: sterile [aseptic] dressings. But, the development of the antiseptic dressing under Lister's direction will eternally have a large historical value".[528] What was the primary difference between the two methods of wound care, and why was Listerism suddenly of historic rather than practical interest? Borelius stated in another article that disinfection was the goal of both methods; however, that asepsis "strives to

---

[525] Michael Worboys also highlights that chemicals were still recommended in English-language surgical textbooks into the early twentieth century. Worboys, *Spreading Germs*, 190.

[526] Instruments were placed in 1:20 carbolic acid solutions half an hour prior to operations, and the area that would be operated on was shaved with a 1:500 sublimate solution and bandage applied to the area several hours prior to the operation. Jacques Borelius, "Antiseptiken på Listers afdelning på Kings College Hospital i London". *Hygiea*. Vol. 51, No. 11, November 1889, 665–669, 667.

[527] Worboys, "The History of Surgical Wound Infection", 223. See also Worboys, *Spreading Germs*, 172; Kisacky, *Rise of the Modern Hospital*, 107.

[528] Jacques Borelius, "Joseph Lister, An address on a new antiseptic dressing' Brit. Med. Journal 1889, nov 9, 1890, jan. 4. Referat af Jacques Borelius". *Hygiea*. Vol. 52, No. 8, August 1890, 589–591, 591. [Detta förband har väl icke och kommer nog icke att få stor praktisk betydelse. De fleste hafva väl nu öfvergått eller äro beredda att öfvergå till de enklaste och säkraste af alla förband, sterilförbandet. Men utvecklingen af det antiseptiska förbandet i Listers egen hand har för evärdliga tider sin stora historiska betydelse.]

remove or reduce the use of antiseptic solutions as much as possible and replace them with meticulous and consequent disinfection by other means".[529] There is also an important lexical distinction in Swedish sources. While antisepsis was often referenced in terms of wound care [*sårbehandling*], asepsis related to the environment in itself and its lack of germs.[530]

At Lister's ward, Borelius observed that "the operator removed his jacket and rolled up his shirt sleeves–linen coats or aprons were not used–the assistant removed his cufflinks, but the arms of his regular jacket were not rolled up, rather hovered endlessly in the immediate vicinity of the site of operation and wound".[531] Unlike Listerist antisepsis, aseptic practice was more than just a method of wound management, but a system of cleanliness that applied to the surrounding environment. This required practitioners to work methodically, to an even greater degree than antiseptic wound care, to ensure the surroundings were germ-free. The difference here is in the work toward germ-free wounds (antisepsis) versus creating germ-free environments (asepsis). Under an aseptic system of cleanliness, the assistant's hovering shirtsleeves, likely his street clothes, could have introduced cross-contamination.[532] It was vital that the entire surgical environment was germ-free. But, this was not always easy to discern.

In addition to environmental concerns, practitioners also grappled with contact infections and what could lead to them. In another article by Borelius, this time from 1893, illustrates this distinction. He noted in the article that anything within the immediate vicinity of the site of operation or a wound, or that comes in contact with this rather large spatial field, could lead to a contact infection. This included the site of the operation, hands from any of the involved practitioners, instruments, sponges, ligatures, drainage tubes, bandages, and even water and other solutions.[533] Mitigating contact infec-

---

[529] Jacques Borelius, "Den aseptiska sårbehandlingen". *Hygiea.* Vol. 55, No. 4, April 1893, 415–429, 416. [Denna metod sträfvar att borttaga eller till det minsta möjliga inskränka bruket af antiseptiska medel och ersätta dem med noggrant och konseqvent genomförda desinfektionsåtgärder af andra slag]

[530] See Chapter 4. See also Anders Åman who distinguishes between antisepsis and asepsis this way in his book on Sweden's public institutes for healthcare. See Anders Åman. *Om den offentliga vården: Byggnader och verksamheter vid svenska vårdinstitutioner under 1800- och 1900-talen. En arkitekturhistorisk undersökning.* Stockholm: LiberFörlag, 1976, 198.

[531] Borelius, "Antiseptiken på Listers afdelning", 667. [Operatören tar utaf sig sin rock och viker upp skjortärmarna–linnerockar eller förkläden användas ej –, asistenten tar utaf sig manschetterna, men ärmarna af hans vanliga rock vikas ej upp, utan sväfva oupphörligt i omedelbar närhet af operationsfältet och såret.]

[532] See Worboys, *Spreading Germs*, 186; Jeanne Kisacky, "Germs are in the Details", 91.

[533] Borelius, "Den aseptiska sårbehandlingen", 419. Regarding hands in particular, see also Jacques Borelius, "Om behandling af frakturer på underbenet". *Hygiea.* Vol. 56, No. 6, June 1894, 578–592; Georg

tions would necessitate the disinfection of bodies, devices, and other things. Regarding the sterilisation of instruments, Borelius observed that instruments used in Lister's ward were "rinsed in water after the surgery was finished, scrubbed [with a brush], dried thoroughly, and put back in the [storage] cabinet".[534] Other technologies than the Listerist system of chemical treatments were proving to be advantageous for disinfection. Asepsis relied heavily on the use of heat, through steam, boiling, or dry heat to disinfect devices and other items used in surgical and other hospital environments.[535] Two articles in particular looked at two variations of one alternative that solved similar problems: disinfection ovens. Though not instrument-specific, these two articles highlight ways that practitioners explored alternatives to Listerism's chemical-heavy method of disinfection, how these apparatuses functioned, and their effectiveness.

As Jeanne Kisacky points out in her research on the history of the modern hospital, practitioners had some difficulty drawing the line in what items in the surgical space had to be sterilised and what did not.[536] However, it was not just a matter of determining what needed to be sterilised. Practitioners were unsure at first to what extent sterilisation employing heat treatment worked. An article by physician Pontus Söderberg from 1893, describes the use of Seraphim Hospital's disinfection oven. The oven was 1.65 meters high inside, 1.48 meters wide and 2 meters tall, with a rack that could be pulled out to either hang objects from or place them on. Söderberg noted that there was an iron rack that soft items such as cushions, could be placed on, but after use, it was found to imprint rust spots on the fabric, whereby the iron bars were outfitted with wood.[537] The apparatus was connected to the hospital's boiler, which supplied steam, and a closed system of pipes so that the items in the disinfector could dry, and the oven was outfitted with pressure gauge, and a thermometer, which could take readings up to 100 degrees Celsius. First, the

Hellström, "Sjunde Allmänna Svenska Läkarmötet i Lysekil". *Hygiea*. Vol. 57, No. 9, September 1895, 304–332.

See Thomas Schlich, "Negotiating Technologies in Surgery: The Controversy about Surgical Gloves in the 1890s". *Bulletin of the History of Medicine*. Vol. 87, No. 2, Summer 2013, 170–197, for a historical perspective. Schlich notes that gloves played into the element of control over the surgical environment, where the surgeon's hands and their interaction with instruments, chemicals and the patient were sources of risk; but that gloves also were a potential impediment to the dexterity of the surgeon.

[534] Borelius, "Antiseptiken på Listers afdelning", 668. [Instrumenten sköljas efter operationens slut i vatten. [sic] borstas, torkas väl och inläggas derefter i skåpet.]

[535] Worboys, *Spreading Germs*, 186.

[536] Kisacky, *Rise of the Modern Hospital*, 108.

[537] Pontus Söderberg, "Några desinfektionsförsök å Serafimerlasarettets desinfektionsugn". *Hygiea*. Vol. 55, No. 1, January 1893, 1–14, 1–2.

machine would heat up with the help of steam, then the heat from the steam would pressure-treat the items inside the apparatus and the steam vent would close off, with steam only heating the machine's element, which would dry the items.[538]

Söderberg then presented several trials with various combinations of dirt, bacteria, fabrics, and paper to determine how long the different steps of this type of disinfection would take. Importantly, as an article from 1890 highlighted, killing both particles visible and invisible to the eye was the purpose of these apparatuses and the systems they employed.[539] These kinds of experiments had been encouraged by surgeon Richard Wawrinsky, who stated that "the question of practical importance related to the use of high temperatures as a means of disinfection is what kinds of things can be exposed to heat without being destroyed. This question cannot be solved only through experiments in laboratories, but unquestionably requires practical experience".[540] But, as Söderberg's trials indicate, practitioners needed to understand how heat sterilisation worked and the device's necessary settings, depending on material and microbe. And, as the quote by Wawrinsky above highlights, this needed to be discerned through practical trials closer to real-life situations, rather than through laboratory experiments, like those conducted by Koch.

According to the article by Söderberg, the person in charge of disinfection, Söderberg mentioned a machinist, would need to take into consideration that once the machine's thermometer reached 100 degrees, the objects in the apparatus also had to reach that temperature, which would take additional time.[541] These apparatuses were discussed in *Hygiea* concerning materials for wound care, like bandages, more than instruments. The trials conducted with Seraphim Hospital's oven above included cloth, not surgical instruments or other items made from metal. Placing surgical instruments in the care of a machinist would have reduced the surgeon's control over the disinfection of their instruments, and physicians were still fundamentally uncertain about to what extent steam and heat disinfection worked.

---

[538] Söderberg, "Några desinfektionsförsök", 3.

[539] Jacques Borelius. "Om Hennebergs desinfektor för sterilsering af förbandsmaterial m. m". *Hygiea*. Vol. 52, No. 9, September 1890, 677–680, 680.

[540] R. Wawrinsky. "Om desinfektion efter smittosamma sjukdomar. Föreläsning å Karolinska Institutet den 4 oktober 1890". *Hygiea*. Vol. 52, No. 11, November 1890, 798–828, 819. [Af praktisk betydelse med afseende på höga värmegraders användande såsom desinfektionsmedel är frågan om, hvad slags föremål som kunna utsättas för hetta utan att förderfvas. Denna fråga kan icke lösas ensamt genom laboratorieexperiment, utan kräfver onekligen praktisk erfarenhet.]

[541] Söderberg, "Några desinfektionsförsök", 13.

Another article about a disinfection apparatus, written by Borelius, from 1890 examined a German machine called "Henneberg's Disinfector". This apparatus operated on similar principles as the above except it was not pressurised and was intended for the sterilisation of materials for dressing wounds. Borelius noted that the free-flowing steam that this apparatus used to disinfect, disinfected just as well as pressurised machines but had the distinct advantages of being less complicated, cheaper, and constituted no explosion risk. Like Seraphim Hospital's disinfection oven, it too had problems with rust; however, this time in the boiler portion.[542] Although Borelius mentioned it was a less costly alternative to pressurised machines, the apparatus cost around 400 kronor, or less, depending on whether it produced its own steam or utilised the hospital's boiler.[543] In other words, this technology was not marketed or designed for the individual physician to purchase. Outside of cost, it required space and infrastructure, if it was connected to the facility's boiler, to operate.

Apparatuses like these, given their cost and size, were a growing number of similar devices more intended for large-scale institutional use, rather than individual, of which I will being to go into more detail about below.[544] Still, an article by T. H. Pennington on the persistence of Listerist antisepsis additionally details that at the Ziegelstrasse Clinic in Berlin, that used Henneberg's apparatus, instruments were additionally disinfected in a carbolic acid solution before use, pointing to the persistence of chemicals in disinfection technologies.[545] Thomas Schlich illustrates that practitioners found it difficult to gauge whether germs were absent after aseptic treatment in his study on glove usage in German territories. On the other hand, the harsh chemicals commonly used in antiseptic methods "killed germs indiscriminately".[546] The above research on Seraphim Hospital's disinfection oven was one step in understanding the lives of microbes and how to remove them from an object or space, but the use of antiseptic solutions helped practitioners in determining when an object was disinfected because they already knew that these solutions worked.

---

[542] Ibid., 679.

[543] Borelius, "Hennebergs desinfektor", 678. See also note 3 pg. 680.

[544] See also mention of a disinfection oven at Fredriks Hospital in Copenhagen see [Anon.], "Mindre Meddelelser". *Hospitals-Tidende*. Vol. 37, No 33, 15 August 1894, 824. The Hennebergs apparatus in Borelius' article was at Sahlgrenska Hostpital in Gothenburg, Sweden, see pg. 680.

[545] Pennington, "Listerism, its Decline and its Persistence", 40.

[546] Schlich, "Negotiating Technologies in Surgery", 176.

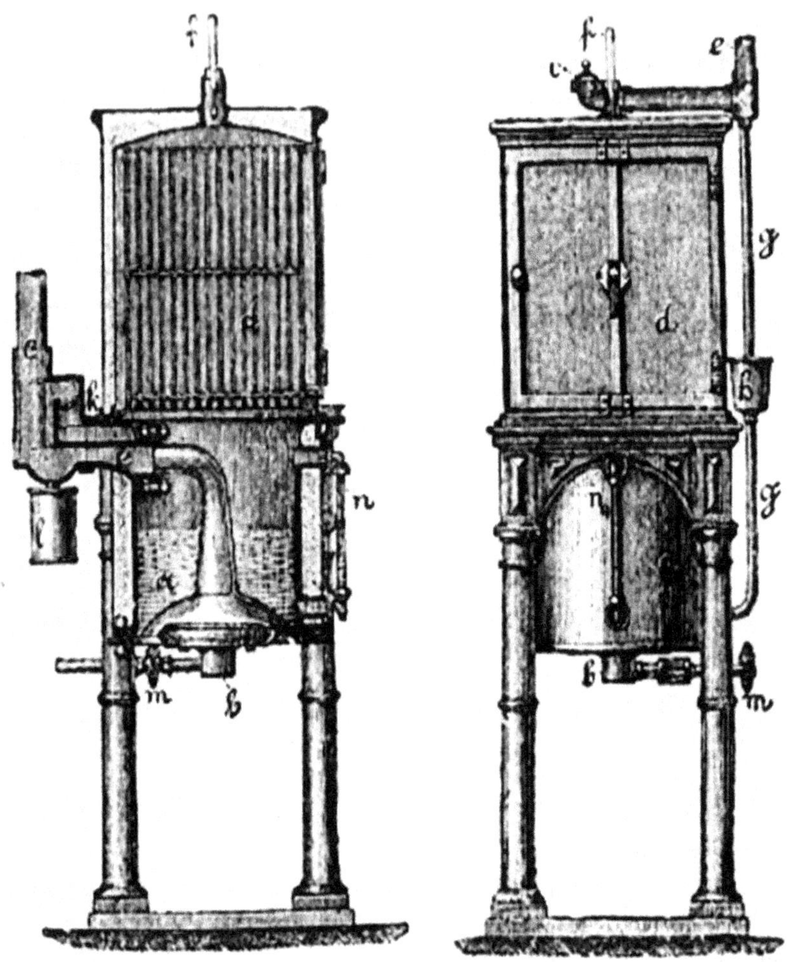

Fig. 23. Henneberg's disinfector. Jacques Borelius. "Om Hennebergs desinfektor för sterilsering af förbandsmaterial m. m.". *Hygiea.* Vol. 52, No. 9, September 1890, 677.

Keeping instruments clean according to aseptic principles was not entirely straightforward, as Swedish sources show. With antisepsis, it was easy for practitioners to know when something had been disinfected. The articles about the two disinfection apparatuses were only discussed for use on soft goods like linens and bandages, not for instruments. Furthermore, during Borelius' time observing Lister in London, he noted that the instrument handles in the theatre had shafts of wood, which meant that "disinfection in boiling water or with steam is not used–that is not possible anyway because the shafts, handles, etc., are wooden".[547] I mentioned in the previous chapter that Sabbatsberg Hospital's surgical instruments were altered after intra-peritoneal operations to assist cleaning by replacing ivory and wooden shafts with ones of iron.[548] Still another article, this one from 1895, mentioned trocar use for draining fluid in the lungs and how their construction could cause problems leading to infection, advocating for instruments of simpler construction, or even syringes, because they were easy to clean and sterilise according to aseptic praxis.[549] Schlich points out that the distinction might lie in a difference of condition and the ability to control it. Antisepsis predetermined that germs were present, and surgeons actively disinfected the object in question; asepsis stipulated the absence of germs altogether, which was more difficult to determine and control.[550]

Schlich's point about control is corroborated in other articles that indicate that asepsis and antisepsis were used fluidly in Sweden and Denmark. Swedish surgeon R. Wawrinsky remarked in *Hygiea* that "a single appropriate method for disinfection has still not been invented and in my opinion will probably never be invented. We must [...] learn to individualise and use different means in different cases".[551] And this was not just the case for devices and other objects used in surgery but could be medically necessary as well. An article from 1894 in *Ugeskrift* by Danish surgeon Oscar Bloch remarked that practitioners following aseptic methods could not avoid antiseptic solutions anyway. Bloch argued that in certain circumstances, such as with abscesses, rinsing with antiseptic solutions was a necessity.[552] One of his primary arguments for the continued use of antiseptic solutions was contact infections. Lister's method tackled this problem with the use of the carbolic acid spray, but this could be done with other chemical solutions like chloral water, carbolic acid, or sublimate.[553] Bloch highlighted that the insertion of

---

[547] Borelius, "Antiseptiken på Listers afdelning", 668. [Desinfektion i kokande vatten eller ånga användes ej–en sak, som för öfrigt ej låter sig göra, då skaft, handtag och dylikt äro af trä.]

[548] F. W. Warfvinge. *Årsberättelse från Sabbatsbergs sjukhus i Stockholm för 1884.* Stockholm, 1885, 116.

[549] Ivar Svensson, "Om punktion af pleuritiska exsudat". *Hygiea.* Vol. 57, No. 8, August 1895, 122–153, 138.

[550] Schlich, "Negotiating Technologies in Surgery", 183–184.

[551] Wawrinsky, "Om desinfektion", 828. [En för alla fall lika lämplig desinfektionsmetod är för öfrigt ännu icke uppfunnen och lärer enligt min åsigt heller aldrig blifva uppfunnen. Vi måste, såsom jag redan ofvan påpekat, lära oss at individualisera och att i olika fall slå in på olika vägar.]

[552] Oscar Bloch, "Smaanoter fra den kirurgiske Praksis". *Ugeskrift for Læger.* Series 5, Vol. 1, No. 50, 14 December 1894, 1175–1185, 1176.

[553] [Anon.], "Kontakt- og Luft-Infektion i den praktiske Kirurgi; Kümmel (Hamborg) (Beil. zum Centrabl. für Chirurgie 1885. Nr. 24. Meddelt paa den 14de tyske Kirurg-Kongres)". *Hospitals-Tidende.* Vol. 28, No. 29, 22 July 1885, 691–698, 693–694. The chemicals used were dependent on what was being

objects inside the patient during surgical procedures would put the patient at a higher risk of infection and that surgeons should be particularly mindful of this. However, he encouraged practitioners to proceed with caution, *nil nocere* [do no harm] was referred to not once, but twice, and argued for the continuing use of antiseptic chemicals in mitigating infection.[554] Under certain circumstances, like the above, the use of antisepsis and its reliability gave practitioners some measure of control over the procedure and its outcome. This illustrates that the fluid relationship between antisepsis and asepsis was enacted in different ways, depending on practical circumstances. Physicians knew they were eliminating germs by using them and maintained a degree of control over the process when using antiseptic methods.

Another example of difficulties with asepsis and control was the introduction of pre-packaged bandages that were marketed as sterile. In an article in *Ugeskrift*, Danish physician Oscar Hecksher questioned whether or not these bandages were sterile and if their sterility had a best-before date. He also took issue with poor packaging and poor labelling. The assurance that these items arrived well-packaged and sterile was especially advantageous for physicians in the countryside because few physicians had time to sterilise bandages themselves, according to Hecksher.[555] The two articles by Hecksher and Bloch highlight that physicians were still unsure of the sterility of objects not treated chemically, and that chemicals could serve as a practical guarantee for physicians in discerning an object's sterility. It was difficult to discern the quality of pre-packaged articles and they placed control outside of the physician's hands. The previous chapter illustrated that physicians often made antiseptic bandages and dressings themselves, which put them in control of the process. But the absence of germs was less apparent with asepsis or pre-packaged sterilised articles and gave them less control over the situation. The use of antiseptic and aseptic practices overlapped in their implementation at this time. These two methods were used fluidly so that physicians could maintain control over the quality of the objects used in practice and ensure that the materials they were using were free from contamination.

disinfected. Hands should be washed with a chemical soap and then treated with a chemical solution consisting of thymol, boric acid, salicylic acid or "sterilised water"; whereas the operation wound should be frequently irrigated with a sublimate solution. Instruments depended on their composition–materially as well as aesthetically–but the author recommended carbolic acid, sublimate or thymol solutions.

[554] Bloch, "Smaanoter", 1175–1185.

[555] Oscar Heckscher, "Om Mangler ved Indpakningen af sterile Forbindstoffer". *Hospitals-Tidende*. Vol. 38, No. 4, 23 January 1895, 113–115.

The Instrument Maker's Model Surgical Suite

The move to asepsis was a respatialisation of practice and an encouragement to think institutionally. The sterility of the surgical space would have been difficult to maintain outside institutional settings. For one, the apparatuses for disinfection highlighted above were expensive, required space, and were reliant on specific infrastructural technologies like boilers. Furthermore, surgical spaces necessitated other spatial concerns. For example, Kisacky highlights that American institutions during the dawn of asepsis in the 1890s started to include "complex spatial sequences" to ensure decontamination. This was not only respective to the decontamination of the operating room itself but of objects and people entering the sterilised space.[556] In other words, surgical spaces beyond the operating room functioned as a set of locks to guarantee decontamination upon arrival and were a means of controlling the conditions of the surgical space and its occupants.

This required thinking institutionally. This point is illustrated in an article from 1893 in *Hygiea*, by ophthalmologist Johan Widmark quoted the German ophthalmologist Julius Hirschberg. He quoted Hirschberg, stating that "an aseptic institution is better than an antiseptic method of wound management".[557] The two larger hospitals in Stockholm at the time followed the pavilion system, which included several separate ward buildings.[558] At one of them, Seraphim Hospital, after its renovation was completed in 1893, the surgical ward was connected to the main hospital building via a corridor. At the other, Sabbatsberg Hospital, which was completed in 1879, the surgical ward was a completely separate building. In terms of management, the surgical wards at both hospitals could be treated as enclosed entities. The pavilion system was one means of spatial control. By containing the operating facilities in specific spaces away from the wards, the surgical wards themselves might be able to better fulfil the statement Widmark quoted.

---

[556] Kisacky, *Rise of the Modern Hospital*, 141.

[557] Johan Widmark, "Om kokain och desinfektion af ögat vid starroperationer". *Hygiea*. Vol. 57, No. 9, September 1895, 189–239, 193. [»En aseptisk anstalt är bättre än en antiseptisk sårbehandling»]

[558] For more information on the development of the pavilion system see Kisacky, *Rise of the Modern Hospital*, 22–25. Kisacky highlights the pavilion system, hospital design and ventilation on pgs. 41–50. Wolfram Kock details the discussions about expansion of Seraphim Hospital, which include discussions about the housing of patients, ventilation and improving standards in order to raise the hospital's general standard. Wolfram Kock. *Kungl. Serafimerlasarettet, 1752–1952: En studie i svensk sjukvårdshistoria*. Jönköping: H. Halls Boktr. A.-B., 1952, 149–155. Kock also notes that in 1868, a committee for the renovation and expansion of Seraphim Hospital referred to the expansion of the pavilion system in Great Britain and in continental Europe, but that the city council in Stockholm preferred the older corridor system for financial reasons (139).

Control of the conditions of surgical spaces affected the number and types of surgical procedures that were carried out. Articles about novel surgeries appeared frequently in medical serials. For example, in *Hygiea*, at least 27 of the original articles published between 1890 and 1893 were specifically about novel surgeries. To give a better sense of the magnitude, approximately 26 original articles were published per volume, with one yearly volume published in 1890 and two per year in 1891–1893. This means that the number of articles on novel surgeries published over four years would fill a volume of *Hygiea* by themselves. Thomas Schlich highlights in his book on the development of organ transplantation that surgeons would rarely have left accounts of novel operations unpublished.[559] This means that the volume of these articles can be a good indicator of what kinds of procedures were being carried out, modified, and developed. In addition to this, reports detailing the numbers of surgeries undertaken at wards across the country were published in *Hygiea* throughout the period examined. These reports represented both larger hospitals as well as smaller ones, located in smaller centres in the countryside. Reports like these give a general overview of what kinds of surgeries and how many were performed in the country.[560]

By comparing similar articles from the 1880s about surgical procedures at Sabbatsberg Hospital in Stockholm, we can see that the amount and types of surgeries had changed significantly in just under a decade. For example, in 1881, 404 surgical procedures in total were performed at Sabbatsberg Hospital in Stockholm, with no specific mention of outpatient procedures.[561] This indicates that outpatient procedures may have been included in the total number of surgeries. Just eight years later, the same hospital accounted for 1059 operations, not including numbers for outpatient procedures in 1889.[562]

---

[559] Thomas Schlich. *The Origins of Organ Transplantation: Surgery and Laboratory Science, 1880–1930*. Rochester: Rochester University Press, 2010, 11.

[560] See for example W. Karström, "Kirurgisk kasuistik från Wexiö lasarett". *Hygiea*. Vol. 53, No. 3, March 1891, 243–276; Jules Åkerman, "Kirurgisk kasuistik från Malmöhus läns sjukvårdsinrättningar i Lund". *Hygiea*. Vol. 54, No. 10, October 1892, 299–325; Alrik Lindh, "Kirurgisk kasuistik från Sahlgrenska sjukhuset i Göteborg". *Hygiea*. Vol. 54, No. 11, November 1892, 410–419; Anders Hansson, "Kasuistik från Warbergs lasarett". *Hygiea*. Vol. 55, No. 4, April 1893, 402–406. For a historical overview and a closer look at the relationships between risk and suffering in nineteenth-century surgery, see Martin S. Pernick, "The Calculus of Suffering in Nineteenth-Century Surgery". *The Hastings Centre Report*. Vol. 13, No. 2, April 1983, 26–36.

[561] Ivar Svensson, "Operationer verkstälda å Sabbatsbergs sjukhus under år 1881". *Hygiea*. Vol. 44 No. 7, July 1882, 378–383, 382

[562] E. V. Bolinder, "Operationer verkstälda å Sabbatsberg sjukhus' kirurgiska afdelning under år 1889". *Hygiea*, Vol. 52, No. 6, June 1890, 409–417, 413. Mortality was 3.5%. Tracheotomies for croup and diphtheria not included in mortality statistics, 16 out of 31 of these cases were fatal; however, removing

According to these reports, both outpatient services, i.e., smaller, less invasive procedures, and invasive surgeries, such as ovariotomies, laparotomies, and hernia strangulation, increased. This is one indication of the intimate connections between technological and spatial changes in surgical practice. Kisacky also highlights this relationship, noting that outdated surgical facilities could limit the kinds of procedures carried out and that renovations, on the other hand, could encourage practitioners to undertake riskier surgeries.[563]

The change in space is significant in that it altered the possibility of disinfection techniques, which will be discussed in relation to Max Stille's model surgical suite. Different surgical spaces introduced measures that increased the surgeon's control over the spaces they operated in and placed stricter requirements on the hygiene of the occupants and objects in the space. Micheal Worboys highlights this element of control in cleaning practices, where "aseptic practitioners aimed to sterilise surgical instruments, ligatures, dressings, tables, floors and walls of the operating room, which was redesigned for the ease of disinfection, and to keep surgeons' hands and patients' tissues germ-free too".[564] Aseptic practice maintained a germ-free state. However, with antisepsis, germs were implied to occupy a given space and were subsequently removed by chemical means. The spatial conditions of cleanliness were not always easy to discern and to some degree depended on the materials and design in the space. Annemarie Adams also points to control in her study of architectural spaces for surgery through history, noting that design and material gave surgeons more control over the sensuous impressions in surgical space, but also gave surgeons an associated environment to exact control over.[565] Surgeons did not experience their

these statistics was likely due to disease mortality. See for example Thure Hellström, "Om diagnosticerandet af difteri". *Hygiea*. Vol. 58, No. 9, September 1895, 240–303. See also Gretchen A. Condran, "The Elusive Role of Scientific Medicine in Mortality Decline: Diphtheria in Nineteenth- and Early Twentieth-Century Philadelphia". *Journal of the History of Medicine and Allied Sciences*. Vol. 63, No. 4. October 2008, 484–522. Wolfram Kock also notes in his book *Kungliga Serafimerlassarettet 1752–1952* that the majority of operations through the 1870s were on the extremities, see page 186.

[563] Kisacky, *Rise of the Modern Hospital*, 144.

[564] Worboys, "The History of Surgical Wound Infection", 223.

[565] Annemarie Adams, "Surgery and Architecture: Spaces for Operating", in *The Palgrave Handbook of the History of Surgery*, Thomas Schlich (ed.), 261–281. London: Palgrave Macmillan, 2018, 277. Adams and Kisacky have pointed out that the construction of requisite spaces for surgical practice gave surgeons a domain of control and helped raise the status of the profession. See also Kisacky, *Rise of the Modern Hospital*, 142–144. Rosemary Wall and Christine Hallet also highlight the role of nursing in the professionalisation of surgery, where nurses played an essential role in upholding and maintaining surgical and post-operative environments, especially moving into the age of germ-free surgery. Rosemary Wall and Christine E. Hallet, "Nursing and Surgery: Professionalisation, Education and

increased control over space as entirely unproblematic, however, as it also entailed increased responsibility. Two articles that I mentioned in the previous chapter about the implementation of Listerism highlighted the increased burden on surgeons over correct procedures, even. This could divert their attention from the task at hand.[566] At the same time, the increased responsibility and control also gave way to the growing possibility for delegation, as these two articles also highlighted, with the presence of assistants in the room. This was particularly the case once surgeons, students, and nurses became more comfortable with the results and processes of certain procedures.[567] And, rather than stand for the cost of some of their associated devices, this shift necessitated institutional responsibility for furnishing and supplying surgeons with their associated tools.

In 1894, Max Stille opened a model-surgical suite in an older building used by the firm on the island-borough of Kungsholmen in Stockholm. Max had officially taken over the Stille business the previous year after his father Albert passed away but had already been involved in the firm's operations for several years. The intention of Stille's model suite was "to illustrate for those interested in the subject how Mr. Stille thought a surgical suite should be organised to correspond completely to the requirements that should be placed upon such an important part of larger healthcare facilities".[568] The last three words delineate who potential customers were. Stille's suite was not a projection intended for individual surgeons, even if they might have had a

Innovation", in *The Palgrave Handbook of the History of Surgery*, Thomas Schlich (ed.), 153–174. London: Palgrave Macmillan, 2018. For the role of institutions in professional development more broadly see Joseph F. Kett. *The Formation of the American Medical Profession: The Role of Institutions, 1780–1860*. New Haven: Yale University Press, 1968.

[566] W. Netzel, "Utdrag ur bref från Dr M. Salin". *Hygiea*. Vol. 41, No. 2, February 1879, 98–104; O. F. Hallin, "Om lasarettsväsendet i Sverige 1880". *Hygiea*. Vol. 43, No. 11, November 1881, 601–632; Valdemar Holmer, "Om Resektion af Knæleddet I kroniske Knæledssygdomme". *Hospitals-Tidende*. Vol. 15, No. 45, 6 November 1872, 177–179.

[567] Stephanie Snow looks briefly at delegation with respect to the growing familiarity with and safety of anaesthesia, moving through the nineteenth century. Stephanie J. Snow, "Surgery and Anaesthesia: Revolutions in Practice", in *The Palgrave Handbook of the History of Surgery*, Thomas Schlich (ed.), 195–214. London: Palgrave Macmillan, 2018. Researchers have also examined the history of surgical delegation within a legal framework of risk and negligence. See Claire Brock, "Risk, Responsibility and Surgery in the 1890s and Early 1900s". *Medical History*. Vol. 57, No. 3, 2013, 317–337; Torsten Riotte, "Medical Negligence in Nineteenth-Century Germany", in *Progress and Pathology: Medicine and Culture in the Nineteenth Century*, Melissa Dickson, et. al. (eds.), 56–77. Manchester: Manchester University Press, 2020.

[568] [Anon.], "En mönster-operationssal". [Afsigten dermed är att visa dem, som äro för sådana ämnen intresserade, huru hr Stille tänkt sig en operationssal skulle vara inrättad för att fullt motsvara de anspråk som böra ställas på en så ytterst vigtig del af större sjukvårdsanstalter.]

stake in swaying hospital administration.[569] It was intended for institution settings and buyers. Still, Stille's suite illustrated both his awareness of and interest in developments involving the use of devices they manufactured for their buyers. But his interest was also, naturally, commercial, and the suite served as a showroom for devices produced by his firm. Shortly after he opened his model suite in Stockholm, he was off to Rome for the Eleventh International Medical Congress where he also set up a similar suite with accompanying instruments.[570]

Stille's suite projected his vision of what a surgical suite should be, but also allegedly offered advantages for practitioners by improving some of the technical features of the space according to technological and medical developments in the period. In addition to this, it served as a showroom for the firm's instruments and other medical devices, which were displayed there. A newspaper article from 1894 about the suite describes it as follows:

> The suite is both unusually large and unusually bright [...] with daylight from above, by means of a roof lantern, as well as two large windows [...] The entire suite can be cleaned from top to bottom in just a few minutes. In this spacious suite, an exhibit of the kinds of devices and instruments that can be used in various kinds of operations are displayed.[571]

Newspaper articles do not provide much information about material choices Stille made in the construction of his model suite. However, the suite itself was near the surgical venues at Seraphim Hospital. The surgical pavilion at Seraphim Hospital was newly built, finished in 1893, and was on a street adjacent to Stille's exhibit. Seraphim Hospitial's surgical pavilion was separate from the hospital itself and included several smaller rooms for sterilisation, storage, etc., as well as one smaller surgical suite and a surgical amphitheatre that could seat one hundred people.[572] Because of the Stilles' long-

---

[569] Kisacky notes the importance of physician input in the planning involved in the aseptic design of the Lying-In Hospital in New York. See Kisacky, "Germs are in the Details", 88. Kisacky also discusses the relationships between hospital design and physician input in her book *Rise of the Modern Hospital*, where physicians were not always involved in the process, but that collaborative efforts between architects and physicians helped inform architects of practical requirements. Kisacky, *Rise of the Modern Hospital*, 102–104; 116; 176–177.

[570] [Anon.], "En mönster-operationssal".

[571] [Anon.], "En mönster-operationssal". [Salen är bade ovanligt stor och ovanligt ljus… får dager ovanifrån, genom en lanternin, och dessutom från två väldigt fönster… Hela salen renspolas från ofvan till nedan på ett par minuter. I denna rymliga sal är ordnad en utställning af allt hvad som i instrument- och redskapsväg gerna kan komma i fråga att användas vid utförande af olika slags operationer.]

[572] Kock, *Kungliga Serafimerlassarettet*, 214–5.

standing connections with the Karolinska Institute, also nearby at the time, some degree of mutual influence might be the case here.[573] At any rate, it was clear that Stille had some relation to both the challenges and requirements for modern surgical spaces. The suite allegedly tackled two significant practical problems, thorough cleaning and lighting. I will address these two challenges by relating them to Seraphim Hospital and more general developments in the construction of hospital facilities and surgical spaces during the 1880s and 1890s.

The newspaper quote above highlights that "the entire room can be cleaned from top to bottom in just a few minutes".[574] The ease of cleaning the space quickly would have been a hygienic advantage for surgical procedures, in particular aseptic ones. But, it would also have ensured the suite could be used with little downtime. Although the article does not mention the suite's material composition, an illustration of the suite, pictured in figure 24, gives us some clues. One feature visible in figure 24 is the tiled or terrazzo floor. Tiled or terrazzo floors over other materials like wood would have offered natural advantages. Problems cleaning the untreated wood floors at Seraphim Hospital had been noted as far back as the 1830s. After scrubbing the floors, the water seeped under the deafening boards and increased the room's humidity. The floorboards were later painted to mitigate the problem.[575] Before the construction of the hospital's surgical pavilion, the surgical facilities were in an attic without proper lighting, drainage, or water. The operating table was a whitewashed wooden table with leather cushions.[576] By the 1890s, wood had been increasingly replaced with materials like terrazzo or tile. Kisacky notes that while wood was previously the most common material in hospital interiors, its porosity, even if varnished and sealed, was increasingly understood as a receptacle for germs.[577] Based on this, the image of the suite in figure 24 likely has few wooden features in its furnishings or overall details.

---

[573] I have not examined archival documents pertaining to the construction of the new surgical pavilion at the hospital. Although there was a degree of collaboration and exchange between Stille and physicians, there is no direct indication of collaboration with the architect behind the hospital expansion, Axel Kumlien, architect for the National Board of Health (*Medicinalstyrelsen*). Nor was Stille's model suite solely an architectural endeavour.

[574] [Anon.], "En mönster-operationssal". [hela salen renspolas från ofvan till neden på ett par minuter.]

[575] Kock, *Kungliga Serafimerlasarettet*, 125.

[576] John Berg. *Några synpunkter på antiseptikens genombrottstid av den som upplevat den: Föredrag i Svenska läkarsällskapet 17 mars 1931*. Off-print, *Hygiea*, Vol. 93. Stockholm, 1931.

[577] Kisacky, "Germs are in the Details", 90.

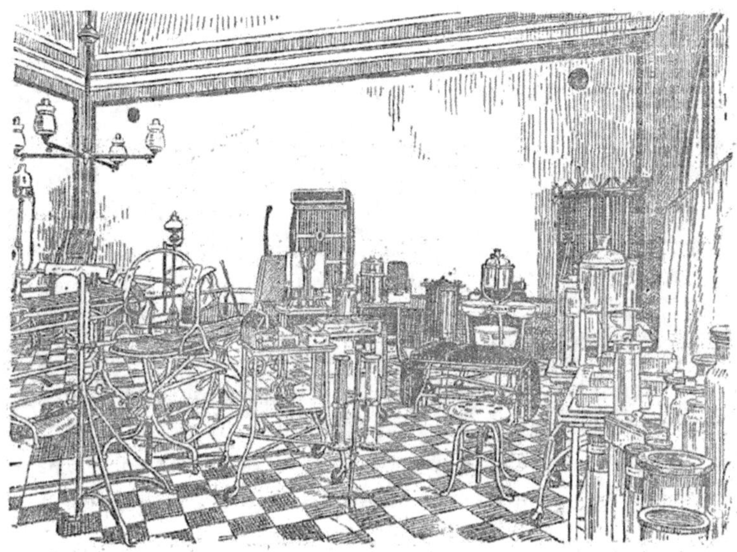

Fig. 24. Stille's display room/model suite. In this image, it looks more like a display room than a model suite. The illustration is dated nine years after the room first opened. In which case, the purpose of the room might have shifted over nearly a decade. [Anon.], "Bilder från svenskt industri- och näringslif. Alb. Stilles kirurgiska instrumentfabrik". *Aftonbladet*. 21 February 1903.

The material considerations to accommodate the thorough cleaning of hospital spaces changed by the 1890s. An article by Ivar Svensson in *Hygiea* from 1895 detailed one of these methods of cleaning. In this disinfection procedure for a room, he recommended the "removal [of] all soft and dust-collecting furniture in the thereafter close space, boil water in large, open vessels so that not only the air is overwhelmed with humidity, but that the intense steam completely soaks even the [remaining] furniture, the walls, the floors, and the ceiling".[578] The type of treatment suggested by Svensson would have required special spatial and material accommodations to be carried out frequently. If this procedure was to be performed routinely, the removal of specific furniture items might eventually be deemed superfluous. Instead, they would be replaced with furnishing that could stay in the room during treatment. Furthermore, Svensson's method was to ensure the room's air was "free from microorganisms" in particular, not necessarily the surfaces of the

---

[578] Svensson, "Om punktion af pleuritiska exsudat", 140. [utflytta alla mjuka och dammande möbler, i den derefter afstängda lokalen koka vatten i stora öppna kärl så länge, att icke blott luften blir öfvermättad med fuktighet, utan äfven genom den rikliga ångbildningen möbler, väggar, golf och tak blifva helt våta]

space.[579] However, Kisacky points out similar procedures were used in Austria and the United States to clean the room itself, including its surfaces, and not just the air in it.[580] Svensson's focus on air might be a miasmatic hold-over and a means to explain the complex relationship between spatial features, infection, and hospital hygiene practices. The surgical procedure he is describing in the article involves the insertion of an instrument into the pleural cavity in order to drain fluid from the lungs that could have been caused by an infection (exudative pleural effussions). In this procedure, the patient would have likely already been septic. Surgeons would have had to be particularly cautious when caring for septic patients, for the sake of the patient and themselves. Furthermore, the treatment of septic patients would have required additional disinfection procedures in the surgical or hospital space, in particular afterwards. Even if, by 1895, physicians might have better understood bacteriology and methods to reduce the spread of infection, "bad air" might still have been a means of rationalising the process.[581]

Given that Stille's model suite could be cleaned in just a few minutes, the materials used were no doubt more impermeable than wood, which might explain the higher cost and the interest. The process described by Ivar Svensson above would have taken a significant amount of time and labour, which Svensson noted himself. He stated that "the more time a room treated in such a way is closed, the closer it is to being absolutely free from micro-organisms".[582] But, soft and dust-collecting furnishings also had to be removed from the room prior to treatment, and presumably returned after-wards. Stille's suite, on the other hand, might have had a sloping floor for drainage and materials and furnishings that could withstand water, like the floor that appears to be tiled and the smooth, simple furnishings pictured in figure 24. If the suite could be cleaned so quickly, it was likely because it could be hosed down. Kisacky describes an American gynaecological suite that could be cleaned in a similar fashion, and that being able to hose down the room was a relatively common feature in the 1890s.[583] Seraphim Hospital's new surgical pavilion also employed the same method of hosing down the

---

[579] Svensson, "Om punktion af pleuritiska exsudat", 140. [fri från mikroorganismer]

[580] Kisacky, *Rise of the Modern Hospital*, 139.

[581] Ulrika Graninger notes something similar, stating that physicians still had on their "miasma glasses" [*miasmatiska glasögon*] even after bacteriology was generally accepted by Swedish physicians. See Graninger, *Från osynligt till synligt*, 230.

[582] Svensson, "Om punktion af pleuritiska exsudat", 140. [Ju flera timmar ett så behandlat rums luft får vara i hvila, desto närmare är den absolut fri från mikroorganismer]

[583] Kisacky, *Rise of the Modern Hospital*, 139.

rooms following surgical procedures.[584] Certainly, this would offer adventages over the process described by Svensson, which would require the space to be closed for some time to ensure thorough treatment. This would drastically limit the room's use. For the sake of comparison, after its expansion, Seraphim Hospital had just two operating rooms in its surgical pavilion.[585] Closing one for an extended amount of time following every surgical procedure would be costly and reduce the number of surgical procedures that could be performed.

An additional feature that Stille's model suite addressed was lighting. Given the daylight hours and weather during winter in the Nordic countries, keeping spaces well-lit would have been a challenge; something that I have already acknowledged in the second chapter regarding examinations with lensed instruments. The article about the suite mentioned a roof lantern and the unusual nature of the suite in terms of how well-lit it was.[586] This would have given the suite a daylighting feature. It would have also cast fewer shadows on the bodies of patients: something advantageous for surgical procedures. Figure 24 also includes a large window on the right of the image, which would have given additional light. Thomas Schlich points out that lighting conditions were one of the practical reasons why surgery was relocated to a specific space in the first place, as a favourable, and hopefully well-lit, visual field was important to surgeons.[587] As I have already noted, the growing number of surgical procedures performed–many of them complex–moving through the 1890s would have made well-lit spaces all the more important. Like Stille's space, Seraphim Hospital's surgical amphitheatre also boasted a roof lantern and large windows to let in light.[588] This was not new, though. Different means of mitigating lighting issues are a historical feature of medical spaces. For example, the anatomical theatre at Uppsala University, which was completed in 1663, was built as a cupola, with windows around the perimeter so that the room was as well-lit as possible.[589]

---

[584] Kock, *Kungliga Serafimerlasarettet*, 215.

[585] Ibid., 214–215.

[586] [Anon.], "En mönster-operationssal".

[587] Schlich, "Surgery, Science and Modernity", 236.

[588] Kock, *Kungliga Serafimerlasarettet*, 215.

[589] Hjördis Kristenson's doctoral thesis examines scientific buildings during the nineteenth century and connects the anatomical theatre with developments in surgical amphitheatres during the eighteenth and nineteenth centuries. Kristenson relates the construction of new amphitheatres by surgical societies such as the *École de Chirurgie* in Paris as monuments in the service of science. These new amphitheatres bore similiarites to the anatomical ones of the sixteenth and seventeenth centuries. See Hjördis Kristenson. *Veteskapens byggnader under 1800-talet: Lund och Europa*. Stockholm: The Swedish Museum of Architecture, 1990, 37–76.

However, Stille's room differed significantly from amphitheatre-style surgical spaces. As figure 24 illustrates, Stille's model suite had no tiered seating sloping toward the surgeon and their team at centre stage. That does not mean that spectators were impermissible in similar spaces, only that other arrangements might have been made to accommodate them. Though Stille's suite looks cramped and devoid of wall space that might accommodate viewers, it was also a showcase for his firm's instruments, so it likely is not a completely accurate representation of a functional surgical suite furnished by Stille. Rather, it served as a suggestive image of what one could look like according to different alternatives and/or needs. Adams states that seating still could be and was arranged in similar suites, around the outside of the room, and some even offered viewing galleries.[590] Stille's suite might not have been designed with spectators in mind, either. Seraphim Hospital's new surgical pavilion included two rooms: one designed for spectators with seating and a smaller room without seating. Kisacky notes that some surgeons in the same period banished spectators from their smaller operating rooms and that, at any rate, crowds had dwindled by the turn of the century.[591]

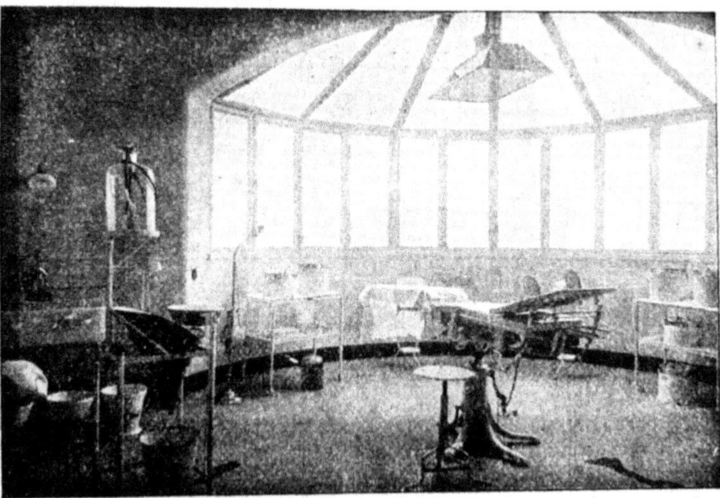

Fig. 25. An image of a surgical suite at a Danish hospital furnished by Camillus Nyrop's Establishment that illustrates the lighting of these facilities better, with large windows providing natural light. No year is provided, but the image is likely from around 1910. Camillus Nyrops etablissement. *Illustreret Katalog.* Copenhagen: Nielsen & Lydiche, [n.d.], vi.

---

[590] Adams, "Surgery and Architecture", 270.
[591] Kisacky, *Rise of the Modern Hospital*, 142.

Stille's suite implemented architectural techniques to maximise advantageous lighting conditions for surgeons to practice and removed the spectacle that surgical amphitheatres such as the amphitheatre in Uppsala, the newly built surgical amphitheatre at Seraphim Hospital a short distance away and similar spaces offered. Adams points to general trends in hospital architecture during the late nineteenth and early twentieth centuries that premiers the closed-off, contained, and highly defined space with a specific purpose in hospital architecture.[592] Stille's model suite is an example of this, but Seraphim's newly built amphitheatre seemed to follow the older style, perhaps due to the hospital's relationship with the education of physicians at the medical school at Karolinska Institute. This would have necessitated seating and a proper visual field for the instruction of students. Stille's suite might also represent a different style of hospital facility. Kisacky highlights a difference between American and European approaches in hospital design in the 1880s and 1890s. She states that European architects worked with an already-established framework of public building types, using the example of poor houses and orphanages. American architects, on the other hand, worked directly with medical professionals in making their requirements a reality.[593] In this sense, Stille's model-suite follows the latter tendency in being closely connected with the needs of practitioners.

At any rate, Stille was selling a concept. And the concept sold: Stille was commissioned to furnish operating suites in St. Petersburg in 1903, nine years following the initial opening of his model suite.[594] One of these suites was at a gynaecological clinic with an order amounting to over 100 000 kronor, "even though his offer was 30 000 kronor higher than the other proposals".[595] This was a significant amount of money. For the sake of comparison, the total salary costs for physicians, officials, a priest, and a caretaker at Seraphim Hospital in 1894 was 15 150kr.[596] In addition to St. Petersburg, an article from 1903 in the Swedish newspaper *Aftonbladet* that profiled Stille's business remarked that Stille sold packaged solutions for

---

[592] Adams, "Surgery and Architecture", 274.

[593] Kisacky, *Rise of the Modern Hospital*, 116,

[594] [Anon.], "I förbifarten". *Stockholmstidningen*, 17 January 1903. See also, [Anon], "Ryskt uppdrag åt svensk". *Sydsvenska dagbladet*. 18 January 1903.

[595] [Anon.], "Bilder från svenskt industri- och näringslif. Alb. Stilles kirurgiska instrumentfabrik". *Aftonbladet*. 21 February 1903. [trots at hans anbud med cirka 30,000 kr. öfversted de andra kostnadsförslagen.]

[596] SE/RA/42025 Riksarkivet, Serafimerlasarettet, B 4 A 1: Ekonomiska berättelser 1852–1938.

operating suites to northern and southern Germany and Switzerland.[597] These solutions were markedly for institutions and not individuals.

Adams states that physicians, in designing and modifying surgical spaces, showed "considerable architectural sophistication".[598] This could be said for Stille as well. Though his suite was a model one, perhaps not ready-to-go and functional as is, it was still more than just a showroom. Rather, it was his projection of what a model space for surgical procedures might look like. Stille's suite was both a physical manifestation of the needs of practitioners and his ideas in tandem with the changing demands of the industry producing furnishing for medical facilities and instruments. Instruments required less personal attention from instrument makers, could be machine forged and were easier to produce *en masse*. Mechanisation in the 1890s began replacing some steps in the manufacturing process, though finishing work was still often done by hand. Furthermore, the growth of the mass production of surgical instruments in Germany refocused some of the cross-border trade of instruments, where they could increasingly be sold by wholesalers abroad and were economical alternatives.[599] However, Stille offered an alternative to this mass production, as devices from his firm were still handmade.[600] The following section will look more closely at one of them–namely, his operating and examination tables.

Operating Tables and Aseptic Standards

Jeanne Kisacky highlights that while rounded corners in operating rooms had long-been standards in hospital settings, asepsis and germ theory strengthened these standards.[601] Although she is speaking primarily about the architectural qualities of surgical spaces, this standard can be seen in furnishings

---

[597] [Anon.], "Bilder från svenskt industri- och näringslif".

[598] Adams, "Surgery and Architecture", 271.

[599] James Edmonson. *American Surgical Instruments: An Illustrated History of Their Manufacture and a Directory of Instrument Makers to 1900*. San Francisco: Norman Publishing, 1997, 135-6. Though Edmonson does not make specific mention of Sweden or Denmark, due to the American focus of his book, other sources lift the purchase of prefabricated instruments from Germany by both Stille and Ch. O. Werner, like in a report for the National Institute for Working Life [*Arbetslivscentrum*] (pg. 35). A catalogue from Camillus Nyrop's Establishment also mentions this problem in its short preface. See Peter Gullers. *Verktygsmakare & operatörer: Några aspekter på den kirurgiska instrumenttillverknings svenska historia*. Report 37. Stockholm: Arbetslivscentrum, 1982; and Camillus Nyrops Etablissement. *Illustreret Catalog*. Copenhagen: Nielsen & Lydiche, [n.d.], xiii.

[600] According to a catalogue from Camillus Nyrop's Establishment, probably from the first decade of 1900, instruments from this workshop were handmade as well. The page the citation is on is not paginated. Camillus Nyrops Etablissement. *Illustreret Catalog*.

[601] Kisacky, *Rise of the Modern Hospital*, 120.

as well. Part of Stille's draw could have been that his furnishings for surgical spaces were "as far as the eye could discern, put together with rounded joints so that they were easy to clean and devoid of dirt traps".[602] Looking at figures 24 and 25, one can see the clean, rounded edges of the furnishings, mostly devoid of ornamentation. Except for a few, smooth cushions on gurneys and a chair, there are no soft-looking objects in the room. A stark contrast to the image in figure 22, which depicts a minor surgical procedure. One of the features of Stille's surgical suite was the different beds for patients that were on display. These included his patented and award-winning operating table, a stretcher that could be transported on rails, and a sickbed that could be placed on wheels.[603] Stille's tables were a fixture in his model surgical suite, presented as an innovation in the press, and in an article that he penned in *Hygiea*.[604]

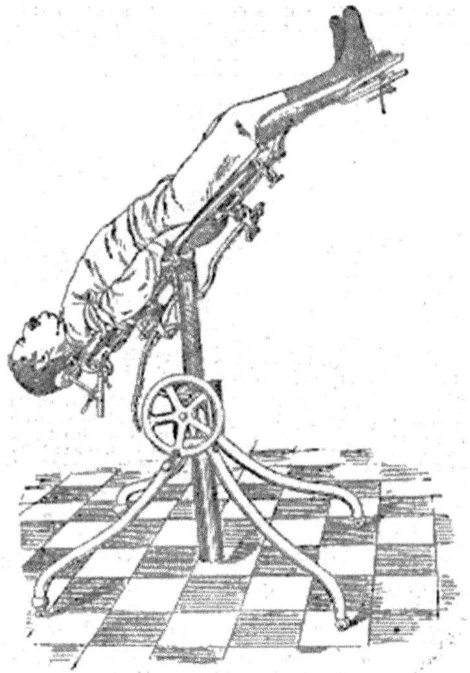

Fig. 26. One of Stille's operating tables. [Anon.], "Bilder från svenskt industri- och näringslif. Alb. Stilles kirurgiska instrumentfabrik". Aftonbladet. 21 February 1903.

---

[602] [Anon.], "Bilder från svenskt industri- och näringslif".
[603] [Anon.], "En mönster-operationssal".
[604] [Anon.], "Erkännande från Amerika åt svensk industri"; [Anon.], "Stilles operationssal vid läkarkongressen i Rom".

One reason behind the popularity of Stille's beds and tables might have been their relationship with practical demands. Much like the operating theatre, Stille's tables were often described in terms of practicality. The relationship to practical problems, or highlighting practicalities, was noted in its descriptions. In one of the Swedish Society of Medicine's meetings in 1894, it was described as follows:

> Mr. Stille exhibited an examination table constructed by his workshop, to be used in the physician's examination room. The apparatus, using a lever, can be raised to 90 cm in height and lowered to 60 cm. The bed consists of four connected parts, where both the outer [parts] can be folded down. The apparatus then takes up a mere 105 cm; by drawing up the gables, it is 196 cm in length. Both middle parts can also be raised and lowered separately. The apparatus is therefore useful as both an examination table as well as a massage table and can even function as a gynaecological operating table by using the corresponding stirrups. Covered in strong gutta-percha, its price is 200kr.[605]

The table was not only multi-purpose, even superseding general and gynaecological examinations: it could also be used for massage. Moreover, it could be made more compact if desired, but long enough to reasonably accommodate most patients. The apparatus to raise and lower the gurney would have likely made the device more comfortable for the practitioner to use, and the devices to raise and lower the outer connected parts probably made it more comfortable for the patient.

With the length and complexity of surgical procedures growing and a bevy of tools to assist in examinations–like the ones studied in the second chapter– the length of these procedures was increasing.[606] In which case, a device to serve the comfort of both practitioners and patients might mitigate at least one problem: comfort. Though it is difficult to ascertain whether this specific table and its accompanying devices were patented conclusively, Stille took several patents with similar descriptions. Stille's tables were new in terms of their material composition, design, and construction. These factors com-

---

[605] *Förhandlingar vid Svenska läkarsällskapets sammankomster*, 11 December 1894. [Hr STILLE förevisade en å hans verkstad förfärdigad *undersökningsbädd*, afsedd att begagnas i läkarens mottagningsrum. Apparaten kan medelst en häfstång höjas till 90 cm:s höjd och sänkas till 60 cm. Sjelfva bädden består af 4 st. sammanhängande delar, hvaraf de båda yttersta kunna nedfällas. Apparaten upptar då en längd af endast 105 cm; genom gaflarnes uppfällande blir densamma 196cm. i längd. De båda midteldelarne kunna äfven hvar för sig höjas och sänkas. Apparaten lämpar sig således såväl till undersöknings- som massagebädd och kan äfven genom användande af dithörande fotstöd användas såsom gynekologiskt operationsbord. Dess pris är, klädd med starkt guttaperkatyg, kr. 200.]
[606] See Chapter 2.

bined meant his tables could fit in better in an aseptic surgical suite, compared to some of the alternatives. Furthermore, while they were praised in newspapers and presented by Stille, there was merit to both the praise and Stille's zeal in presenting them. To properly ascertain the innovation of Stille's table, I will relate it to some of the other alternatives that were marketed in Sweden and Denmark in the latter half of the nineteenth century.

Camillus Nyrop's book *Bandager og Instrumenter*, from 1864, offers a look at three alternatives, pictured below in figures 27, 28 and 29. All three would have been familiar to contemporaries, including Stille. The chair in figure 27 would have been used for procedures on the head, throat and chest, according to Nyrop. It was constructed in a way that would mitigate "the operator and his assistants working from an extremely stooped position", which would have been the case had the patient been positioned in an unadjustable bed.[607] The chair also included leather straps to restrain "unruly" patients, which would have been useful for procedures without anaesthesia. It also had leather supports and cushions to support the patient's head, and accommodate for "shorter people and children".[608] Patients could also be transported lying down in the chair by adjusting the foot support. Much like Stille's table, the chair was adjustable to some degree and could suit a variety of different patients. It was designed for procedures involving the head, throat, and chest, so its use might have been limited to these.

Nyrop offered another example, this time a mechanical sick bed from Belgium with adjustable supports to position the patient according to need in fourteen different positions, see figure 28. Nyrop added that the cog apparatus added an extra measure of safety as the original Belgian apparatus consisted of just ropes and cords. This modification was made by another Danish bandagist, and Nyrop noted that he had made some additional modifications himself, though he does not mention exactly what.[609] The next bed in figure 29 was labelled as a "fracture bed". It included special foot supports to assist with wound care and immobilisation, but Nyrop also noted that it was modelled after a "general surgical bed".[610] The bed, however, was equipped with two lower "legs" at the foot end, designed for the patient's legs.

---

[607] Camillus Nyrop. *Bandager og Instrumenter afbildede og beskrevne med en tilføi et Prisfortegnelse.* Copenhagen: G.E.C. Gad, 1864, 218. [en almindelig Seng ved sin Brede alltid foraarsager ved at tvinge Operateuren og hans Medhjælpere til at intage en meget bøiet Stilling]

[608] Nyrop, *Bandager og Instrumenter*, 219. [Læderpude… kan anbriges paa Sædet, for at mindre Folk og Børn kunne kommet il at naae op til den tidligere omtalte Hovedpude.]

[609] Ibid., 179.

[610] Ibid., 221. [Sengen er en almindelig saa kaldet chirurgisk Seng]

These "legs" could be moved apart with a slat that could be opened, which made tending to the injured leg easier for the attendant or medic.[611]

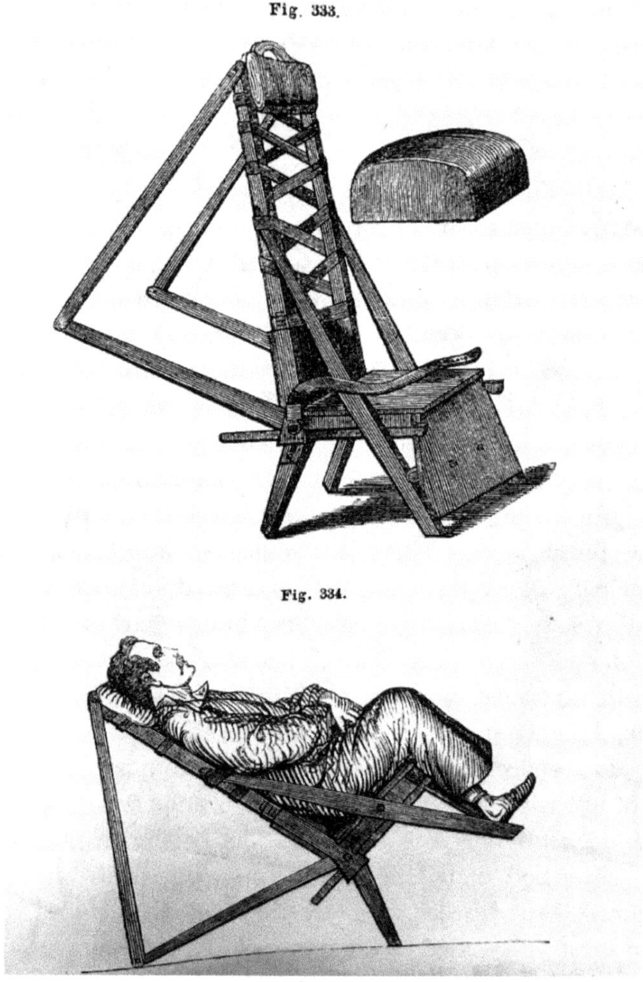

Fig. 27. "Jäger's operating chair" [Jägers Operationsstol] from Camillus Nyrop. Bandager og Instrumenter afbildede og beskrevne med en tilføi et Prisfortegnelse. Copenhagen: G.E.C. Gad, 1864, 219.

Materially speaking, all three alternatives were made primarily of wood and the chair included leather straps. This would have had some limitations. They

___

[611] Ibid., 222.

would have been difficult to clean, in accordance with asepsis. The fracture bed would fit nicely in the room pictured in figure 22; however, the design would have been out of place in Stille's model suite in figure 24, even if the fracture bed was modelled after a surgical table. The lack of rounded corners on all three would not have as easily accommodated cleaning as Stille's table in figure 26. The joints on all three could be receptacles for germs and difficult to keep clean. The chair, with its system of restraints, probably predated the prevalence of anaesthesia, where restraining patients would have been a necessity. By the time Stille's table was constructed, practitioners were comfortable with anaesthesia in surgical settings, and its use was comparatively safe.[612] Furthermore, all three were only adjustable to a degree, and longer procedures or examinations would have put the physician and/or patient in an awkward position, if they were intended for longer procedures at all. The former two examples were designed more for convalescence. Nyrop's devices served different purposes and were from a different era with different needs.

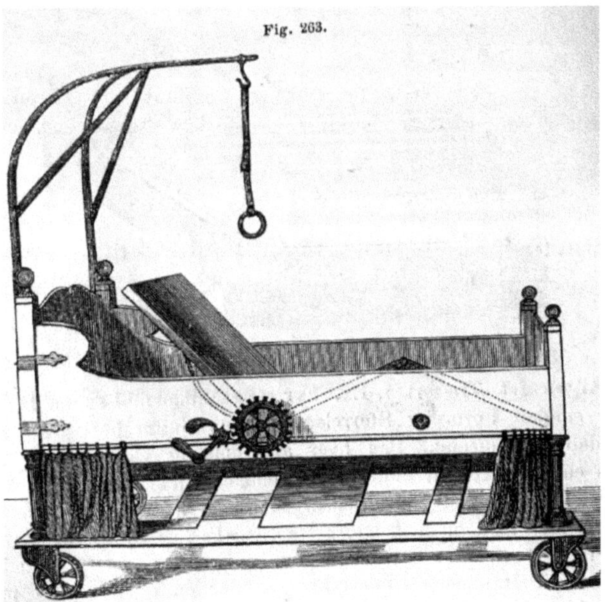

Fig. 28. "Mechanical sick bed" Camillus Nyrop. *Bandager og Instrumenter afbildede og beskrevne med en tilføi et Prisfortegnelse.* Copenhagen: G.E.C. Gad, 1864, 178.

---

[612] Stephanie Snow highlights that the reliability of anaesthesia toward the turn of the century meant lead to an increased number of surgical procedures on a wider variety of patient groups and that the obstruction of pain with its use eliminated one of the more significant surgical risks. Snow, "Surgery and Anaesthesia", 205.

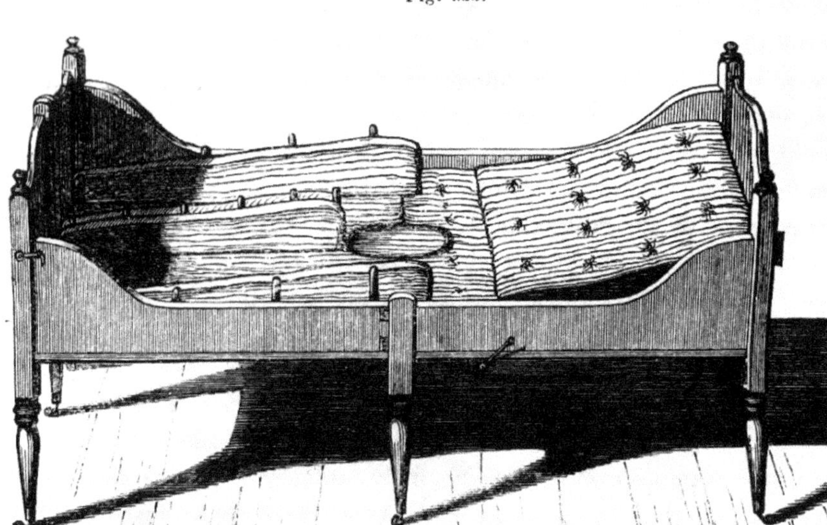

Fig. 29. "Stein's fracture bed" [Steins Fracturseng], Camillus Nyrop, Bandager og Instrumenter afbildede og beskrevne med en tilføi et Prisfortegnelse. Copenhagen: G.E.C. Gad, 1864, 220.

Nyrop's beds were from the 1860s, and by the 1890s they were outdated. By this time, physicians had taken to the challenge of tackling some of the problems that Nyrop had highlighted in his presentation of the chair and the two beds. In 1890, Swedish physician Carolina Widerström noted in the Society of Medicine's meeting minutes that she had "let gymnastics carpenter Ekstrand construct a slab as large as the operating table's that could be screwed together [...] Another slab was placed on top of this one [...] This moveable piece can be raised and lowered with support from the same apparatus as our normal gymnastic plinths".[613] Another physician, S. Lindström, explained the benefits of a customisable upholstered "bed" for examinations in an article from 1894. The bed could be raised and lowered, rotated and installed in different positions, see figure 30. Lindström also acknowledged that he constructed it after recognising there was a demand

---

[613] *Förhandlingar vid Svenska läkarsällskapets sammankomster*, 11 March 1890. [Jag lät derför gymnastiksnickaren Ekstrand härstädes göra en skifva, lika stor med operationsbordets, hvarå den fastskrufvas... Ofvanpå denna skifva ligger en annan... Denna ställbara del höjes och sänkes med stöd af samma apparat som våra vanliga gymnastikplintar]

for something similar. The advantages of this "bed" were that the physician could easily change its position according to need, and that it served the comfort of both patient and doctor. Importantly, it differed from "a normal [examination table] that admittedly works according to intention but instead has the inconvenience of seeming repulsive and frightening for patients".[614] He noted specifically that it was designed to be used in circumstances where the physician did not need to be meticulous concerning "antisepsis".[615] This bed would have fit in well amongst the décor in figure 22.

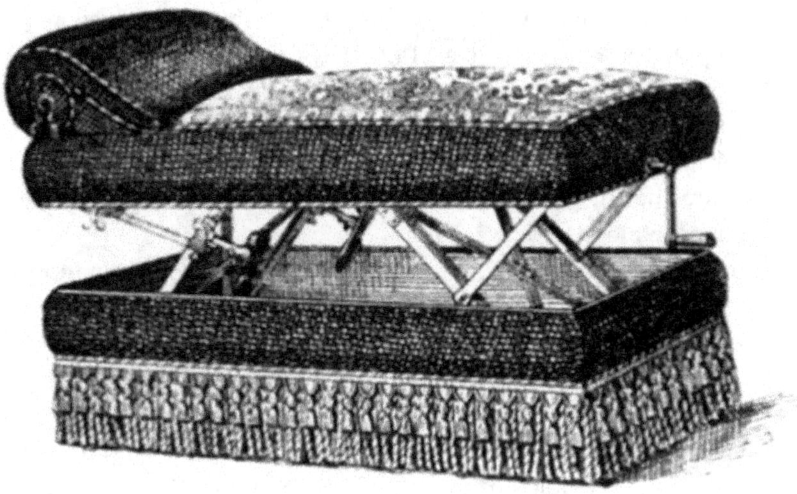

Fig. 30. Lindström's bed. S. Lindström, "En ny medicinsk möbel". *Hygiea*. Vol. 56, No. 4, April 1894: 364–366, 364.

These five pieces of medical furniture are examples of how problems, perceived or otherwise, were tackled practically, from the standards and professional conditions of the era they were constructed in. They all assisted in situating the physician and patient in more comfortable positions. They accounted for the sensibilities of patients. As Lindström remarked, patients might be disturbed by the clean lines and stripped-down aesthetic of a normal examination table, like the one in figure 30. His, on the other hand, looked more like a sofa than an examination table and might have better suited a

---

[614] S. Lindström, "En ny medicinsk möbel". *Hygiea*. Vol. 56, No. 4, April 1894, 364–366, 364. [ett vanligt bord, som visserligen fyller ändamålet, men i stället har den olägenheten att verka frånstötande och afskräckande på patienterna]
[615] Lindström, "En ny medicinks möbel", 365.

private practice, where a homelier atmosphere prevailed into the twentieth century.[616] As the above cases highlight, there were multiple ways of handling technological problems, some of which physicians were tasked to resolve themselves. Stille's tables follow this trend and he was quick to tie them to practical demands in literature where they were presented to physicians.

The table was legitimised professionally by underlining encouragement from patrons and the most likely professional group to be interested in them: physicians. Stille did not presume that the table served specific needs, rather he was encouraged by his target audience: those actually using the tables. Another table from Stille's workshop, this one heatable, offered yet another example of practical emphasis. In an 1897 article in *Hygiea*, Stille underlined several important features. One of these features was that "the upper part of the table is adjustable according to need and can therefore be used as head support, or in the lowered position, can serve as support for the shoulders. This apparatus has the additional advantage of not drenching the patient's neck and head in blood and lavage fluid". [617]

Covering the patient in blood and lavage fluid during an operation was certainly impractical, both for the practitioner and patient, but the gurney offered additional advantages as well. It was portable, required less space than other tables, could be screwed to the floor for stability, and could "be positioned in all the positions one wishes [and] the stirrups are even of a new design and positioned so that they cannot lead to compression of the blood vessels in the knees or folds of the groin".[618] These functions served practitioners, but also patients. I have mentioned previously that the nature of operations changed throughout the latter part of the nineteenth century and one key change was the increasing length of procedures. As such, the long-term positioning of patients in ways that could have detrimental effects worked against practical considerations. The new functions of the table Stille presented were likely because of "encouragement from several operators", as

---

[616] See for example Karin Johannisson, "Kliniken: medicinens praktik", in *Medicinen blir till vetenskap: Karolinska Institutet under två århundraden*, Karin Johannisson, Ingemar Nilsson and Roger Qvarsell (eds.), 43–83. Stockholm: Karolinska Institutet University Press, 2010; Christopher Crenner. *Private Practice: In the Early Twentieth-Century Medical Office of Dr. Richard Cabot*. Balitmore: Johns Hopkins University Press, 2005.

[617] Max Stille, "Operationsbord för laparotomier och gynekologiska operationer". *Hygiea*. Vol. 59, No. 2, February 1897, 289–290, 290. [Den öfre delen af plattan är ställbar efter behag och kan således lämpas såsom hufvudgärd samt tjena till stöd för axlarne vid det sänkta läget. Genom denna anordning vinnes äfven att patientens hals och hufvud ej nedsölas af blod och sköljvätska.]

[618] Stille, "Operationsbord", 290. [kan detta bord ställas i alla önskade lägen, benhållarne härtill äro äfven af ny konstruktion och så inrättade, att desamma ej förorsaka någon hoptryckning af blodkärlen i knä- eller ljumskvecken.]

the heatable element was.[619] By this time, Stille-made surgical tables, going by the positive Swedish press, would have sold tables in Europe, the Middle East and North America, and, given the contact the firm's father and son proprietors had with physicians throughout the latter half of the nineteenth century, they were presumably open for suggestions from their patrons.

The newspaper article from 1903 in *Aftonbladet* about Stille's firm also discussed Stille's operating tables. It mentioned that his firm manufactured and sold several different models–from simpler varieties to more complicated tables–with varying price tags. The most expensive was the one pictured in figure 26, which was Stille's "newest and most advanced [...] constructed together by Professor Schuchard [sic] in Stettin and manufacturer Stille".[620] I have mentioned the Stilles' contact with Swedish physicians several times in previous chapters; however, Max Stille's work with Karl August Schuchardt, a German surgeon and gynaecologist based in Stettin, now Szczecin, also indicates that he worked with foreign physicians as well, highlighting the reach and scope of his instruments. The article remarked that in addition to his work with Schuchardt, his tables were sold widely outside of Sweden, and it also gives clues to who was purchasing them.

Regarding Stille-Schuchardt table, the article noted that "there are not many Swedish surgeons who consider themselves able to afford it [Stille's table]".[621] That table in particular would set the buyer back 1200 kronor and, according to the article, Stille's cheapest alternative was still 500 kronor.[622] The article noted that this was significantly more expensive than the most expensive German-made alternative, which cost just 175 kronor.[623] To compare the cost with the aforementioned furniture made or commissioned by Lindström and Nyrop, there was a significant difference in price between Stille's furniture and theirs. Lindström's bed cost 180 kronor, though the price could vary depending on upholstery choice and footrest–it was 130 kronor if the buyer chose a model without a footrest.[624] The mechanical sick bed pictured in Nyrop's *Bandager og Instrumenter* (figure 28) cost 350 Danish rigsdaler–approximately 700 kronor after the currency reform in 1873– which would have been considerably expensive given *Bandager og*

---

[619] Ibid., 289. [På uppmaning af flera operatörer har jag sökt konstruera ett lätt uppvärmbart operationsbord]

[620] [Anon.], "Bilder från svenskt industri- och näringslif". [det nyaste och mest fulländade af de Stilleska operationsborden... konstrueradt af prof. Schuchard (sic) i Stettin och fabrikör Stille gemensamt.]

[621] Ibid. [det är ej många svenska kirurger som ansett sig ha råd att skaffa sig det]

[622] Ibid.

[623] Ibid.

[624] Lindström, "En ny medicinsk möbel", 366.

Instrumenter was published in the 1860s and 1870s.[625] A city physician [*stadsläkare*] in Sweden, earned 700 riksdaler riksmynt per month in 1865, and for the sake of furniture comparison, a divan cost 42 kronor in 1900.[626] Stille's tables would have been a significant investment for an individual physician.

With that in mind, it seems clear that Stille's tables were not made for the individual physician. Given the "package deal" Stille presented with his theatre, and his successes in selling the concept abroad, it seems unlikely that the intended consumers for many of his tables–operating tables in particular–were individual physicians. The same could be said for the sick bed from *Bandager og Instrumenter* (figure 28), with its considerable cost; however, Lindström's divan-like bed was less costly and would work well alongside the furniture in the doctor's office pictured in figure 22. Lindström's divan was mindful of the private practice; Stille's tables were mindful of the institutional practice. Moreover, Stille's tables conformed with the aseptic system of cleanliness, with their smooth corners and invisible, or at least clean, joints.[627] As figures 24 and 26 illustrate, they were stripped of unnecessary detail and aesthetically plain. Their appearance was not designed first and foremost to make patients feel comfortable. Rather, the importance of exacting cleanliness trumped aesthetic sensibilities. The Stilles' longstanding work alongside physicians in Sweden, and clearly outside of the country as well in the Schuchardt case, meant that in terms of research and development on the technical side, Max Stille was aware of scientific developments in the profession as well. Toward the turn of the century, this was increasingly becoming the case for instruments more generally, where they were made as "plain and smooth as possible… made of one piece of steel, all niches and crevices being avoided wherever possible. Scissors and forceps are made so that the two parts may be readily separated and joined again".[628]

---

[625] Denmark used *rigsdaler* until 1873; whereby, it was replaced with the gold krone. One rigsdaler was worth two kroner after the reform, putting the mechanical bed at around 700 kroner. Sweden and Denmark entered a currency union in 1873, which pegged the two currencies at 1:1. See Ingrid Henriksen and Niels Kærgård, "The Scandinavian Currency Union 1875–1914", in *International Monetary Systems in Historical* Perspective Reis J. (eds.), 91-112. London: Palgrave Macmillan, 1995.

[626] Lars O. Lagerqvist. *Vad kostade det? Priser och löner, från medeltid till våra dagar.* Lund: Historiska Media, 2011, 140 & 143. 1 riksdaler riksmynt was 100 öre between 1855 and 1873. After the Scandinavian Currency Union, 1 krona was 100 öre, see Ibid., 68.

[627] [Anon.], "Bilder från svenskt industri- och näringslif". See also Kisacky, *Rise of the Modern Hospital,* 120.

[628] Nicholas Senn. *Practical Surgery for the General Practitioner.* Philadelphia: W. B. Saunders & Co., 1902, 174.

Stille emphasised practicalities in his article and these were highlighted in presentations of his work. He worked closely with physicians, and practical gains likely served at least two purposes. Firstly, practicality could be a means of selling the device: its advantages and practicalities served as advertisement as much as it did for the aforementioned patented hernia truss in the previous chapter. The tables were multi-purpose, one did not cover the patient's head in bodily fluids, they could be made more compact and were portable. These qualities would have mitigated storage issues. They were also made easy to clean, which conformed better to the increasingly reliance on the aseptic system of cleanliness in institutional settings. Secondly, by making it seem practical and highlighting work with physicians, however cursory, in its design, Stille could have alleviated some of the tensions of being new. This played into the importance of control, where novelty could be unpredict-able.[629] Solutions to these problems were not new, either. *Hygiea* offers several indications that other physicians had been experimenting with solutions to some of the problems that were allegedly solved by Stille's innovation.

Concluding Remarks

Antiseptic wound care was a surgical technology that could be carried out in nearly any space, whilst asepsis was a surgical technology that treated cleanliness more systematically. This systematisation of surgery required special rooms, methods and apparatuses that were quite different to the ones encountered in the previous chapter. This chapter has examined the early years of aseptic practice and its relation to surgical spaces and devices in Sweden. During the 1880s and 1890s, aseptic and antiseptic practices over-lapped. Physicians were positive to asepsis, as it solved some of the problems encountered with antiseptic chemicals; however, the matter of control over the sterilisation process meant that chemicals were still used occasionally as a guarantee. By this time, practitioners were familiar with how chemicals worked and using them actively destroyed germs. This was easier to control than determining whether a space, object, or body was germ-free. Aseptic and antiseptic technologies were used fluidly and simultaneously. Their imbrication highlights that strict asepsis was more of an ideal at this time, at least based on the ability for practitioners to control the cleanliness of their environment and the understanding of steam cleaning. Because asepsis had bearing on the surrounding environment, asepsis and antisepsis required different spatial configurations, and the respatialisation of practice was part

---

[629] See Frampton, "Defining Difference", 66.

of the proliferation of asepsis. Much of this chapter has centred around the work of Swedish instrument maker Max Stille, in particular on a model surgical suite and his firm's operating and examination tables. Both Stille's model surgical suite and his operating and examination tables conformed with surgical respatialisation and introduced devices that conformed to the aseptic system of cleanliness.

Part of this process was tied to the greater institutionalisation of medical practice and surgery in particular. These changes conform with overall practical changes in surgery and the establishment of specific surgical spaces in institutional settings. In conjunction with respatialisation and institutionalisation, the nature of surgical procedures changed, and the number of surgical procedures grew. Surgery became less associated solely with emergency situations and more invasive. Surgery also came to be associated with a specific space in an institutional setting. This spatial configuration of aseptic surgery called for particular material considerations, and Stille's model surgical suite followed trends in creating stripped-down surgical spaces that were easy to clean and well-lit. Because asepsis was a system of cleanliness that demanded control over an environment, spaces required different materials and architectural considerations than before. Beyond the space itself, the furnishings also required attention to different design and material expressions. These features have been little examined in the history of surgery in Sweden and played an increasingly significant role in surgical spaces. The contraposition between Stille's tables and those made with different spaces in mind illustrate the different material requirements associated with surgical space in the age of asepsis. With smooth, rounded corners, minimised joints, and materials that accommodated quick and easy cleaning, surgical spaces began establishing their requisite symbolism that gave surgeons a domain of control.

6. Conclusion

The aim of this thesis was to shed light on practical changes in nineteenth-century Swedish and Danish medicine. This has been accomplished by studying four cases. The first case highlighted the use of mirrored and lensed instruments in examinations of the throat, nose, and eyes, and the practical discussions around their implementation. In the second case, I have studied the fluid landscape of Danish orthopaedics by centring the work of surgical instrument maker Camillus Nyrop and three discussions he partook in in *Ugeskrift for Læger*. For the third case, I looked at the introduction of Listerism in Sweden and Denmark framed alongside the practical challenge of finding a safe alternative for amputation. Here, I highlighted the practical challenges that physicians identified with this method of wound care. The fourth case builds on some of the challenges introduced with Listerism and takes a closer look at the development of asepsis and its respatialisation of surgical practice.

By looking more closely at the ways that devices were enacted in medical texts, I have been able to highlight that the introduction of ophthalmoscopes, rhinoscopes, and laryngoscopes were dependent on the cultivation of technique. But this process also required the consolidation of a requisite knowledge bank, or thought style, so that practitioners could understand what they were looking at and why it was important. Previous research has highlighted the importance of cultivating visual perception in physiology. However, this was clearly the case for more everyday medical practice as well, as the use of these three devices has shown. Visual perception could also be hindered by poor quality lenses and other mitigating factors like dark spaces and bad weather. The effect of darkness on the utility of laryngoscopes, ophthalmoscopes, and rhinoscopes compelled practical indications like conducting exams when the sun was high. And if the sun was not high, the introduction of lighting equipment and reflectors helped assist physicians in discerning what they were looking at. Even though visual perception and requisite knowledge of the inside structures of the body were important, they were not the whole picture. These variables highlight the importance of looking at how the use of devices unfolds in practice.

Bandagists, a group of orthopaedic practitioners that constructed and applied trusses, braces, and bands to treat musculoskeletal disorders, were an important part of the fabric of Danish orthopaedics throughout the nineteenth century. During that period, they were unlicensed, but as I have shown in the third chapter, their work existed alongside that of physicians and was accepted. By studying the work of surgical instrument maker and bandagist Camillus Nyrop, it is clear that differences within orthopaedic practice coexisted during this period. However, coexistence also implied occasional friction. The frictions between Nyrop, Levy, and Drachmann as well as the prevailing problem of itinerant practitioners are illustrative of this. Practitioners had different conceptions of favourable treatment and included both licensed and unlicensed members. Rather than a climate of disagreement between sharply demarcated professions, unlicensed practice was relatively tolerated and both physicians and bandagists operated on a similar playing field within orthopaedic practice. Indeed, the tensions between Nyrop, Drachmann, and Levy appeared to be primarily due to divergent practice rather than direct issues with Nyrop's professional status and training.

The problem of theory, which has often been prioritised over practice in historical studies of medicine, is particularly noteworthy in the case of Listerist antisepsis. Listerism has been framed by historians previously in relation to developments in germ theory and bacteriology. However, when it was enacted in practice during the late 1860s and 1870s in Sweden and Denmark, practitioners were less concerned with the method's theoretical underpinnings than they were for the method's results, as I have shown. The method gave good clinical results, and it mitigated a significant practical problem; that of wound infection. Articles about Listerism, much like Lister's own articles, were focused on the performance of Listerism, and even in Swedish and Danish articles authors were keen to detail how to perform Listerist surgery under different circumstances. Relating Listerism to practical matters included devices. New protocol for cleaning devices and new devices themselves were introduced, including the infamous carbolic acid sprayer. This also involved discussions about mitigated problems and altering both practice and device to streamline use. Fundamentally, practitioners who were well-versed in the method were encouraged to make modifications, according to practical need. Articles about Listerism in the three journals I have examined offered practical, rather than theoretical, explanations. Listerism was deployed in practice in different ways and this is illustrated by attending to practical matters, the locally situated nature of Listerist practice and its adaptations.

Moving through the 1880s, Listerism and other antiseptic practices began overlapping with another method of mitigating infection: asepsis. The significant difference between antisepsis and asepsis was their approach to microbes. Antisepsis on the one hand acknowledged the presence of microbes in a given space and uses chemicals to kill them. On the other hand, asepsis anticipated a space without microbes at all. On the practical level, whether or not a space was microbe-free was difficult to ascertain, which led to the coexistence of the two methods. Asepsis also implied a more systematic approach to ensuring that a space was microbe-free that involved thorough cleaning with steam and hot water. Indeed, many of the initial articles discussing practical asepsis involved cleaning more specifically, rather than wound management. Furthermore, as the analysis of surgical instrument maker Max Stille's work on a model surgical suite and an operating table shows, the aseptic system of cleanliness required new spatial considerations. It also introduced different sets of problems and concerns regarding the design and material construction of devices. The case highlights the interrelations between device, knowledge, and practice and the importance of technical cunning in the development of aseptic surgery in Sweden.

Cases for Non-Universality in the History of Medicine

In the concluding chapter of the anthology *Devices and Designs: Medical Technologies in Historical Perspective*, Stuart Blume queried whether or not medical practice can be reframed as scientific, but not committed to universality. He highlights this in action by using two examples, cochlear implants and polio vaccines, where scientists, governing bodies, and clinicians drew different conclusions about their safety and utility, despite analysing the same bodies of scientific evidence.[630] One way of approaching this is through closer examination of the enactments of objects with the help of actor-network theory, as I have done. By re-examining the role of context in our studies, we might come closer to practical multitudes. Annemarie Mol notes for example that "if practices are foregrounded there is no longer a single passive object in the middle, waiting to be seen from the point of view of seemingly endless series of perspectives. Instead, objects come into being [...] And since the object of manipulation tends to differ from one practice to another, reality multiplies".[631]

By scrutinising cases where devices were discussed, I have been better able to examine the practical circumstances to which they pertain. This has not entailed a decontextualisation, but rather a recontextualisation. At times,

---

[630] Stuart Blume, "The Politics of Endpoints", in *Devices and Designs: Medical Technologies in Historical Perspective*, Carsten Timmermann and Julie Anderson (eds.), 249–272. Basingstoke: Palgrave Macmillan, 2006.

[631] Annemarie Mol. *The Body Multiple: Ontology in Medical Practice*. Durham, NC: Duke University Press, 2003, 5.

outside circumstances involved in a given practice have been less interesting than the clinical implications of device use, based on journal articles. This has allowed for a more literal examination of the journal articles in question where practices were not immediately reduced to outside contexts. Kristin Asdal highlights the literal examination of historical texts, suggesting that framing texts around outside contexts can be reductive.[632] Significantly, these contexts may not have even been crucial for historical actors, and in my study, keeping this in mind when studying practice has been particularly important.

I suggest that this might be significant in analysing the practical concerns of medical practitioners in historical materials, because we already know the scientific outcome. Furthermore, because of the rapid change during the nineteenth century, some of the practices that turn up in journal articles are unfamiliar. In the case of Listerist antisepsis for example, framing the introduction of the method within the context of bacteriology is problematic, as I have shown. Rather, the science of germ theory was not something all practitioners understood, and in fact, looking at Listerist practice in Sweden and Denmark in the context of bacteriology is anachronistic. Moving closer to the level of practice, rather than framing this work alongside theoretical developments, has shown that practitioners worked through uncertainty. Even if practitioners could not clarify the theoretical basis of a practice, they could, and did, explain how to perform it under different circumstances, what modifications to make and why, and highlight the given method's clinical results. At the same time, recontextualisation rather than decontextualisation has been an important factor in examining practice. For instance, locally specific circumstances impacted practical matters. As I have pointed out, things like weather and lighting conditions affected practice and were matters that practitioners accounted for in articles in medical journals. This is a further argument for studies of practice that are locally oriented.

Rather than reducing medical texts to their contexts, by shifting focus to the level of practice and how the objects of study are enacted in practice, we might get a better picture of the choices practitioners made, their understanding of clinical results, relationships with their surroundings and the differences between actors within medicine. I have also highlighted this in the case of Danish orthopaedics, where divergent practices coexisted in nineteenth-century medicine, despite friction. Rita Felski suggests that con-

---

[632] Kristin Asdal, "Contexts in Action–And the Future of the Past in STS". *Science, Technology, and Human Values*. Vol. 37, No. 4, April 2012, 379–403, 387.

texts can work like "boxes" and encase historical phenomena.[633] With nine-teenth-century Danish orthopaedics, confining the work of physicians and bandagists as distinct and demarcated professions would have missed the nuance and particularities in practice, where practitioners largely coexisted.

The argument for recontextualisation is perhaps stronger concerning international scholarship in the history of medicine. One of the prevailing problems is the dominance of scholarship, in particular in English, examining specific circumstances in Britain, the United States, Germany and German-speaking territories, and France. This calls attention to specific sets of circumstances that have, to some degree, been sketched as overviews.[634] Lorraine Daston and Peter Galison note that overviews can help illuminate the outlines of phenomena but that phenomena can manifest differently on the local level.[635] The overarching prevalence of certain national histories of medicine still entails challenges for historians working outside these contexts, especially in English-language scholarship, as others have identified.[636]

Studies that highlight further engage with local specificity might assist in challenging this, in particular those that examine the proliferation and spread of medical techniques and technologies. Thomas Schlich argues that part of dominance of British, North American, French and German studies is because "much of the dynamism in late modern surgery originates in these regions".[637] However dynamism entails force or energy. Part of the dynamism of late modern surgery must lay in local adaptation, not only in technological development. To better understand this dynamic, one suggestion may be to continue to shift focus from the question of *who* established a technique to that of *how* the given technique was enacted in practice. Histories that examine practical manifestations of technologies and the mechanics behind how practices were adopted, modified and translated locally are a significant part of the dynamic of nineteenth-century medicine.

Thomas Schlich's comment about where technological momentum originates is still important to consider, given the proliferation of medical

---

[633] Rita Felski, "Context Stinks!". *New Literary History*. Vol. 42, No. 4, Autumn 2011, 573–591.

[634] See William F. Bynum. *Science and the Practice of Medicine in the Nineteenth Century*. Cambridge: Cambridge University Press, 1994, xiii; Lorraine Daston and Peter Galison. *Objectivity*. New York: Zone Books, 2010, 47; Thomas Schlich, "Introduction: What Is Special About the History of Surgery", in *The Palgrave Handbook of the History of Surgery*, Thomas Schlich (ed.), 1–24. London: Palgrave Macmillan, 2018, 3.

[635] Daston and Galison. *Objectivity*, 47.

[636] See Frank Huisman, "Transcending the Language Barrier: Medical History in a Globalizing World". *European Journal for the History of Medicine and Health*. Vol. 78, 2021, 15–20

[637] Schlich, "Introduction", 3.

knowledge and deep interest in international developments that are clear in Swedish and Danish journals. All four case studies have examined trans-national phenomena, but with eyes on locally situated practices. However, it is not the origin stories themselves that might be most interesting, but how technologies, devices, and knowledge spread and were adapted locally. The international transfer of medical knowledge has motivated my engagement with previous research that studies these origins, originators, and circumstances beyond Sweden and Denmark. This does not necessarily entail fluid or unproblematic adaptation. Rather, studying the practical implementation of this knowledge can give a better sense of local diversion and adaptation. It might not indicate significant divergence either, but this needs to be determined through locally situated scholarship that studies the sets of circumstances involved in the proliferation of a technique or technology in nineteenth-century medicine.

Reconnecting to Blume's question about a non-universal understanding of medical science, historical studies that further engage with difference might add more nuance here. Rather than framing the diffusion of medical knowledge as a smooth transfer between divergent sites, greater local specificity needs to be attended to, in particular in English-language scholarship.[638] I argue that the ANT approach that I have used might assist scholars in examining these themes in the future, as it has served as a fruitful means of attending to how medical knowledge has unfolded in practice. This has highlighted both local circumstances, such as weather, and the information practitioners themselves deemed important, like clinical results. Speaking on the dominance of certain narratives in the history of medicine, Huisman argues that "there is a much more complex and sophisticated story to be told about the 'modernisation' of medicine [and] this can only happen when we

---

[638] Just a few examples of positive research trends in this area are Pratik Chakrabarti. *Bacteriology in British India: Laboratory Medicine and the Tropics*. Rochester: Boydell & Brewer, 2012; Sabrina Minuzzi, "'Quick to say Quack': Medicinal Secrets from the Household to the Apothecary's Shop in Eighteenth-Century Venice". *Social History of Medicine*. Vol. 32, No. 1, February 2019, 1–33; Projit Bihari Mukharji. *Doctoring Traditions: Ayurveda, Small Technologies, and Braided Sciences*. Chicago: The University of Chicago Press, 2016; Thomas Schlich, "Farmer to Industrialist: Lister's Antisepsis and the Making of Modern Surgery in Germany". *Notes and Records of the Royal Society of London*. Vol. 67, No. 3, 20 September 2013, 245–260; Thomas Schlich, "Negotiating Technologies in Surgery: The Controversy about Surgical Gloves in the 1890s". *Bulletin of the History of Medicine*. Vol. 87, No. 2, Summer 2013, 170–197; Peter Twohig, "Innovating Expertise: X-Ray and Laboratory Workers in the Canadian Hospital, 1920–1950", in *Devices and Designs: Medical Technologies in Historical Perspective*, Carsten Timmermann and Julie Anderson (eds.), 74–94. Basingstoke: Palgrave Macmillan, 2006.

develop regional and national self-awareness."[639] My study will hopefully contribute to this aim.

There are some themes that I have not discussed in any significant detail, but that may be interesting to study further in the future. One theme is a deeper exploration of the dynamic between unlicensed and licensed practitioners in Denmark, but also in Sweden. The work of Camillus Nyrop and other Danish bandagists, including itinerant ones, requires further study. Their presence in not only Denmark, but also Sweden and their relationships with physicians, local communities, and other bandagists offers an interesting case for further examination of the fluid landscape of nineteenth-century Nordic medicine. Studying whether or not regional differences existed in the reception and acceptance of bandagists could also be worthwhile. A hypothesis could be that their role outside of larger communities might have been different. Furthermore, their transnational itinerancy might offer insight into the fabric of medicine beyond national borders. This falls in line with calls to re-examine the role of place in the history of medicine, and could be a case for further engaging with regional and national discrepancies.[640]

Another theme that merits further study is that of hospital environments and the shift in responsibility for procurement brought on by the aseptic system of cleanliness detailed in the fifth chapter. I have but only discussed some of the spatial changes in hospital settings, mostly by centring surgical space in relation to the introduction of asepsis. A look at the relationships between the systematisation of infection control exemplified by asepsis and changes within the organisational politics of medicine moving into the twentieth century is merited. This theme might also be fruitful to study from an epistemological standpoint related to the universal transmogrify of modern medicine and an investigation of the hospital's representation of claims of universality.

---

639 Huisman, "Transcending the Language Barrier", 19.
640 See for example Sarah Hodges, "'The Global Menace'". *Social History of Medicine.* Vo. 25, No. 3, August 2012, 719–728.

Sammanfattning

Avhandlingens syfte är att undersöka förändringar i svensk och dansk medicin mellan 1855 och 1897, genom att studera medicinska redskap och hur de har beskrivits och diskuterats framför allt i svenska och danska läkartidskrifter. I närläsning av läkartidskrifterna har jag valt att fokusera på hur några av periodens teknologiska förändringar diskuterades med avseende på praktisk tillämpning.

Forskningen om 1800-talets medicinhistoria har länge präglats av ett antal metaberättelser om teknologisk framgång och utveckling. Fältet har dessutom styrts av forskning som har fokuserat på ett fåtal regioner, nämligen Storbritannien och den engelskspråkiga världen, tyskspråkiga regioner och Frankrike. Forskningen har också präglats av generella antaganden och varit av övergripande karaktär. Under de senaste decennierna har dock flera forskare pekat på behovet av att undersöka lokala miljöer och omständligheter, och studera andra områden i Europa och världen. Min forskning ligger i linje med det och med andra studier som har nyanserat och lyft fram hur teknologier har överförts praktiskt och betonat vikten av lokala sammanhang.

Arbetet styrs därutöver av fyra frågeställningar. Jag har velat undersöka hur förhållanden mellan instrument, praktik och kunskap har manifesterat sig i läkartidskrifter; studera vilka faktorer som påverkade användningen och spridningen av medicinska teknologier under perioden; lyfta fram hur medicinska teknologier presenterades i relation till professionella förväntningar och utmaningar; samt studera på vilka sätt medicinska teknologier användes i relation till användarnas och tillverkarnas karriärer.

En viktig inspirationskälla för studiens teoretiska och metodologiska ramverk är aktör-nätverksteori (ANT). Detta angreppsätt har använts framför allt utifrån Annemarie Mols fokus på iscensättning [*enactment*] och fluiditet [*fluidity*] men också Kristin Asdals och Ingunn Mosers problematisering av kontext inom historiska studier. Utifrån ANT-perspektivet är det viktigt att lyfta fram den mångfacetterade verklighet som medicinska teknologier används eller tas i bruk i. Det innebär en problematisering av metaberättelser om medicinska framgångar och ett fokus på de lokala omständligheterna kring en teknologis praktiska användning och tillämpning.

Avhandlingens huvudsakliga källmaterial är de svenska och danska läkartidskrifterna *Hygiea, Ugeskrift for Læger* och *Hospitals-Tidende*. Utöver detta ges en överblick över medicinsk press i Sverige och Danmark under 1800-

talets senare hälft samt en redogörelse för ländernas mest framträdande kirurgiska instrumentmakare.

Avhandlingen består av fyra kapitel i vilka jag undersöker fyra olika teknologiska och redskapsmässiga förändringar under 1800-talets andra hälft. Dessa är lins- och spegelinstrument för undersökning av kroppens inre; det ortopediska landskapet i Danmark; antiseptisk sårbehandling enligt Joseph Lister; och slutligen aseptikens påverkan på kirurgins praktik.

I avhandlingens andra kapitel, som följer direkt på inledningen, studerar jag instrument för undersökningar av öga, näsa och hals–oftalmoskop, rinoskop och laryngoskop–och relationerna mellan instrumentens bruk och kultiveringen av sinnesintryck. Instrumenten gav läkare ny möjlighet att kunna studera kroppens inre. I kapitlet visar jag att det var avgörande för läkare att både lära sig att använda instrumenten i fråga och att förstå varför kroppens inre strukturer som betraktades med instrumenten var betydelsefulla. I denna del av analysen utgår jag från Ludwik Flecks distinktion mellan att betrakta och att se, där seende kopplas till förekomsten av ett kollektivt tänkande [*tankekollektiv*]. För att kunna utföra undersökningar med instrumenten behövde läkare utveckla sin skicklighet även i andra avseenden. Konkreta tips om instrumenten och hur de användes meddelades i läkartidskrifter, som ett sätt att överföra vad Michael Polanyi kallar för tyst kunskap [*tacit knowledge*]. Det kunde röra sig om hur instrumenten kunde användas för att undvika att åsamka patienten smärtor eller om hur väder, ljusförhållande och linsernas kvalitet påverkade undersökningarnas förutsättningar. Föresatsen i kapitlet är att lyfta fram sambanden mellan teoretisk och praktisk kunskap i förhållande till lokala omständigheter som var betydelsefulla för användningen av dessa instrument.

I det tredje kapitlet studerar jag det danska ortopediska landskapet under 1860- till 1880-talen. Annemarie Mols begrepp *coexistence of difference* som pekar på hur skillnader och olikheter samexisterar är ett viktigt analytiskt verktyg i detta kapitel. Olika sätt att arbeta, som vi i efterhand har hänfört till olika eller rent av rivaliserande professioner och kunskapstraditioner, kunde inte sällan samexistera och överlappa varandra på praktiknivå. I kapitlet lyfter jag fram en ännu icke-formaliserad yrkesgren, de så kallade bandagisterna. Bandagisterna fyllde en viktig funktion som behandlare av ortopediska åkommor i det danska medicinska landskapet under en period och var generellt en accepterad profession som ibland arbetade tillsammans med läkare. För att förstå hur samexistensen fungerade och hur relationerna mellan bandagist och läkare såg ut undersöker jag den danske kirurgiska instrumentmakaren och bandagisten Camillus Nyrop.

En central poäng i kapitlet är att den gängse professionaliseringsberätt-elsen leder fel i fallet Nyrop. Nyrop var en väl respekterad utövare som också sysslade med ortopedi i någon mån. Trots att han saknade formell medicinsk utbildning blev han en respekterad individ i Danmarks medicinska landskap och kunde göra karriär. Även om Nyrop kom i konflikt med ett fåtal läkare handlade konflikterna mer om skilda behandlingsmetoder än Nyrops professionella status. Till viss del kunde Nyrop och läkare samlas under vad som identifierades som ett behov av att reglera en viss typ av bandagister, som var ambulerande och betraktades som mindre seriösa utövare. Men reglering uteblev, och läkare och bandagister av olika slag, inklusive Nyrop, fortsatte att samexistera. Undersökningen utmynnar i slutsatsen att polariseringen mellan de som saknade formell utbildning och utbildade läkare inte är applicerbar på en dansk 1800-talskontext.

Det fjärde kapitlet ger en överblick av antiseptisk sårbehandling i Sverige och Danmark såsom den kom att utformas framför allt av den brittiska kirurgen Joseph Lister och sedan anpassas till svenska och danska förhåll-anden. Analysen utgår från de diskussioner som fördes i Sverige och Danmark om vikten av att utveckla ett säkert och framgångsrikt sätt att behandla allvarliga skador som ofta krävde amputation. Även här är för-medlingen av tyst kunskap enligt Michael Polanyi ett viktigt verktyg i analysen. En effektivare sårbehandling ansågs kunna minska behovet av amputation och lindra patientens lidanden. Redan samma år som Lister skrev sin första artikel om sin metod publicerades redogörelser för den i Danmark, och året därpå i Sverige. Antiseptisk sårbehandling gav nya möj-ligheter för läkare att behandla komplexa och infekterade sår, något som kunde dämpa behovet av att amputera kroppsdelar för att rädda liv. Införandet av antiseptisk sårbehandling har ofta förknippats med utveck-lingen inom bakteriologisk teori. Genom en närläsning av svenska och danska artiklar om metoden visar jag dock att antiseptiken framför allt motiverades av dess framgångsrika kliniska resultat och att dess teoretiska underbyggnad för läkare i allt väsentligt var sekundär.

Den antiseptiska framgången skapade också problem. Den kemiska lösningen som rekommenderas av Lister, karbolsyra, var frätande för instru-menten och retande för huden, och läkare var därför måna om att undersöka alternativ. Ett sådant alternativ var den aseptiska metoden. I det femte kapitlet undersöks introduktionen av aseptik, som inleddes vid slutet på 1880-talet. Till skillnad från antiseptisk sårbehandling krävde aseptiken ett mer systematiskt tillvägagångsätt kring hygien och renlighet. Samtidigt upplevde läkare att det var svårt att bedöma om aseptisk behandling, med ånga och värme snarare än kemikalier, faktiskt gjorde instrument, ytor och hud rena. Ett resultat av undersökningen i detta kapitel är att antiseptiska och aseptiska praktiker överlappade varandra och användes sida vid sida.

Med Annemarie Mols begrepp iscensättning [*enactment*] och fokus på mångfacetterade verkligheter [*multiples*] visar jag att den systematiska syn som aseptiken krävde var sammankopplad med kirurgins fysiska miljö på ett mer omfattande sätt än vad antiseptiken var. För att betona aseptikens systematiska krav studerar jag den svenska kirurgiska instrumentmakaren Max Stilles arbete. Jag analyserar den mönsteroperationssal och det operationsbord som Stille utvecklade i syfte att bättre tillgodose den aseptiska praktiken. Operationssalen ger exempel på miljöförändringar och redskapsförändringar som lämpade sig för aseptiken. Rummet kunde spolas rent under kort tid med vatten, redskapen var lätta att rengöra, likaså operationsbordet som också saknade kanter och skarvar, något som kunde dölja mikrober. Gemensamt för Stilles sal och bord var att de nu riktade sig till en annan kundkrets: sjukhusen. Ett viktigt resultat av undersökningen är att en förskjutning av ansvar krävdes för att realisera aseptiken på en systematisk nivå: från att den medicinska praktiken främst var läkarens angelägenhet till att vara institutionens.

Avslutningsvis sammanfattar jag avhandlingen i det sjätte kapitlet och knyter an till en av de inledande diskussionerna om vikten av att fortsätta bedriva studier med fokus på lokala omständigheter. Mina fyra delstudier belyser att införande av medicinska praktiker tar form i relation till lokala förhållanden varmed de nyanserar de gängse metaberättelserna om professionalisering och medicinvetenskapens linjära utveckling. Genom att titta närmare på praktiska beskrivningar i medicinska tidskrifter poängterar jag att allt från praktisk övning till väderförhållande haft inverkan på hur förändring gick till och hur nya instrument togs i bruk inom de fyra medicinska områden som jag har undersökt: lins- och spegelinstrument, dansk ortopedi, Listerism och asepsis. Jag visar dessutom ett nyanserat professionslandskap där kirurgiska instrumentmakare och bandagister har varit delaktiga aktörer i utformandet av medicinsk praktik. Vidare visar jag att kliniska erfarenheter hade större betydelse för aseptikens genombrott i Sverige och Danmark än teoretiska landvinningar.

Slutligen pekar jag ut två intressanta forskningsområden som kan vara värda att undersöka vidare. Den första är dynamiken mellan bandagister och andra icke-licenserade utövare av medicin, och läkare i både Danmark och Sverige. Framför allt är ett större fokus på landsbygden viktigt eftersom ett glesare utbud av legitimerade läkare kan ha påverkat deras mottagandet och eventuella samarbeten med läkare. Den andra är att undersöka förändringen i sjukhusmiljöer runt sekelskiftet 1900 och deras inköp av och ansvar för instrument som föranleddes av aseptikens mer systematiska tillvägagångsätt. En givande ingång skulle kunna vara att väva in förändringen med sjukhuset som projektionsyta för medicinens anspråk på universalitet.

I avhandlingen lyfter jag alltså fram vikten av att ta hänsyn till praktik i medicinhistoriska studier och uppmanar till att i större utsträckning se tidskriftsartiklar som förmedlare av praktiska rön, tyst kunskap och invändningar. Läkartidskrifter är inte bara förmedlare av teoretisk kunskap utan bör ses som informativa källor för det medicinska hantverket.

Acknowledgements

I am forever indebted to a great number of people for their support during this process. You are far too many to name and I risk forgetting someone. I apologise for that. But, truly, a warm and profound thank you to everyone who has answered a fraught text, given me a call (or let me call!) and helped in any way during these last four and a half years.

I want to extend immeasurable gratitude to my students, past, present, and future. Being able to teach you has been one of the greatest joys of this process, and you have taught me, and will teach me, more than most anything else. Plsease keep reaching for the stars and never abandon your critical eye!

Thank you to my supervisors, Peter Josephson and Leif Runefelt. Thank you for your support, critical comments, and fielding my never-ending barrage of questions.

My gratitude goes to my colleagues, both at Södertörn, but elsewhere as well. I would like to thank the members of the Scientific Instrument Commission in particular, who provided both a warm welcome and a wonderful forum for intellectual exchange. I will never forget the hospitality I received as a newcomer. Truly, thank you all. I would also like to thank my colleagues in the history of ideas at Södertörn University, fellow PhD students, and colleagues from Saco-S and SULF. In particular, thank you to Lena Lennerhed, Marie Jonsson, Jenny Gustafsson, Liza Jakobsson (big thank you for proofreading my Swedish summary, Liza!), Kateryna Zorya, Jane Ruffino, Martin Johansson, Vasileios Petrogiannis, Gilda Hoxha, My Klockar Linder, Synne Myrebøe, Riikka Taavetti, Tintin Hodén, Lovisa Olsson, Oscar von Seth, Mats Dahllöv, Anders Ullholm, Helena Bergman, Henrik Bohlin, David Östlund, Anders Burman, Magnus Rodell, and many, many more. Solange Hamrin and Erik van Ooijen, you both encouraged me to start studying again. Thank you, Mattias Jeschko-Edberg, for always putting things into perspective.

Thank you to my opponents at my 50% and 90% seminars, Jenny Beckman and Sven Widmalm. Your critical eyes helped me orient my research better and shape my study.

Warm gratitude to Julia Falk, Joel Johansson, Peter Lundberg, and Roland Meisel for both the higher and lower seminars. Your friendship over the years has been invaluable and I am eternally grateful for it.

It is unlikely that I would have interested myself in this subject at all if I hadn't interned briefly at Medicine and Heritage at the Karolinska Institute.

Warm thank you to Eva Åhrén, Anna Lantz, Olof Ljungström, Daniel Normark, Ann Gustavsson, Dan Jibreus, Gertie Johansson, Maria Josephson, Hjalmar Fors, Marie Oscarsson and Lars Helin. Being able to work directly with collections in an intellectual stimulating and friendly environment truly shaped my interest in the history of medicine, medical devices, and collections.

Without the help and support of library and archive staff, none of this would have been possible. Thank you for answering my strange questions, helping me find material, and digging up old, hospital ledgers. A special thank you to Jon Robson for the help with my manuscript and cover art.

Several foundations have provided me with economic support for this thesis. As a doctoral student in the Baltic and East European Graduate School, I would like to thank The Foundation for Baltic and East European Studies for funding my work. Further economic support has generously been granted by *Helge Ax:son Johnsons stiftelse* and *Stiftelsen J A Letterstedts resestipendiefond*. Sophiahemmet has additionally provided me access to portions of their archive.

Finally, and most importantly, I would like to thank my family. Kim, your unwavering support during this period has been invaluable. Thank you for keeping me grounded. Garm, you may be a dog, but you know more about historical medical devices than most anyone else at this point. Thank you for always being the first to listen to and judge my conference presentations, and I am truly sorry for putting you through so many Zoom calls during naptime. Mom, Ian, Meylina, Mia, and Scout, you all inspire me. Thank you for always believing in me. I can't wait to see you all again.

Kristin Halverson
Sköndal, Sweden
March 31, 2022

Bibliography

Unpublished Sources

Rigsarkivet
07809. Nyrop, Camillus, instrumentmager, bandagist.

Riksarkivet
Karolinska institutet 1813–1980 SE/RA/420128/02
D I 1: Inventarieförteckningar 1859–1892
Sabbatsbergs sjukhus administrativ arkiv SE/SSA/0252/A
D 2: Inventarieförteckningar
G 1 B: Inventariehuvudböcker
G 2: Kassaböcker
Serafimerlasarettet SE/RA/420251
B 4 A 1: Ekonomiska berättelser 1852–1938
B 4 B 1: Årsrapporter 1859–1938
G 1 A 97–147: Huvudböcker 1850–1900
G 6 BC 1–3: Månadsräkenskaper redovisade kontovis
Sophiahemmet SE/RA/740111
G 1 A 1–14: Huvudbok 1883–1899

Stockholm stadsarkiv
Hall- och manufakturrätten SE/SSA/0099
B 3: Fabriksberättelser

Stockholms stadsmuseum
Josabeth Sjöberg, Inventarienummer SSM 502493

Svenska Läkarsällskapet
Förhandlingar vid Svenska läkarsällskapets sammankomster 1850–1900.

Uppsala University
Medicinska fakulteten
D II: Inventarie- och arkivförteckningar
G I: Räkenskaper

Tekniska museet
F F956. Handlingar rörande Albert Stille, Kirurgisk Instrumentfabrik, AB Stille-Werner, Stockholm, Teknik- och industrihistoriska arkivet.

Published Sources

Books

Berg, John. *Några synpunkter på antiseptikens genombrottstid av den som upplevat den: Föredrag i Svenska läkarsällskapet 17 mars 1931*. Off-print, *Hygiea*, Vol. 93. Stockholm, 1931.

Camillus Nyrops etablissement. *Illustreret Catalog*. Copenhagen: Nielsen & Lydiche, [n.d.].

Drachmann, A. G. *Om Rygradens Sidekrumning med særligt Hensyn til dens Diagnose, Ætlologi og Behandling*. Copenhagen: C. A. Reitzel, 1852.

Hansen [Grut], Edmund. *Kort Fremstilling af den i praktiske Øiemed anvendelie Undersøgelse med Øienspeilet og af de ved denne Undersøgelse indvundne Resultater*. Diss. Copenhagen University, 1857.

Hygiea: Register öfver banden elfva (1849)–Tjugutvå (1860). P. A. Norstedt & Söner, 1863.

Hygiea: Register öfver banden XXIII (1861)–XXXII (1870). Stockholm: P. A. Norstedt & Söner, 1874.

Nyrop, Camillus. *Bandager og Instrumenter afbildede og beskrevne med en tilføi et Prisfortegnelse*. Copenhagen: G.E.C. Gad, 1864.

Ruppaner, Antoine. *The Principles and Practice of Laryngoscopy & Rhinoscopy in Diseases of the Throat and Nasal Passages*. New York: A. Simpson & Co., 1868.

Senn, Nicholas. *Practical Surgery for the General Practitioner*. Philadelphia: W. B. Saunders & Co., 1902.

Sundberg, Carl. *Läkarvetenskapen och dess samhällsbetydelse under det nittonde århundradet*. Stockholm: P. A. Nordsted & Söners Förlag, 1920.

Söderbaum, Per. *Listers antiseptiska method*. Diss. Uppsala University, 1877.

Udsigt over Udstillingen af indenlandske Industrie-Producter. Bianco Lund & Schneider, 1837.

Ugeskrift for Læger: Sag- og Navneregister til Ugeskrift for Læger. Förste Række I–X Bind og anden Række I–XXXI Bind (1839–1860). Copenhagen: C. A. Reitzels Forlag, 1860.

Ugeskrift for Læger: Sag- og Navneregister til Ugeskrift for Læger. Anden Række XXXII–XLIII Bind og Tredje Række I–XXVIII Bind (1860–1879). Copenhagen: C. A. Reitzels Forlag, 1880.

Virchow, Rudolf. *Cellular Pathology*. Trans. Frank Chance. London: John Churchill, 1860.

Warfvinge, F. W. *Årsberättelse från Sabbatsbergs sjukhus i Stockholm för 1884*. Stockholm, 1885.

Medical Journals

[Anon.], "Behandlingen af komplicerede Benbrud. Efter Richard Volkmann (klin. Vorträge 117–118)". *Ugeskrift for Læger*. Series 3, Vol. 24, No. 17, 6 October 1877, 249–256, 253–4.

[Anon.], "Berättelse om Undervisningen vid Kongl. Carolinska Medico-Kirurgiska Institutet Under år 1855". *Hygiea*, Vol. 18, No. 1, January 1856, 3–15.

[Anon.], "Berättelse om Undervisningen vid Kongl. Karolinska Mediko-Kirurgiska Institutet: Under läsåret 1857–58". *Hygiea*. Vol. 20, No. 9, September 1858, 513–520.

[Anon.], "Berättelse om Undervisningen vid Kongl. Karolinska Medico-Kirurgiska Institutet under läsåret 1863–64". *Hygiea*. Vol. 27, No. 1, January 1865, 3–18.

[Anon.], "Claude Bernards nyere Undersögelser om Blodets Egenskaber (Af et Brev fra Paris.)". *Ugeskrift for Læger*. Series 2, Vol. 28, No. 18, 10 April 1858, 265–277.

[Anon.], "Disputats". *Ugeskrift for Læger*. Series 2, Vol. 27, No. 16, 3 October 1857, 248.

[Anon.], "Dødsfald". *Ugeskrift for Læger*. Series 4, Vol. 9, No. 1, 5 January 1884, 23.

[Anon.], "Dødsfald i Udlandet". *Hospitals-Tidende*. Vol. 36, No. 45, 8 November 1893, 1116.

[Anon.], "Endoskopien". *Ugeskrift for Læger*. Series 2, Vol. 42, No. 29, 17 Juni 1865, 449–458.

[Anon.], "Erfaringer om Brugen af Strubespeilet". *Ugeskrift for Læger*. Series 2, Vol. 30, No. 18, 9 April 1859, 273–280.

[Anon.], "Et Tilfælde af Chloroformdød: Klinisk Foredrag, af Prof. Billroth (Wien. med. Wchschrift 1868, Nr. 46, 47, 48 og 49)". *Ugeskrift for Læger*. Vol. 6, No. 5, 25 July 1868, 65–77.

[Anon.], "Forgiftning med Karbolsyre: Efter Dr. Machin (Brit. med. journ. Marts 1868.–L'un. méd. 1868. Nr. 108)". *Ugeskrift for Læger*. Series 3, Vol. 6, No. 20, 17 October 1868, 295–296.

[Anon.], "Forord". *Hospitals-Tidende*. Vol. 1, No. 1, January 6, 1858, 1.

[Anon.], "Journalistik". *Hospitals-Tidende*. Vol. 16, No. 40, 1 October 1873, 159–160.

[Anon.], "Karbolsyreforgiftning". *Ugeskrift for Læger*. Series 3, Vol. 13, No. 25, 25 May 1872, 403–404.

[Anon.], "Kloral som antisepticum. Efter Dujardin-Beaumetx og Hirne (L'un. méd. 1873. Nr. 62 og Nr. 63)". *Ugeskrift for Læger*, Series 3, Vol. 16, No. 12, 6 September 1873, 177–181.

[Anon.], "Kontakt- og Luft-Infektion I den praktiske Kirurgi; Kümmel (Hamborg) (Beil. zum Centrabl. für Chirurgie 1885. Nr. 24. Meddelt paa den 14de tyske Kirurg-Kongres)". *Hospitals-Tidende*. Vol. 28, No. 29, 22 July 1885, 691–698.

[Anon.], "Koppernes pathologiske Anatomi". *Ugeskrift for Læger*. Series 2, Vol. 40, No. 28–29, 18 June 1864, 433–449.

[Anon.], "Lagenbech: Det permanente varme Vandbad (Prager Vierteljahrschr. 1856. 3 Bd.)". *Ugeskrift for Læger*. Series 2, Vol. 25, No. 6, 26 July 1856, 73–85.

[Anon.], "Mindre Meddelelser". *Hospitals-Tidende*. Vol. 37, No. 33, 15 August 1894, 824.

[Anon.], "Nordisk kirurgisk förenings samforskning angående kirurgisk narkos". *Hygiea*. Vol. 59, No. 2, February 1897, 291–292.

[Anon.], "Officielt". *Hospitals-Tidende*. Vol.26, No. 52, 26 December 1883, 1248.

[Anon.], "Om Anvendelsen af Karbolsyren I Chirurgien". *Hospitalds-Tidende.* Vol. 12, No. 21, 26 May 1869, 82–83.

[Anon.], "Om Anæmie foraarsaget ved Formindskelse af Blodets Æggehvideholdighed og deraf fölgende Vattersot". *Ugeskrift for Læger.* Series 2, Vol. 13, No. 7, 17 August 1850, 97–110.

[Anon.], "Om Blodets Koagulation (B. Richardson: The cause of the coagulation of the blood anm. i The brit. and for. med. chir. review. Juli 1858)". *Ugeskrift for Læger.* Series 2, Vol. 29, No. 6, 31 July 1858, 74–84.

[Anon.], "Om de paa Nervestammernes Ender ved amputerede Lemmer forekommende Knuder Prof. Wdel. Zeitschr. d. k. k. Gellesch. D. Aertze zu Wien. Jan. 1855". *Ugeskrift for Læger.* Series 2, Vol. 25, No. 5, 26 January 1856, 65–73.

[Anon.], "Om de specifiske fremkaldende Aarsager til Epidemier". *Ugeskrift for Læger.* Series 2, Vol. 20, No. 20–21, 20 May 1854, 295–323.

[Anon.], "Om farlige Følger af den ophthalmoscopiske Ungersøgelse [sic] af Øiet". *Hospitals-Tidende.* Vol. 2, No. 32, 10 August 1859, 127–128.

[Anon.], "Om Hjerteforkamrenes Funktion". *Ugeskrift for Læger.* Series 2, Vol. 18, No. 17, 30 April 1853, 249–260.

[Anon.], "Om nogle Desinfektionsmidler (Wilson: Pharmacol. Journ. Decbr. 1852, Schmidts Jahrb. 1853, Nr. 6)". *Ugeskrift for Læger.* Series 2, Vol. 20, No. 3–4, 28 January 1854, 62–63.

[Anon.], "Om operative Behandling af Kroup". *Ugeskrift for Læger.* Series 2, Vol. 30, No. 6, 29 January 1859, 73–85.

[Anon.], "Om Resektion af de större Led (The brit. and for. med. chir. review. October 1857)". *Ugeskrift for Læger.* Series 2, Vol 28, No. 1–2, 2 January 1858, 1–23.

[Anon.], "Om Resektion af de större Led (The brit. and for. med. chir. review. October 1857)". *Ugeskrift for Læger.* Series 2, Vol 28, No. 3, 9 January 1858, 25–33.

[Anon.], "Om Resektion af de större Led (The brit. and for. med. chir. review. October 1857)". *Ugeskrift for Læger.* Series 2, Vol 28, No. 4, 16 January 1858, 41–53.

[Anon.]. Om Speculum laryngis og dets Anvendelsesmethode". *Ugeskift for Læger.* Series 2, Vol. 30, No. 5, 22 January 1859, 66–9.

[Anon.], "Om uforsigtig Anvendelse af Ophtalmoskopet (Desmarres i Gazette des Hôpiteaux. 1859. Nr. 67.)". *Ugeskrift for Læger.* Series 2, Vol. 32, No. 21, 5 May 1860, 325–327.

[Anon.], "Pathologisk Physiologi–Cellularpathologi". *Ugeskrift for Læger.* Series 2, Vol. 30, No. 13–14. 12 March 1859, 193–202.

[Anon.], "Resektionsspørgsmaalet". *Ugeskrift for Læger.* Series 3, Vol. 9, No. 3, 8 January 1870, 35–37.

[Anon.], "Rhinoskopi: Efter Szermak [sic] (W. Wschr. 16de Febr. 1861)". *Ugeskrift for Læger.* Series 2, Vol. 34, No. 15, 23 March 1861, 225–231.

[Anon.], "Tracheotomi for et fremmed Legeme I Luftröret". *Ugeskrift for Læger.* Series 2, Vol. 21, No. 15, 14 October 1854, 235–238.

[Anon.], "Vatforbinding. Efter Hervey (Arch. gén. de méd. Dcbr. 1871–Juni 1872)". *Ugeskrift for Læger*. Series 3, Vol. 15, No. 11, 1 March 1873, 161–172.

Berg, John, "Minnesteckning: Max Stille". *Hygiea*. Vol. 68, No. 4, April 1906, 358–363.

—. "Några ord om subkutana osteomier i allmänhet och behandling af genu valgum i synnerhet". *Hygiea*. Vol. 41, No. 11 & 12, November/December 1879, 721–731.

—. "Resebref från Dr John Berg. Uppläst i Medicinska Föreningen den 28 Februari 1880". *Hygiea*. Vol. 42, No. 5, May 1880, 286–291.

Björkén, J., "Bentumör i sinus frontalis". *Hygiea*. Vol. 26, No. 1, January 1864, 17–27.

Bloch, Oscar, "Om den forskellige Saarbehandling i forskellige kirurgiske Services". *Hospitals-Tidende*. Series 2, Vol. 3, No. 18, 3 May 1876, 273–283.

—. "Om den forskellige Saarbehandling i forskellige kirurgiske Services". *Hospitals-Tidende*. Series 2, Vol. 3, No. 19, 10 May 1876, 289–294.

—. "Om den forskellige Saarbehandling i forskellige kirurgiske Services". *Hospitals-Tidende*. Series 2, Vol. 3, No. 20, 17 May 1876, 305–310.

—. "Smaanoter fra den kirurgiske Praksis". *Ugeskrift for Læger*. Series 5, Vol. 1, No. 50, 14 December 1894, 1175–1185.

Bolinder, E. V., "Operationer verkstälda å Sabbatsberg sjukhus' kirurgiska afdelning under år 1889". *Hygiea*, Vol. 52, No. 6, June 1890, 409–417.

Borelius, Jacques, "Antiseptiken på Listers afdelning på Kings College Hospital i London". *Hygiea*. Vol. 51, No. 11, November 1889, 665–669.

—. "Den aseptiska sårbehandlingen". *Hygiea*. Vol. 55, No. 4, April 1893, 415–429.

—. "Joseph Lister, An address on a new antiseptic dressing' Brit. Med. Journal 1889, nov 9, 1890, jan. 4. Referat af Jacques Borelius". *Hygiea*. Vol. 52, No. 6, June 1890, 589–591.

—. "Om behandling af frakturer på underbenet". *Hygeia*. Vol. 56, No. 6, June 1894, 578–592.

—. "Om Hennebergs desinfektor för sterilsering af förbandsmaterial m. m.". *Hygiea*. Vol. 52, No. 9, September 1890, 677–680.

Boye, J., "Et Tilfælde af Ovariotomi med heldigt Udfald". *Hospitals-Tidende*. Vol. 10, No. 12, 16 October 1867, 165–167.

Brünniche, Andreas, "Til Belysning af den I Efteraaret 1875 her I Byen forekomme Epidemi af Dysenteri". *Hospitals-Tidende*. Vol. 19, No. 23, 7 June 1876, 354–357.

Budde, V., [unititled]. *Ugeskrift for Læger*. Series 4, Vol. 8, No. 6, 4 August 1883, 80–81.

Böttiger, G., "Om Etherisationen. Tal, hållet vid franska Wetenskaps-Academiens Årssammankomst d. å., af VELPEAU". *Hygiea*. Vol. 12, No. 6, June 1850, 350–364.

—. "Om Etherisationen. Tal, hållet vid franska Wetenskaps-Academiens Årssammankomst d. å., af VELPEAU". *Hygiea*. Vol. 12, No. 7, July 1850, 411–415.

Carlsson, H. J., "Utdrag ur en till Kgl. Sundhets-Collegium afgifven berättelse om en, med understöd af statsmedel företagen vetenskaplig resa". *Hygiea*. Vol. 12, No. 7, July 1850, 393–410.

Cederschjöld, F. A., "Ett nytt Perforatorium". *Hygiea*. Vol. 12, No. 9, September 1850, 531–534.

Drachmann, A. G., [untitled]. *Ugeskrift for Læger.* Series 2, Vol. 15, No. 6–8, 16 August 1851, 127–128.

—. "Om den Langgaardske orthopædiske Anstalt". *Ugeskrift for Læger*, Series 2, Vol. 6, No. 26, 29 May 1847, 405–416.

—. "Om Skoliosens Behandling: Nogle Bemærkninger i Anledning af Prof. Nyrops Udtalelser i «Bandager og Instrumenter» 3die Bd. 1ste Hefte. 1872". *Ugeskrift for Læger.* Series 3, Vol. 13, No. 22, 11 May 1872, 337–345.

—. "Om Virksomheden som kirurgisk Instrumentmager og Bandagist". *Ugeksrift for Læger.* Series 4, Vol. 5, No. 23, 20 May 1882, 345–349.

Drachmann, A. G. And Schøidte, Immanuel, "Beretning om Institutet for medicinsk og ortopædisk Gymnastik fra 1ste Maj 1868 til 30te April 1869". *Ugeskrift for Læger*, Series 3, Vol. 9, No. 13, 12 March 1870, 193–198.

—. "Beretning om Institutet for medicinsk og ortopædisk Gymnastik fra 1ste Maj 1868 til 30te April 1869". *Ugeskrift for Læger*, Series 3, Vol. 9, No. 14–15, 19 March 1870, 209–225.

Edholm, Edward, "Lehrbuch der Militär-Hygiene, bearbeitet von Dr C. Kirchner, mit 75 Holzschnitten und 6 lithografirten Tafeln. 445 sid. Erlangen 1869". *Hygiea.* Vol. 31, No. 8, August 1869, 359–366.

Ekström, F. A., "Ögonspegelns bruk vid diagnosen af sjukdomar i ögats inre delar". *Hygiea.* Vol. 16, No. 11, November 1854, 649–656.

Engdahl, E., "Om eteriseringen". *Hygiea.* Vol. 39, No. 9, September 1877, 489–505.

—. "Om eteriseringen". *Hygiea.* Vol. 41, No. 4, April 1879, 227–232.

Hallin, O. F., "Om lasarettsväsendet i Sverige 1880". *Hygiea.* Vol. 43, No. 11, November 1881, 601–632.

Hannover, Adolph, "Resektioner fra Krigen 1864 i den danske Armes Underklasser". *Ugeskrift for Læger.* Series 3, Vol. 7, No. 12–13, 6 March 1869, 169–195.

Hansson, Anders, "Kasuistik från Warbergs lasarett". *Hygiea.* Vol. 55, No. 4, April 1893, 402–406.

Heckscher, Oscar, "Om Mangler ved Indpakningen af sterile Forbindstoffer". *Hospitals-Tidende.* Vol. 38, No. 4, 23 January 1895, 113–115.

Hellström, Georg, "Sjunde Allmänna Svenska Läkarmötet i Lysekil". *Hygiea.* Vol. 57, No. 9, September 1895, 304–332.

Hellström, Thure, "Om diagnosticerandet af difteri". *Hygiea.* Vol. 58, No. 9, September 1895, 240–303.

Holmer, Valdemar, "Om Resektion af Knæleddet i kroniske Knæledssygdomme". *Hospitals-Tidende.* Vol. 15, No. 43, 23 October 1872, 169–171.

—. "Om Resektion af Knæleddet i kroniske Knæledssygdomme". *Hospitals-Tidende.* Vol. 15, No. 44, 30 October 1872, 173–175.

—. "Om Resektion af Knæleddet i kroniske Knæledssygdomme". *Hospitals-Tidende.* Vol. 15, No. 45, 6 November 1872, 177–179.

—. "Om Resektion af Knæleddet i kroniske Knæledssygdomme". *Hospitals-Tidende*. Vol. 15, No. 46, 13 November 1872, 181–184.

—. "Om Resektion af Knæleddet i kroniske Knæledssygdomme". *Hospitals-Tidende*. Vol. 15, No. 47, 20 November 1872, 185–186.

Howitz, F., "Et Tilfælde af Ovariotomi". *Hospitals-Tidende*. Vol. 7, No. 12, 23 March 1864, 45–47.

Huss, Magnus, "Sällsyntare sjukdomsfall. *Hygeia*. Vol. 18, No. 8, August 1856, 525–555.

Hülphers, H., "Om luftstrup-spegeln, laryngoskopet". *Hygeia*. Vol. 20, No. 8, August 1858, 469–474.

Ibsen, Eugen, "Om Magniumlysets Anvendelse ved Laryngoskopi. *Ugeskrift for Læger*. Series 2, Vol. 43, No. 24, 18 November 1865, 392–394.

Karström, W., "Kirurgisk kasuistik från Wexiö lasarett". *Hygiea*. Vol. 53, No. 3, March 1891, 243–276.

Kjellman, F., "Om operationen af näspolyper. *Hygiea*. Vol. 43, No. 6, June 1881, 281–286.

Kullberg, A., "Den tredje internationella medicinska kongressen i Wien 1873. Om karantäner mot kolera". *Hygiea*. Vol. 35, No. 11, November 1873, 658–673.

Landgren, G. A., "Om amputation med tibio-tarsalleden och förenkling af operationssätt dervid". *Hygiea*. Vol. 13, No. 5, May 1851, 285–288.

Langell, A. A., "Bidrag till läran om auskultationen af fel i hjertats valver och mynningar". *Hygeia*. Vol. 19, No. 10, October 1857, 683–700.

—. "Om Ileo-typhus och Typhus exanthematicus å Allmänna och Sahlgrenska sjukhuset i Göteborg". *Hygiea*. Vol. 32, No. 9, September 1870, 441–451.

Larsen, P. C., "Prof. Listers antiseptiske Forbinding". *Hospitals-Tidende*. Vol. 11, No. 32, 5 August 1868, 126–127.

Levy, Sigfred, "Om Kjæderbrokbaand (Efter Emil Edel. Arch. f. klin. Chir. XXII. 3)". *Ugeskrift for Læger*. Series 3, Vol. 26, No. 28, 14 December 1878, 433–435.

—. "Om Kjædebrokbaand". *Ugeksrift for Læger*. Series 3, Vol. 27, No. 2, 11 January 1879, 21–22.

—. "Om Kjædebrokbaand". *Ugeksrift for Læger*. Series 3, Vol. 27, No. 5, 25 January 1878, 62.

—. "Om Virksomheden som kirurgisk Instrumentmager og Bandagist". *Ugeksrift for Læger*. Series 4, Vol. 5, No. 23, 20 May 1882, 349–353.

Lindh, Alrik, "Kirurgisk kasuistik från Sahlgrenska sjukhuset i Göteborg". *Hygiea*. Vol. 54, No. 11, November 1892, 410–419.

Lindström, S., "En ny medicinsk möbel". *Hygiea*. Vol. 56, No. 4, April 1894, 364–366.

Lister, Joseph, "Address in Surgery Delivered at the Thirty-Ninth Annual Meeting of the British Medical Association, Held in Plymouth, August 8th, 9th, 10th and 11th, 1871. 26 August 1871". *British Medical Journal*. Vol. 2, No. 556, 26 August 1871, 225–233.

—. "An Address on the Catgut Ligature". *British Medical Journal*. Vol. 1, No. 1055, 5 February 1881, 183–185.

—. "An Address on the Treatment of Wounds". *The Lancet*. Vol. 118, No. 3038, 19 November 1881, 863–866.

—. "Den antiseptiske Metode". *Hospitals-Tidende*. Vol. 14, No. 47, 22 November 1871, 186–188.

—. "Observations on the Ligature of Arteries under the Antiseptic System". *Lancet*. Vol. 93, No. 2379, April 1869, 451–455.

—. "On the Antiseptic Principle in the Practice of Surgery". *The British Medical Journal*. Vol. 2, No. 246, 21 September 1867, 246–248.

—. "On a New Method of Treating Compound Fracture, Abscess, &c., with Observations on the Conditions of Suppuration. Part I". *The Lancet*. Vol. 89, Issue 2272, 16 March 1867, 336–339.

—. "On a New Method of Treating Compound Fracture, Abscess, &c. Part II". *The Lancet*. Vol. 89, Issue 2274, 30 March 1867, 95–96.

Lovén, Christian, "Om Begreppen Retning och Retbarhet, af Prof. Rudolf Virchow (Archive für pathologishe Anatomie und Physiologie und für klinische Medicin Bd. XIV (neue Folge Bd. IV) Hft. 1 ausgegeben in August 1858.)". *Hygiea*. Vol. 20, No. 5, May 1859, 277–294.

Naumann, G., "Om antiseptisk behandling af brännsår". *Hygiea*. Vol. 40, No. 6, June 1878, 282–286.

Netzel, W., "Utdrag ur bref från Dr M. Salin". *Hygiea*. Vol. 41, No. 2, February 1879, 98–104.

Nyrop, Camillus, "En Indsigelse". *Ugeskrift for Læger*. Series 3, Vol. 14, No. 18–19, 26 October 1872, 306–307.

—. "En Replik". *Ugeskrift for Læger*. Series 3, Vol. 13, No. 25, 25 May 1872, 405–407.

—. "I Anledning af Hr. Professor Drachmanns Udtalelser I Nr. 13 og 14. 15 af «Ugeskr. F. Læger» d. A". *Ugeskrift for Læger*. Series 3, Vol. 9, No. 29, 18 June 1870, 449–461.

—. "Kjæderbrokbaand". *Ugeskrift for Læger*. Series 3, Vol. 26, No. 30, 28 December 1878, 469–472.

—. "Om Kjædebrokbaand". *Ugeksrift for Læger*. Series 3, Vol. 27, No. 3 & 4, 18 January 1879, 52–53.

—. "Om Virksomheden som kirurgisk Instrumentmager og Bandagist". *Ugeskrift for Læger*. Series 4, Vol. 5, No. 21, 6 May 1882, 313–326.

—. "Om Virksomheden som kirurgisk Instrumentmager og Bandagist". *Ugeksrift for Læger*. Series 4, Vol. 5, No. 28–29, 17 June 1882, 433–437.

Paulli, E., "Undersögelsen af Nethinden i det levende Öie". *Ugeskrift for Læger*. Series 2, Vol. 17, No. 23, 4 December 1852, 353–364.

Philipsen, Harald, "Om antiseptisk Forbinding. Efter Prof. Joseph Lister i Glasgow («The Lancet», 21de Septbr. 1867)". *Ugeskrift for Læger*. Series 3, Vol. 4, No. 25, 28 November 1867, 381–390.

Rasmussen, Anton, "Bekjendtgjørelse." *Ugeskrift for Læger*. Series 3, Vol. 3, No. 12, 2 March 1867, 183.

—. "Dr. Richardsons anæsthesiske Doucheapparat". *Ugeskrift for Læger*. Series 3, Vol. 3, No. 11, 23 February 1867, 175.

—. "Patteflasker med Metalsugerør". *Ugeskrift for Læger*. Series 2, Vol. 41, No. 17, 8 October 1864, 70–71.

—. "Simplifikation af Wintrichs Pandespeil". *Ugeskrift for Læger*. Series 3, Vol. 2, No. 25, 24 November 1866, 390.

Ravn, N. E., "Et Tilfælde af Strubehoste helbredet ved Tracheotomi". *Ugeskrift for Læger*. Series 2, Vol. 21, No. 16, 21 October 1854, 241–253.

Rosborg, C. A., "Hjertats fettsjukdomar, af Richard Quain, M. D.". *Hygiea*. Vol. 15, No. 1. January 1853, 32–46.

Rossander, Carl, "Hans Ranke: Ueber das Thymol und seine Benutzung bei der antiseptischen Behandlung der Wunden". *Hygiea*. Vol. 40, No. 4, April 1878, 205–208.

—. "Nya områden för den antiseptiska sårbehandlingen". *Hygiea*. Vol. 40, No. 6, June 1878, 315–324.

—. "Nya områden för den antiseptiska sårbehandlingen". *Hygiea*. Vol. 40, No. 7, July 1878, 345–368.

—. "Nya områden för den antiseptiska sårbehandlingen". *Hygiea*. Vol. 40, No. 10, October 1878, 529–541.

—. "Nya områden för den antiseptiska sårbehandlingen". *Hygiea*. Vol. 40, No. 11–12, December 1878, 605–625.

—. "Nya områden för den antiseptiska sårbehandlingen IV fortsättning". *Hygiea*. Vol. 41, No. 2, February 1879, 85–98.

—. "R. Volkmann: Die Behandlung der complicirten Fracturen. Klinische Vorträge N:o 117 och 118 (R. Volkmann: Die Behandlung der complicirten Fracturen. Klinische Vorträge N:o 117 and 118)". *Hygiea*. Vol. 40, No. 4, April 1878, 200–205.

—. "Sonnenburg: Zur Diagnose und Therapie der Carbolintoxicationen. Deutsche Zeitschrift für Chirurgie. Band. 9, sid. 356". *Hygiea*. Vol. 40, No. 9, September 1878, 499–501.

Santesson, Carl, "Ett fall af död efter Chloroform; jemte en öfversigt af alla hittills kända likartade olyckshändelser". *Hygiea*. Vol. 12, No. 10, October 1850, 599–624.

Sköldberg, Sven, "Fall af Ovariotomi, III". *Hygiea*. Vol. 29, No. 11, November 1867, 479–481.

—. "Fall af Ovariotomi, VIII". *Hygiea*. Vol. 31, No. 7, July 1869, 316–318.

Snellman, Gerhard, "Beskriftning öfver den i Kemi Socken Terwola Capell gångbara Skått-Sjukan". *Hygiea*. Vol. 12, No. 1, January 1850, 39–47.

Sondén, M., "Diskussion om antiseptica, Berliner kiln. Wochenschr. N:o 17. 1878". *Hygiea*. Vol. 40, No. 5, May 1878, 254–255.

Stenberg. Sten, "Kemisk undersökning af leucocythæmiskt blod". *Hygiea*. Vol. 20, No. 2. February 1858, 83–89.

Stille, A. M. [Max], "Operationsbord för laparotomier och gynekologiska operationer". *Hygiea*. Vol. 59, No. 2, February 1897, 289–290.

Struckmann, C. R., "Et Instrument for Ikke-Kirurger". *Ugeskrift for Læger*. Series 4, Vol. 5, No. 1–2, January 7, 1882, 1–5.

Svalin, O. A., "Om den fibroplastiska tumören; diskussion rörande diagnostiken af svulster, hvilka blifvit ansedde som kräftartade". *Hygiea*. Vol. 15, No. 1, January 1853, 24–32.

Svensson, Ivar, "Om punktion af pleuritiska exsudat". *Hygiea*. Vol. 57, No. 8, August 1895, 122–153.

—. "Från kirurgiska afdelningen af Sabbatsbergs sjukhus". *Hygiea*. Vol. 43, No. 7, July 1881, 321–381.

—. "Operationer verkstälda å Sabbatsbergs sjukhus under år 1881". *Hygiea*. Vol. 44, No. 7, July 1882, 378–383.

Sätherberg, Herman, "Gymnastik och Ortopedi. Belysningar och meddelanden". *Hygiea*. Vol. 24, No. 1, January 1862, 3–27.

—. "Gymnastik och Ortopedi. Belysningar och meddelanden". *Hygiea*. Vol. 24, No. 3, March 1862, 65–85.

—. "Årsberättelse från Gymnastiskt Ortopediska Institutet för år 1859". *Hygiea*. Vol. 23, No. 5, May 1861, 257–262.

Söderberg, Pontus, "Några desinfektionsförsök å Serafimerlasarettets desinfektionsugn". *Hygiea*. Vol. 55, No. 1, January 1893, 1–14.

Trautner, T. M., "Om Bandagistvirksomheden". *Ugeskrift for Læger*. Series 4, Vol. 5, No. 22, 13 May 1882, 343–344.

Trier, Frederik, "A. Rasmussens medikopneumatiske Anstalt i Kjøbenhavn". *Ugeskrift for Læger*. Series 2, Vol. 41, No. 10, 27 August 1864, 152–158.

—. "Nogle Tilfælde af Blodgang som Hospitalssygdom". *Hospitals-Tidende*. Vol. 19, No. 31, 2 August 1876, 481–489.

Törnblom, Alrik, "Notiser i den kirurgiska journallitteraturen". *Hygiea*. Vol. 34, No. 3, March 1872, 144–159.

Wawrinsky, R., "Om desinfektion efter smittosamma sjukdomar. Föreläsning å Karolinska Insitutet den 4 oktober 1890. Af dr R. Wawrinsky". *Hygiea*. Vol. 52, No. 11, November 1890, 798–828.

Warfvinge, F. W., "Redogörelse för sjukvården och ekonomien inom Sabbatsbergs sjukhus under år 1879". *Hygiea*. Vol. 42, No. 4, April 1880, 241–255.

Westermark, F., "Om vaginofixation af den retroflekterade uterus". *Hygiea*. Vol. 56, No. 2, Feburary 1894, 159–170.

Wiborgh, A., "Om antiseptisk förbandstyg". *Hygiea*. Vol. 40, No. 8, August 1878, 413–416.

Widmark, Johan, "Om kokain och desinfektion af ögat vid starroperation". *Hygiea*. Vol. 57, No. 9, September 1895, 189–239.

Wistrand. Alfred Hilarion, "Sammandrag af års-rapporterna från Kongl. Allmänna Garrisons-Sjukhuset I Stockholm för åren 1846–1850, jemte summarisk redogörelse för Sjukvården å Sjukhusets medicinska afdelning under loppet af år 1850". *Hygiea*. Vol. 16, No. 7, July 1851, 385–414.

Åkerman, Jules, "Kirurgisk kasuistik från Malmöhus läns sjukvårdsinrättningar i Lund". *Hygiea*. Vol. 54, No. 10, October 1892, 299–325.

Newspapers

[Anon.], "A. Den industrielle Afdeling af Udstillingen". *Lolland-Falsters Stifts-Tidende*. 31 May 1863.

[Anon.], "Bilder från svenskt industri- och näringslif. Alb. Stilles kirurgiska instrumentfabrik". *Aftonbladet*. 21 February 1903.

[Anon.], "Den danske Afdeling af Udstillingen i London". *Fyens Stiftstidende*. 22 August 1862.

[Anon.], "En mönster-operationssal". *Dagens Nyheter*. 28 Feburary 1894.

[Anon.], "Elektricitet är lif". *Sölvesborgsposten*. 15 April 1874.

[Anon.], "Erkännande från Amerika åt svensk industri". *Smålandsposten*. 9 Feburary 1894.

[Anon.], *Fædrelandet*. 15 January 1856.

[Anon.], *Fædrelandet*. 2 June 1862.

[Anon.], "I förbifarten". *Stockholmstidningen*, 17 January 1903.

[Anon.], "I sista minuten". *Upsala Nya Tidningen*. 21 August 1895.

[Anon.], "Industriudstillingen i Malmø". *Lolland-Falsters Stifts-Tidende*. 17 September 1861.

[Anon.], "Inrikes". *Najaden*. 31 January 1840.

[Anon.], "Lagskipning". *Öresundsposten*. 1 April 1874.

[Anon.], "Lock-outen hos fabrikör Stille. *Upsala Nya Tidningen*. 21 August 1895.

[Anon.], "Lockouten kos [sic] Stilles". *Socialdemokraten*. 23 August 1895.

[Anon.], "Om senaste försöket att vanställa ortopedien och hos allmänheten inplanta fördomar mot ortopediska institutet". *Aftonbladet*. 30 December 1857.

[Anon.], "Om senaste försöket att vanställa ortopedien och hos allmänheten inplanta fördomar mot ortopediska institutet". *Aftonbladet*. 5 January 1858.

[Anon], "Ryskt uppdrag åt svensk". *Sydsvenska dagbladet*. 18 January 1903.

[Anon.], "Særskilte Bekjendtgjørelser". *Tillæg til den Berlingske politiske og Avertissements-Tidende*. 11 May 1849.

[Anon.], "Stilles operationssal vid läkarkongressen i Rom". *Stockholms Dagblad*. 22 April 1894.

[Anon.], "Werldsutställning i Wien". *Aftonbladet*. 28 May 1873.

Heskier, P., [Advertisement]. *Horsens Folkeblad*. 12 January 1877.

—. [Advertisement]. *Horsens Folkebland*. 19 January 1877.

—. [Advertisement]. *Bornholms Tidende*. 14 Feburary 1878.

—. [Advertisement]. *Sorø Amtstidende*. 14 February 1879.

—. [Advertisement]. *Lolland-Falsters Folketidende*. 22 February 1879.

—. [Advertisement]. *Aarhus Amstidende*. 5 November 1881.

—. [Advertisement]. *Stubbekøbing Avis*. 21 February 1882.

—. [Advertisement]. *Svendborg Amtstidende.* 6 September 1882.

—. [Advertisement]. *Kolding Folkeblad.* 11 December 1883.

Nyrop, Camillus, [Advertisement]. *Fredriksborgs Amts Tidende og Adressavis.* 16 May 1865.

—. [Advertisement]. *Göteborgs Handels- och sjöfartstidning.* 4 April 1866.

—. [Advertisement]. *Fædrelandet.* 7 December 1881.

Schiønning [Schiönning], Julius. [Advertisement]. *Nya Kristinehamnposten.* 25 September 1891.

Stille, Albert, [Advertisement]. *Aftonbladet.* 20 October 1845.

—. [Advertisement]. *Aftonbladet.* 6 November 1845.

—. [Advertisement]. *Aftonbladet.* 21 November 1845.

—. [Advertisement]. *Aftonbladet.* 29 November 1845.

—. [Advertisement], *Stockholms Dagblad.* 30 October 1845.

—. [Advertisement], *Stockholms Dagblad.* 6 November 1845.

—. [Advertisement], *Stockholms Dagblad.* 13 November 1845.

—. [Advertisement], *Stockholms Dagblad.* 20 November 1845.

—. [Advertisement], *Stockholms Dagblad.* 27 November 1845.

Patents

Edel, Emil, "Improvement in Trusses". 1877. United States Patent US198586A, filed 14 July 1876, issued 25 December 1877.

Stille, A. M. [Max], "Anordning vid apparater för afbrytande eller rättställande af lemmar à menniskokroppen". 1896. Swedish patent SE7872C1, filed 1 December 1896, issued 15 May 1897.

—. "Anordning vid operationssoffor". 1895. Swedish patent SE6315C1, filed 15 January 1895, issued 7 September 1895.

—. "Anordning vid operationssoffor". 1896. Swedish patent SE6756C1, filed 23 December 1895, issued 11 April 1896, [modification of SE6315C1].

—. "Anordning vid väskor för transport och förvaring af desinfektions- eller steriliseringskärl". 1897. Swedish patent SE7470C1, filed 11 February 1896, issued 16 January 1897.

—. "Bårsäng". 1894. Swedish patent SE5351C1, filed 8 March 1894, issued 11 August 1894.

—. "Instrument för uppklippning af hufvudskålsbenen, gipsbandage och dylikt". 1895. Swedish patent SE6729C1, filed 8 November 1895, issued 21 March 1896.

—. "Kombinerad instrumentkokare och sköljkanna". 1897. Swedish patent SE8415C1, filed 1 April 1897, issued 30 October 1897.

—. "Lyftinrättning vid operationsbord, sjuksängar m.m.". 1893. Swedish patent SE4720C1, filed 5 July 1893, issued 18 November 1893.

Literature

Adams, Annemarie, "Surgery and Architecture: Spaces for Operating", in *The Palgrave Handbook of the History of Surgery*, Thomas Schlich (ed.), 261–281. London: Palgrave Macmillan, 2018.

Alberti, Samuel J. M. M., "Shaping Scientific Instrument Collections: A Historiography". *Journal of the History of Collections*. Vol. 31, No. 3, November 2019, 445–452.

Amelin, Olov. *Medaljens baksida: Instrumentmakaren Daniel Ekström och hans efterföljare i 1700-talets Sverige*. Diss. Uppsala University, 1999.

Amster, Ellen. *Medicine and the Saints: Science, Islam and the Colonial Encounter in Morocco, 1877–1956*. Austin: University of Texas Press, 2013.

Anderson, Julie, et. al. *Surgeons, Manufacturers and Patients: A Transatlantic History of Total Hip Replacement*. Basingstoke: Palgrave Macmillan, 2007.

Arnold, Ken. And Söderqvist, Thomas, "Medical Instruments in Museums: Immediate Impressions and Historical Meanings". *Isis*. Vol. 102, No. 4, December 2011, 718–729.

Asdal, Kristin, "Contexts in Action–And the Future of the Past in STS". *Science, Technology, and Human Values*. Vol. 37, No. 4, April 2012, 379–403.

Asdal, Kristin. And Jordheim, Helge, "Texts on the Move: Textuality and Historicity Revisited". *History and Theory*. Vol. 57, No. 1, March 2018, 56–74.

Asdal, Kristin. And Moser, Ingunn, "Experiments in Context and Contexting". *Science, Technology, and Human Values*. Vol. 34, No. 4, July 2012, 291–306.

Berg, Annika. *Den gränslösa hälsan: Signe och Axel Höjer, folkhälsan och expertisen*. Diss. Uppsala University, 2008.

van Bergen, Leo, "Surgery and War: The Discussions About the Usefulness of War for Medical Progress", in *The Palgrave Handbook of the History of Surgery*, Thomas Schlich (ed.), 389–407. London: Palgrave Macmillan, 2018.

Biagioli, Mario, "From Print to Patents: Living on Instruments in Early Modern Europe". *History of Science*. Vol. 44, No. 2, June 2006, 139–186.

—. "Rights or Rewards?: Changing Frameworks of Scientific Authorship", in *Scientific Authorship: Credit and Intellectual Property in Science*, Mario Biagioli and Peter Galison (eds.), 253–279. New York: Routledge, 2003.

Björk, Elin. *Att bota en prostata: Kastrering som behandlingsmetod för prostatahypertrofi 1893–1910*. Diss. Linköping University, 2019.

Blume, Stuart. *Insight and Industry: On the Dynamics of Technological Change in Medicine*. Cambridge, Mass.; MIT Press, 1992.

—. "The Politics of Endpoints", in *Devices and Designs: Medical Technologies in Historical Perspective*, Carsten Timmermann and Julie Anderson (eds.), 249–272. Basingstoke: Palgrave Macmillan, 2006.

Boox, Mikael, "Svenska frivilliga till Danmark: Krigen 1848–1850 och 1864". *Militärhistorisk tidskrift*. 2004, 13–68.

Bowen, Diana K. et. al., "Sounds and Charrière: The Rest of the Story". *Journal of Pediatric Urology*. Vol 10, 2014, 1106-1110.

Bracegirdle, Brian, "J. J. Lister and the Establishment of Histology". *Medical History*. Vol. 21, No. 2, April 1977, 187–191.

Brieger, Gert H., "From Conservative to Radical Surgery in Late Nineteenth-Century America", in *Medical Theory, Surgical Practice*, Christopher Lawrence (ed.), 216–231. London: Routledge, 1992.

Broberg, Gunnar, "Liten svensk medicinhistoria", in *Til at stwdera läkedom: Tio studier i svensk medicinhistoria*, Gunnar Broberg (ed.), 9–50. Lund: Sekel, 2008.

Brock, Claire, "Risk, Responsibility and Surgery in the 1890s and Early 1900s". *Medical History*. Vol. 57, No. 3, 2013, 317–337.

Brändström, Anders, "The Silent Sick: Life-Histories of 19th Century Swedish Hospital Patients", in *Health and Population During the Demographic Transition Society*, A. Brändström & L. G. Tedebrand (eds.), 343–368. Umeå: Almqvist and Wiksell, 1988.

Bynum, William F. *Science and the Practice of Medicine in the Nineteenth Century*. Cambridge: Cambridge University Press, 1994.

Carneiro, Ana. et al., "Shaping Doctors and Society: The Portuguese Medical Press (1880–1926)". *Media History*. Vol. 25, No. 1, 2019, 23–50.

Carroll, Katherine, "Creating the Modern Physician: The Architecture of American Medical Schools in the Era of Medical Education Reform". *Journal of the Society of Architectural Historians*. Vol. 75, 2016, 48–73.

Chakrabarti, Pratik. *Bacteriology in British India: Laboratory Medicine and the Tropics*. Rochester: Boydell & Brewer, 2012.

Chaloner, E. J., et. al., "Amputations at the London Hospital, 1852–1857". *Journal of the Royal Society of Medicine*. Vol. 94, No. 8, August 2001, 409–412.

Condran, Gretchen A., "The Elusive Role of Scientific Medicine in Mortality Decline: Diphtheria in Nineteenth- and Early Twentieth-Century Philadelphia". *Journal of the History of Medicine and Allied Sciences*. Vol. 63, No. 4. October 2008, 484–522.

Crenner, Christopher. *Private Practice: In the Early Twentieth-Century Medical Office of Dr. Richard Cabot*. Balitmore: Johns Hopkins University Press, 2005.

Danish Medicines Agency. *Medical devices*. 13 February 2019. https://laegemiddel styrelsen.dk/en/devices (Accessed 14 January 2020).

Daston, Lorraine. And Galison, Peter. *Objectivity*. New York: Zone Books, 2010.

Davis, Audrey B., "Historical Studies of Medical Instruments". *History of Science*. Vol. 16, No. 2, June 1978, 107–133.

Drakman, Annelie. *När kroppen slot sig och blev fast: varför åderlåtning, miasmateori och klimatmedicin övergavs vid 1800-talets mitt*. Diss. Uppsala University, 2018.

Edmonson, James M. *American Surgical Instruments: An Illustrated History of Their Manufacture and a Directory of Instrument Makers to 1900*. San Francisco: Norman Publishing, 1997.

—. "History of the Instruments for Gastrointestinal Endoscopy". *Gastrointestinal Endoscopy*. Vol. 37, No. 2, March 1991, 27–56.

Eivergård, Mikael. *Frihetens milda disciplin: Normalisering och social styrning i svensk sinnessjukvård 1850–1970*. Diss. Umeå University, 2003.

—. "Frihet, makt och disciplin: om social styrning i svensk sinnesjukvård", in *Att rätt förfoga över tingen: Historiska studier av styrning och maktutövning*, Johannes Fredriksson and Esbjörn Larsson, 157–171, Uppsala: Opscula historica Upsaliensia, 2007.

Eklöf, Motzi. *Läkarens Ethos: Studier i den svenska läkarkårens identiteter, intressen och ideal, 1890–1960*. Diss. Tema Hälsa och samhälle, Linköping University, 2000.

Feldmann, H., "Der Nasenrachenraum und die Rachenmandel in der Geschichte der Otologie und Rhinologie". *Laryngorhinootologie*. Vol. 78, No. 5, 1999, 280–289.

Felski, Rita, "Context Stinks!". *New Literary History*. Vol. 42, No. 4, Autumn 2011, 573–591.

Fleck, Ludwik, "To Look, To See, To Know", in *Cognition and Fact: Materials on Ludwik Fleck*. Robert S. Cohen and Thomas Schnelle (eds.), 129–151. Dordrecht: D. Reidel Publishing Company, 1986.

Fox, N. J., "Scientific Theory Choice and Social Structure: The Case of Joseph Lister's Antisepsis, Humoral Theory and Asepsis". *History of Science*. Vol. 26, No. 4, December 1988, 367–397.

Frampton, Sally, "Defining Difference: Competing Forms of Ovarian Surgery in the Nineteenth Century", in *Technological Change in Modern Surgery: Historical Perspectives on Innovation*, Thomas Schlich and Christopher Crenner (eds.), 51–70. Rochester: University of Rochester Press, 2017.

—. "Opening the Abdomen: The Expansion of Surgery", in *The Palgrave Handbook of the History of Surgery*, Thomas Schlich (ed.), 175–194. London: Palgrave Macmillan, 2018.

Frampton, Sally. And Wallis, Jennerifer (eds.). *Reading the Nineteenth-Century Medical Journal*. New York: Routledge, 2021.

Gabriel, Joseph M. *Medical Monopoly: Intellectual Property Rights and the Origins of the Modern Pharmaceutical Industry*. Chicago: The University of Chicago Press, 2014.

Gieryn, Thomas. *Cultural Boundaries of Science: Credibility on the Line*. Chicago: The University of Chicago Press, 1999.

Graninger, Ulrika. *Från osynligt till synligt: Bakteriologins etablering i sekelskiftets svenska medicin*. Diss. Linköping University, 1997.

Gullers, Peter. *Verktygsmakare & operatörer: Några aspekter på den kirurgiska instrumenttillverknings svenska historia*. Report 37. Stockholm: Arbetslivscentrum, 1982.

Halverson, Kristin, "Medical Technologies and the Social Strategies of Two Surgical Instrument Makers in Denmark and Sweden, 1870–1900". *Acta medico-historica Rigensia*. Vol. 14, 2021, 101–117.

Hart Hansen, Ole, "Saxtorph, Holmer og Listers antiseptik". *Ugeskrift for Læger*. Vol. 169, No. 35. 24 August 2007, 2863.

van Helden, Albert. And Hankins, Thomas L. (eds.). *Instruments*. Chicago: The University of Chicago Press, 1994.

Henriksen, Ingrid. And Kærgård, Niels, "The Scandinavian Currency Union 1875–1914", in *International Monetary Systems in Historical Perspective*, Reis J. (eds.), 91-112. London: Palgrave Macmillan, 1995.

Hemmungs Wirtén, Eva, "The Patent and the Paper: A Few Thoughts on Late Modern Science and Intellectual Property". *Culture Unbound: Journal of Current Cultural Research*. Vol. 7, 2015, 600–609.

Hodges, Sarah, "The Global Menace". *Social History of Medicine*. Vo. 25, No. 3, August 2012, 719–728.

Huisman, Frank, "Transcending the Language Barrier: Medical History in a Globalizing World". *European Journal for the History of Medicine and Health*. Vol. 78, 2021, 15–20.

Jansson, Måns. *Making Metal Making: Circulation of Workshop Practices in the Swedish Metal Trades, 1730–1775*. Diss. Uppsala University, 2017.

Johannisson, Karin. *Det mätbara samhället: statistik och samhällsdröm i 1700-talets Europa*. Stockholm: Nordstedts, 1988.

—. "Kliniken: medicinens praktik", in *Medicinen blir till vetenskap: Karolinska Institutet under två århundraden*, Karin Johannisson, Ingemar Nilsson and Roger Qvarsell (eds.), 43–83. Stockholm: Karolinska Institutet University Press, 2010.

—. *Kroppens tunna skal: Sex essäer om kropp, historia and kultur*. Stockholm: Pan, 1997.

Johnson, Jennifer, "New Directions in the History of Medicine in European, Colonial and Transimperial Contexts". *Contemporary European History*. Vol. 25, No. 2, May 2016, 387–399.

Jones, Claire L., "A Barrier to Medical Treatment? British Medical Practitioners, Medical Appliances and the Patent, 1870–1920". *British Journal for the History of Science*. Vol. 49, No. 4, December 2016, 601–625.

—. *The Medical Trade Catalogue in Britain, 1870–1914*. London: Pickering & Chatto, 2013.

—. "Surgical Instruments: History and Historiography", in *The Palgrave Handbook of the History of Surgery*, Thomas Schlich (ed.), 235–257. London: Palgrave Macmillan, 2018.

Jülich, Solveig. *Skuggor av sanning: Tidig svensk radiologi och visuell kultur*. Diss. Linköping University, 2002.

Kett, Joseph F. *The Formation of the American Medical Profession: The Role of Institutions, 1780–1860*. New Haven: Yale University Press, 1968.

Kirkup, J. *The Evolution of Surgical Instruments: An Illustrated History from Ancient Times to the Twentieth Century*. Novato, CA: Norman Publishing, 2006.

Kisacky, Jeanne, "Germs are in the Details: Aseptic Design and General Contractors at the Lying-In Hospital in the City of New York, 1897–1901". *Construction History*. Vol. 28, No. 1, 2013, 83–106.

—. *Rise of the Modern Hospital: An Architectural History of Health and Healing, 1870–1940*. Pittsburgh: University of Pittsburgh Press, 2017.

Kock, Wolfram. *Kungl. Serafimerlasarettet, 1752–1952: En studie i svensk sjukvårdshistoria*. Jönköping: H. Halls Boktr. A.-B., 1952.

Kremer, Richard L., "Building Institutes for Physiology in Prussia, 1836–1846: Contexts, Interests and Rhetoric", in *The Laboratory Revolution in Medicine*. Andrew Cunningham and Perry Williams (eds.), 72–109. Cambridge: Cambridge University Press, 2002.

Kristenson, Hjördis. *Vetenskapens byggnader under 1800-talet: Lund och Europa*. Stockholm: The Swedish Museum of Architecture, 1990.

Kärnfelt, Johan, "Ett misslyckat stativ", in *Kunskap i rörelse: Kungl. Vetenskapsakademien och skapandet af det moderna samhället*, Johan Kärnfelt, Karl Grandin and Solveig Jülich (eds.), 475–481. Stockholm; Makadam, 2018.

—. "Vetenskapsakademiens Herschel-teleskop: En instrumentbiografi". *Slagmark*. Vol. 81, 2020, 133–154.

La Berge, Ann, "Medical Microscopy in Paris, 1830–1855", in *French Medical Culture in the Nineteenth Century*, Ann La Berge and Mordechai Feingold (eds.). 296–326. Amsterdam: Editions Rodopi, 1994.

La langue française. [n.a.]. Bandagiste. https://www.lalanguefrancaise.com/dictionnaire/definition/bandagiste (Accessed November 5, 2021).

de Laet. Marianne. And Mol, Annemarie, "The Zimbabwe Bush Pump: Mechanics of a Fluid Technology". *Social Studies of Science*. Vol. 30, No. 2, April 2000, 225–263.

Lagerqvist, Lars O. *Vad kostade det? Priser och läner, från medeltid till våra dagar*. Lund: Historiska Media, 2011.

Larsen, Klas, "Her fødtes dansk underlivskirurgi". *Ugeskrift for Læger*. 25 June 2018. https://ugeskriftet.dk/nyhed/her-foedtes-dansk-underlivskirurgi (Accessed 27 November 2021).

Latour, Bruno. *The Pasteurization of France*. Trans. Alan Sheridan and John Law. Cambridge, Massachusetts: Harvard University Press, 1988.

Law, John, "After ANT: complexity, naming and topology", in *Actor Network Theory and After*, John Law and John Hassard (eds.), 1–14. Oxford: Blackwell Publishing, 1999.

LeVay, David. *The History of Orthopaedics: An Account of the Study and Practice of Orthopaedics from the Earliest Times to the Modern Era*. Lancashire: The Parthenon Publishing Group, 1990.

Lightman, Bernard V. (ed.). *Isis*. Vol. 102, No. 4, December 2011.

Lindberg, Bo. *Obstetriska instrument: en historia om gamla förlossningsinstrument i Medicinhistoriska museet i Uppsala*. Uppsala: Acta Universitatis Upsaliensis, 2020.

Ling, Sofia. *Kärringmedicin och vetenskap: Läkare och kvacksalverianklagade I Sverige omkring 1770–1870*. Diss. Uppsala: Uppsala University, 2004.

Lov nr 431 of 10/06/2003, *Lov om bandagister*.

Meyerson, Åke. *Studier I Serafimerlasarettets instrumentsamling: Utgivna med anledning av lasarettets 200-årsjubileum*. Stockholm: Karolinska Institute's Surgical Clinic at Seraphim Hospital, 1952.

Milm, Stephen, "'A Limb Which Shall Be Presentable in Polite Society': Prosthetic Technologies in the Nineteenth Century", in *Artificial Parts, Practice Lives: Modern*

Histories of Prosthetics, Katherine Ott, et. al. (eds.), 282–299. New York: NYU Press, 2002.

Minuzzi, Sabrina, "'Quick to say Quack': Medicinal Secrets from the Household to the Apothecary's Shop in Eighteenth-Century Venice". *Social History of Medicine.* Vol. 32, No. 1, February 2019, 1–33.

Mol, Annemarie. *The Body Multiple: Ontology in Medical Practice.* Durham, NC: Duke University Press, 2003.

Mukharji, Projit Bihari. *Doctoring Traditions: Ayurveda, Small Technologies, and Braided Sciences.* Chicago: The University of Chicago Press, 2016.

Mößner, Nicola, "Scientific Images as Circulating Ideas: An Application of Ludwik Fleck's Thought Styles". *Journal for General Philosophy of Science/Zeitschrift für allgemeine Wissenschaftstheorie.* Vol. 47, No. 2, September 2016, 307–329.

Nilsonne, Harald, "Poul Guildal: In Memoriam". *Acta Orthopaedic Scandinavica.* Vol. 20, No. 3, 1951, 181–183.

Nilsson, Ingemar, "Vetenskapen: medicinens teori", in *Medicinen blir till vetenskap: Karolinska Institutet under två århundraden*, Karin Johannisson, Ingemar Nilsson and Roger Qvarsell (eds.), 13–41. Stockholm: Karolinska Institutet University Press, 2010.

Nilsson, Ulrika. *Kampen om Kvinnan: Professionalisering och konstruktioner av kön I svensk gynekologi 1860–1925.* Diss. Uppsala University, 2003.

Nyland, Nick. *De praktiserande læger I Danmark, 1800–1910: Træk af det historiske grundlag for almen medicin.* Odense: Audit Projekt Odense, 2000.

Nyrop, C., "Rasmussen, Anton Gustav Casimir". *Dansk biografisk Lexikon.* C. F. Bricka (ed.). 503. Volume 8. Copenhagen: Gyldendalske Boghandels Forlag, 1899.

—. *Camillus Nyrop og det kirurgiske Instrumentmageri i Danmark.* Copenhagen: Nielsen & Lydiche, 1884.

—. *Slægten Nyrop: Nogle biografiske oplysninger.* Copenhagen, Nielsen & Lydiche, 1908.

O'Connor, Erin, "'Fractions of Men': Engendering Amputation in Victorian Culture". *Comparative Studies in Society and History.* Vol. 39, No. 4, October 1997, 742–777.

Ordbog over det danske Sprog. [n.a.]. Bandagist. https://ordnet.dk/ods/ordbog?query=bandagist (Accessed November 5, 2021).

Ottosson, Anders, "The Manipulated History of Manipulations of Spines and Joints? Rethinking Orthopaedic Medicine Through the 19th Century Discourse of European Mechanical Medicine". *Medicine Studies.* Vol. 3, No. 2 December 2011, 83–116.

Pennington, T. H., "Listerism, its Decline and Persistence: The Introduction of Aseptic Surgical Techniques in Three British Teaching Hospitals, 1890–1899". *Medical History.* Vol. 39, No. 1, January 1995, 35–60.

Pernick, Martin S., "The Calculus of Suffering in Nineteenth-Century Surgery". *The Hastings Centre Report.* Vol. 13, No. 2, April 1983, 26–36.

Petersen, Jul., "Anders Georg Drachmann". *Dansk biografisk Lexikon*, IV Bind Clemens-Eynden. Copenhagen: Gyldendalske Boghandels Forlag, 1890.

—. "Camillus Nyrop". *Dansk biografisk Lexikon*. Copenhagen: Gyldendalske Boghandels Forlag, 1898.

Pickstone, John V., "Bones in Lancashire: Towards Long-term Contextual Analysis of Medical Technology", in *Devices and Designs: Medical Technologies in Historical Perspective*, Carsten Timmermann and Julie Anderson (eds.), 17–36. Basingstoke: Palgrave Macmillan, 2006.

—. *Ways of Knowing: A New History of Science, Technology and Medicine*. Chicago: The University of Chicago Press, 2000.

Polanyi, Michael. *The Tacit Dimension*. Garden City, New York: Doubleday & Company, 1966.

Porter, Roy, "Introduction", in *Medical Journals and Medical Knowledge: Historical Essays*. William F. Bynum, Stephen Lock and Roy Porter (eds.), 1–5. New York: Routledge, 2019.

—. "The Rise of Medical Journalism in Britain to 1800", in *Medical Journals and Medical Knowledge: Historical Essays*. William F. Bynum, Stephen Lock and Roy Porter (eds.), 6–28. New York: Routledge, 2019.

Qvarsell, Roger, "Historia och medicin–En studie av svenska medicinhistoriska avhandlingar 1970–2004", in *Medicinhistoria idag: Perspektiv på det samtida svenska forskningsfältet*, Eva Åhrén (ed.), 19–40, Stockholm: Nobel Museum Occasional Papers, 2007.

Reinarz, Jonathan, "Mechanizing Medicine: Medical Innovations and the Birmingham Voluntary Hospitals in the Nineteenth Century", in *Devices and Designs: Medical Technologies in Historical Perspective*, Carsten Timmermann and Julie Anderson (eds.), 37–60. Basingstoke: Palgrave Macmillan, 2006.

Riotte, Torsten, "Medical Negligence in Nineteenth-Century Germany", in *Progress and Pathology: Medicine and Culture in the Nineteenth Century*, Melissa Dickson, et. al. (eds.), 56–77. Manchester: Manchester University Press, 2020.

Riving, Cecilia. *Icke som en annan människa: Psykisk sjukdom i mötet mellan psykiatri och lokalsamhället under 1800-talets andra hälft*. Diss. Lund University, Gidlunds förlag, 2008.

Roberts, Lissa, "Introduction", in *The Mindful Hand: Inquiry and Invention from the Late Renaissance to Early Industrialisation*, Lissa Roberts, et. al. (eds.), 1–7. Amsterdam: Edita KNAW, 2007.

Roberts, Lissa. And Schaffer, Simon, "Preface", in *The Mindful Hand: Inquiry and Invention from the Late Renaissance to Early Industrialisation*, Lissa Roberts, et. al. (eds.), xiii–xxvii. Amsterdam: Edita KNAW, 2007.

Runefelt, Leif. *Den magiska spegeln: Kvinnan och varan i pressens annonser 1870–1914*. Lund: Nordic Academic Press, 2019.

Rørbye, Birgitte. *Mellem sundhed og sygdom. Om fortid, fremskridt og virkelige læger: en narrative kulturanalyse*. Copenhagen: Museum Tusculanmus forlag, 2002.

Sachs, Michael. *Geschichte der operativen Chirurgie, ii; Historische Entwicklung des chirurgischen Instrumentariums.* Heidelberg: Kaden Verlag, 2001.

Schlich, Thomas, "Asepsis and Bacteriology: A Realignment of Surgery and Laboratory Science". *Medical History.* Vol. 56, No. 3, 2012, 308–334.

—. "Farmer to Industrialist: Lister's Antisepsis and the Making of Modern Surgery in Germany". *Notes and Records of the Royal Society of London.* Vol. 67, No. 3, 20 September 2013, 245–260.

—. "Introduction: What Is Special About the History of Surgery", in *The Palgrave Handbook of the History of Surgery,* Thomas Schlich (ed.), 1–24. London: Palgrave Macmillan, 2018.

—. "Negotiating Technologies in Surgery: The Controversy about Surgical Gloves in the 1890s". *Bulletin of the History of Medicine.* Vol. 87, No. 2, Summer 2013, 170–197.

—. *The Origins of Organ Transplantation: Surgery and Laboratory Science, 1880–1930.* Rochester: Rochester University Press, 2010.

—. *Surgery, Science and Industry: A Revolution in Fracture Care, 1950s–1990s.* Basingstoke: Palgrave MacMillan, 2002.

—. "Surgery, Science and Modernity: Operating Rooms and Laboratories as Spaces of Control". *History of Science.* Vol. 45, No. 3, September 2007, 231–256.

Schlich, Thomas. And Crenner, Christopher, "Technological Change in Surgery: An Introduction Essay", in *Technological Change in Modern Surgery: Historical Perspectives on Innovation,* Thomas Schlich and Christopher Crenner (eds.), 1–20. Rochester: University of Rochester Press, 2017.

Schmidgen, Henning, "Pictures, Preparations, and Living Processes: The Production of Immediate Visual Perception (Anschauung) in Late-19th-Century Physiology". *Journal of the History of Biology.* Vol. 37, No. 3, Autumn 2004, 477–513.

Singer, Charles, "Notes on the Early History of Microscopy". *Proceedings of the Royal Society of Medicine.* Vol. 7, 1914, 247–279.

Skagius, Peter. *Den offentliga ohälsan: En historisk studie av barnpsykologi och psykiatri i svensk media, 1968–2008.* Diss. Linköping University, 2020.

Snow, Stephanie J., "Surgery and Anaesthesia: Revolutions in Practice", in *The Palgrave Handbook of the History of Surgery,* Thomas Schlich (ed.), 195–214. London: Palgrave Macmillan, 2018.

Staubermann, Klaus, et. al., "Intangible Heritage: Connecting Astronomical Telescopes and Their Users". *Journal of Astronomical History and Heritage.* Vol. 24, No. 3, September 2021, 776–788.

Stevens, Rosemary. *In Sickness and in Wealth: American Hospitals in the Twentieth Century.* Baltimore: Johns Hopkins University Press, 1999.

Svenska Akademiens ordlista. [n.a.]. Bandagist. https://svenska.se/saol/?sok=bandagist (Accessed November 5, 2021).

Swedish Medical Products Agency. *Medical Devices.* 9 July 2009. https://lakemedels verket.se/english/product/Medical-devices/ (Accessed 14 January 2020).

Sørensen, Torsten, "Træk af ovariotomiens historie: Privathospitalet på Jelling Mark", in *Dansk Medicinhistorisk Årbog*, Nils Rosdahl, et. al. (eds.), 40–55, Viborg: Specialtrykkeriet Viborg A/S, 2008.

Taylor, Jeremy. *The Architect and the Pavilion Plan Hospital: Dialogue and Design Creativity in England, 1850–1914*. London: Leicester University Press, 1997.

Tomes, Nancy J. And Warner, John Harley, "Introduction to the Special Issue on Rethinking the Reception of the Germ Theory of Disease: Comparative Perspectives". *Journal of the History of Medicine and Allied Sciences*.Vol. 52, No. 1, January 1997, 7–16.

Turner, David, "Disability and Prosthetics in Eighteenth- and Early Nineteenth-Century England". *The Routledge History of Disease*, Mark Jackson (ed.), 301–319. New York: Routledge, 2017.

Trangbæk, Else. *Kvindernes idræt: Fra rødder til top*. Copenhagen: Gyldendal, 2005.

Tuck, Eve. And Yang, K. Wayne, "Decolonization is not a metaphor". *Decolonization: Indigeneity, Education & Society*. Vol. 1, No. 1, 2012, 1–40.

Twohig, Peter, "Innovating Expertise: X-Ray and Laboratory Workers in the Canadian Hospital, 1920–1950", in *Devices and Designs: Medical Technologies in Historical Perspective*, Carsten Timmermann and Julie Anderson (eds.), 74–94. Basingstoke: Palgrave Macmillan, 2006.

Tybjer, Karin, "Sharp and Telling: Surgical Collections as Instruments of Medicine, History and Culture". *Journal of the History of Collections*. Vol. 31, No. 3, November 2019, 547–562.

Ueyama, Takahiro. *Health in the Marketplace: Professionalism, Therapeutic Desires, and Medical Commodification in Late-Victorian London*. Palo Alto: Society for the Promotion of Science and Scholarship, 2010.

Vallgårda, Signild, "'...Som et træ til sine grene... ': specialisering af lægestanden fra slutningen af 1600-tallet til 1917", in *Historiens kultur, Fortælling, kritik, metode*, Ning de Coninck-Smith, et. al. (eds.), 81–96. Copenhagen: Museum Tusculanum, 1997.

—. "Who Went to a General Hospital in the Eighteenth and Nineteenth Centuries in Copenhagen?". *European Journal of Public Health*, Vol. 9, No. 2, June 1999, 97–102.

Vallgårda, Signild, et. al. *Sundhedsvæsen og sundhedspolitik*. Copenhagen: Munksgaard, 2010.

Vej nr 123 of 20/07/1995, *Vejledning om uddannelse af bandagister (Til sygehusforvaltninger, social- og sundhedsforvaltninger m.fl.)*.

Wallis, Faith, "Pre-Modern Surgery: Wounds, Words and the Paradox of Tradition", in *The Palgrave Handbook of the History of Surgery*, Thomas Schlich (ed.), 49–70. London: Palgrave Macmillan, 2018.

Wall, Rosemary. And Hallet, Christine E., "Nursing and Surgery: Professionalisation, Education and Innovation", in *The Palgrave Handbook of the History of Surgery*, Thomas Schlich (ed.), 153–174.

Wangenstein, Owen H. *The Rise of Surgery: From Empiric Craft to Scientific Discipline*. Minneapolis: University of Minnesota Press, 1978.

Werrett, Simon. *Thrifty Science: Making the Most of Materials in the History of Experiment*. Chicago: The University of Chicago Press, 2019.

Worboys, Michael, "Joseph Lister and the Performance of Antiseptic Surgery". *Notes and Records of The Royal Society*. Vol. 67, No. 3, September 2013, 199–209.

—. "The History of Surgical Wound Infection: Revolution or Evolution", in *The Palgrave Handbook of the History of Surgery*, Thomas Schlich (ed.), 215–233. London: Palgrave Macmillan, 2018.

—. *Spreading Germs: Disease Theories and Medical Practice in Britain, 1865–1900*. Cambridge: Cambridge University Press, 2000.

World Health Organization. "Medical devices: Medical Device–Full Definition". 2019. http://www.who.int/medical_devices/full_deffinition/en/ (Accessed 18 November 2019).

Åhrén, Eva. *Döden, kroppen och moderniteten*. Diss. Carlssons bokförlag, 2002.

Åman, Anders. *Om den offentliga vården: Byggnader och verksamheter vid svenska vårdinstitutioner under 1800- och 1900-talen. En arkitekturhistorisk undersökning*. Stockholm: LiberFörlag, 1976.

Södertörn Doctoral Dissertations

1. Jolanta Aidukaite, *The Emergence of the Post-Socialist Welfare State: The case of the Baltic States: Estonia, Latvia and Lithuania*, 2004

2. Xavier Fraudet, *Politique étrangère française en mer Baltique (1871–1914): de l'exclusion à l'affirmation*, 2005

3. Piotr Wawrzeniuk, *Confessional Civilising in Ukraine: The Bishop Iosyf Shumliansky and the Introduction of Reforms in the Diocese of Lviv 1668–1708*, 2005

4. Andrej Kotljarchuk, *In the Shadows of Poland and Russia: The Grand Duchy of Lithuania and Sweden in the European Crisis of the mid-17th Century*, 2006

5. Håkan Blomqvist, *Nation, ras och civilisation i svensk arbetarrörelse före nazismen*, 2006

6. Karin S Lindelöf, *Om vi nu ska bli som Europa: Könsskapande och normalitet bland unga kvinnor i transitionens Polen*, 2006

7. Andrew Stickley. *On Interpersonal Violence in Russia in the Present and the Past: A Sociological Study*, 2006

8. Arne Ek, *Att konstruera en uppslutning kring den enda vägen: Om folkrörelsers modernisering i skuggan av det Östeuropeiska systemskiftet*, 2006

9. Agnes Ers, *I mänsklighetens namn: En etnologisk studie av ett svenskt biståndsprojekt i Rumänien*, 2006

10. Johnny Rodin, *Rethinking Russian Federalism: The Politics of Intergovernmental Relations and Federal Reforms at the Turn of the Millennium*, 2006

11. Kristian Petrov, *Tillbaka till framtiden: Modernitet, postmodernitet och generationsidentitet i Gorbačevs glasnost' och perestrojka*, 2006

12. Sophie Söderholm Werkö, *Patient patients? Achieving Patient Empowerment through Active Participation, Increased Knowledge and Organisation*, 2008

13. Peter Bötker, *Leviatan i arkipelagen: Staten, förvaltningen och samhället. Fallet Estland*, 2007

14. Matilda Dahl, *States under scrutiny: International organizations, transformation and the construction of progress*, 2007

15. Margrethe B. Søvik, *Support, resistance and pragmatism: An examination of motivation in language policy in Kharkiv, Ukraine*, 2007

16. Yulia Gradskova, *Soviet People with female Bodies: Performing beauty and maternity in Soviet Russia in the mid 1930–1960s*, 2007

17. Renata Ingbrant, *From Her Point of View: Woman's Anti-World in the Poetry of Anna Świrszczyńska*, 2007

18. Johan Eellend, *Cultivating the Rural Citizen: Modernity, Agrarianism and Citizenship in Late Tsarist Estonia*, 2007

19. Petra Garberding, *Musik och politik i skuggan av nazismen: Kurt Atterberg och de svensk-tyska musikrelationerna*, 2007

20. Aleksei Semenenko, *Hamlet the Sign: Russian Translations of Hamlet and Literary Canon Formation*, 2007

21. Vytautas Petronis, *Constructing Lithuania: Ethnic Mapping in the Tsarist Russia, ca. 1800–1914*, 2007

22. Akvile Motiejunaite, *Female employment, gender roles, and attitudes: the Baltic countries in a broader context*, 2008

23. Tove Lindén, *Explaining Civil Society Core Activism in Post-Soviet Latvia*, 2008

24. Pelle Åberg, *Translating Popular Education: Civil Society Cooperation between Sweden and Estonia*, 2008

25. Anders Nordström, *The Interactive Dynamics of Regulation: Exploring the Council of Europe's monitoring of Ukraine*, 2008

26. Fredrik Doeser, *In Search of Security After the Collapse of the Soviet Union: Foreign Policy Change in Denmark, Finland and Sweden, 1988–1993*, 2008

27. Zhanna Kravchenko. *Family (versus) Policy: Combining Work and Care in Russia and Sweden*, 2008

28. Rein Jüriado, *Learning within and between public-private partnerships*, 2008

29. Elin Boalt, *Ecology and evolution of tolerance in two cruciferous species*, 2008

30. Lars Forsberg, *Genetic Aspects of Sexual Selection and Mate Choice in Salmonids*, 2008

31. Eglė Rindzevičiūtė, *Constructing Soviet Cultural Policy: Cybernetics and Governance in Lithuania after World War II*, 2008

32. Joakim Philipson, *The Purpose of Evolution: 'struggle for existence' in the Russian-Jewish press 1860–1900*, 2008

33. Sofie Bedford, *Islamic activism in Azerbaijan: Repression and mobilization in a post-Soviet context*, 2009

34. Tommy Larsson Segerlind, *Team Entrepreneurship: A process analysis of the venture team and the venture team roles in relation to the innovation process*, 2009

35. Jenny Svensson, *The Regulation of Rule-Following: Imitation and Soft Regulation in the European Union*, 2009

36. Stefan Hallgren, *Brain Aromatase in the guppy, Poecilia reticulate: Distribution, control and role in behavior*, 2009

37. Karin Ellencrona, *Functional characterization of interactions between the flavivirus NS5 protein and PDZ proteins of the mammalian host*, 2009

38. Makiko Kanematsu, *Saga och verklighet: Barnboksproduktion i det postsovjetiska Lettland*, 2009

39. Daniel Lindvall, *The Limits of the European Vision in Bosnia and Herzegovina: An Analysis of the Police Reform Negotiations*, 2009

40. Charlotta Hillerdal, *People in Between–Ethnicity and Material Identity: A New Approach to Deconstructed Concepts*, 2009

41. Jonna Bornemark, *Kunskapens gräns–gränsens vetande*, 2009

42. Adolphine G. Kateka, *Co-Management Challenges in the Lake Victoria Fisheries: A Context Approach*, 2010

43. René León Rosales, *Vid framtidens hitersta gräns: Om pojkar och elevpositioner i en multietnisk skola*, 2010

44. Simon Larsson, *Intelligensaristokrater och arkivmartyrer: Normerna för vetenskaplig skicklighet i svensk historieforskning 1900–1945*, 2010

45. Håkan Lättman, *Studies on spatial and temporal distributions of epiphytic lichens*, 2010

46. Alia Jaensson, *Pheromonal mediated behaviour and endocrine response in salmonids: The impact of cypermethrin, copper, and glyphosate*, 2010

47. Michael Wigerius, *Roles of mammalian Scribble in polarity signaling, virus offense and cell-fate determination*, 2010

48. Anna Hedtjärn Wester, *Män i kostym: Prinsar, konstnärer och tegelbärare vid sekelskiftet 1900*, 2010

49. Magnus Linnarsson, *Postgång på växlande villkor: Det svenska postväsendets organisation under stormaktstiden*, 2010

50. Barbara Kunz, *Kind words, cruise missiles and everything in between: A neoclassical realist study of the use of power resources in U.S. policies towards Poland, Ukraine and Belarus 1989–2008*, 2010

51. Anders Bartonek, *Philosophie im Konjunktiv: Nichtidentität als Ort der Möglichkeit des Utopischen in der negativen Dialektik Theodor W. Adornos*, 2010

52. Carl Cederberg, *Resaying the Human: Levinas Beyond Humanism and Antihumanism*, 2010

53. Johanna Ringarp, *Professionens problematik: Lärarkårens kommunalisering och välfärdsstatens förvandling*, 2011

54. Sofi Gerber, *Öst är Väst men Väst är bäst: Östtysk identitetsformering i det förenade Tyskland*, 2011

55. Susanna Sjödin Lindenskoug, *Manlighetens bortre gräns: Tidelagsrättegångar i Livland åren 1685–1709*, 2011

56. Dominika Polanska, *The emergence of enclaves of wealth and poverty: A sociological study of residential differentiation in post-communist Poland*, 2011

57. Christina Douglas, *Kärlek per korrespondens: Två förlovade par under andra hälften av 1800-talet*, 2011

58. Fred Saunders, *The Politics of People–Not just Mangroves and Monkeys: A study of the theory and practice of community-based management of natural resources in Zanzibar*, 2011

59. Anna Rosengren, *Åldrandet och språket: En språkhistorisk analys av hög ålder och åldrande i Sverige cirka 1875–1975*, 2011

60. Emelie Lilliefeldt, *European Party Politics and Gender: Configuring Gender-Balanced Parliamentary Presence*, 2011

61. Ola Svenonius, *Sensitising Urban Transport Security: Surveillance and Policing in Berlin, Stockholm, and Warsaw*, 2011

62. Andreas Johansson, *Dissenting Democrats: Nation and Democracy in the Republic of Moldova*, 2011

63. Wessam Melik, *Molecular characterization of the Tick-borne encephalitis virus: Environments and replication*, 2012

64. Steffen Werther, *SS-Vision und Grenzland-Realität: Vom Umgang dänischer und „volksdeutscher" Nationalsozialisten in Sønderjylland mit der „großgermanischen" Ideologie der SS*, 2012

65. Peter Jakobsson, *Öppenhetsindustrin*, 2012

66. Kristin Ilves, *Seaward Landward: Investigations on the archaeological source value of the landing site category in the Baltic Sea region*, 2012

67. Anne Kaun, *Civic Experiences and Public Connection: Media and Young People in Estonia*, 2012

68. Anna Tessmann, *On the Good Faith: A Fourfold Discursive Construction of Zoroastripanism in Contemporary Russia*, 2012

69. Jonas Lindström, *Drömmen om den nya staden: stadsförnyelse i det postsovjetisk Riga*, 2012

70. Maria Wolrath Söderberg, *Topos som meningsskapare: retorikens topiska perspektiv på tänkande och lärande genom argumentation*, 2012

71. Linus Andersson, *Alternativ television: former av kritik i konstnärlig TV-produktion*, 2012

72. Håkan Lättman, *Studies on spatial and temporal distributions of epiphytic lichens*, 2012

73. Fredrik Stiernstedt, Mediearbete i mediehuset: produktion i förändring på MTG-radio, 2013

74. Jessica Moberg, *Piety, Intimacy and Mobility: A Case Study of Charismatic Christianity in Present-day Stockholm*, 2013

75. Elisabeth Hemby, *Historiemåleri och bilder av vardag: Tatjana Nazarenkos konstnärskap i 1970-talets Sovjet*, 2013

76. Tanya Jukkala, *Suicide in Russia: A macro-sociological study*, 2013

77. Maria Nyman, *Resandets gränser: svenska resenärers skildringar av Ryssland under 1700-talet*, 2013

78. Beate Feldmann Eellend, *Visionära planer och vardagliga praktiker: postmilitära landskap i Östersjöområdet*, 2013

79. Emma Lind, *Genetic response to pollution in sticklebacks: natural selection in the wild*, 2013

80. Anne Ross Solberg, *The Mahdi wears Armani: An analysis of the Harun Yahya enterprise*, 2013

81. Nikolay Zakharov, *Attaining Whiteness: A Sociological Study of Race and Racialization in Russia*, 2013

82. Anna Kharkina, *From Kinship to Global Brand: the Discourse on Culture in Nordic Cooperation after World War II*, 2013

83. Florence Fröhlig, *A painful legacy of World War II: Nazi forced enlistment: Alsatian/Mosellan Prisoners of war and the Soviet Prison Camp of Tambov*, 2013

84. Oskar Henriksson, *Genetic connectivity of fish in the Western Indian Ocean*, 2013

85. Hans Geir Aasmundsen, *Pentecostalism, Globalisation and Society in Contemporary Argentina*, 2013

86. Anna McWilliams, *An Archaeology of the Iron Curtain: Material and Metaphor*, 2013

87. Anna Danielsson, *On the power of informal economies and the informal economies of power: rethinking informality, resilience and violence in Kosovo*, 2014

88. Carina Guyard, *Kommunikationsarbete på distans*, 2014

89. Sofia Norling, *Mot "väst": om vetenskap, politik och transformation i Polen 1989–2011*, 2014

90. Markus Huss, *Motståndets akustik: språk och (o)ljud hos Peter Weiss 1946–1960*, 2014

91. Ann-Christin Randahl, *Strategiska skribenter: skrivprocesser i fysik och svenska*, 2014

92. Péter Balogh, *Perpetual borders: German-Polish cross-border contacts in the Szczecin area*, 2014

93. Erika Lundell, *Förkroppsligad fiktion och fiktionaliserade kroppar: levande rollspel i Östersjöregionen*, 2014

94. Henriette Cederlöf, *Alien Places in Late Soviet Science Fiction: The "Unexpected Encounters" of Arkady and Boris Strugatsky as Novels and Films*, 2014

95. Niklas Eriksson, *Urbanism Under Sail: An archaeology of fluit ships in early modern everyday life*, 2014

96. Signe Opermann, *Generational Use of News Media in Estonia: Media Access, Spatial Orientations and Discursive Characteristics of the News Media*, 2014

97. Liudmila Voronova, *Gendering in political journalism: A comparative study of Russia and Sweden*, 2014

98. Ekaterina Kalinina, *Mediated Post-Soviet Nostalgia*, 2014

99. Anders E. B. Blomqvist, *Economic Natonalizing in the Ethnic Borderlands of Hungary and Romania: Inclusion, Exclusion and Annihilation in Szatmár/Satu-Mare, 1867–1944*, 2014

100. Ann-Judith Rabenschlag, *Völkerfreundschaft nach Bedarf: Ausländische Arbeitskräfte in der Wahrnehmung von Staat und Bevölkerung der DDR*, 2014

101. Yuliya Yurchuck, *Ukrainian Nationalists and the Ukrainian Insurgent Army in Post-Soviet Ukraine*, 2014

102. Hanna Sofia Rehnberg, *Organisationer berättar: narrativitet som resurs i strategisk kommunikation*, 2014

103. Jaakko Turunen, *Semiotics of Politics: Dialogicality of Parliamentary Talk*, 2015

104. Iveta Jurkane-Hobein, *I Imagine You Here Now: Relationship Maintenance Strategies in Long-Distance Intimate Relationships*, 2015

105. Katharina Wesolowski, *Maybe baby? Reproductive behaviour, fertility intentions, and family policies in post-communist countries, with a special focus on Ukraine*, 2015

106. Ann af Burén, *Living Simultaneity: On religion among semi-secular Swedes*, 2015

107. Larissa Mickwitz, *En reformerad lärare: konstruktionen av en professionell och betygssättande lärare i skolpolitik och skolpraktik*, 2015

108. Daniel Wojahn, *Språkaktivism: diskussioner om feministiska språkförändringar i Sverige från 1960-talet till 2015*, 2015

109. Hélène Edberg, *Kreativt skrivande för kritiskt tänkande: en fallstudie av studenters arbete med kritisk metareflektion*, 2015

110. Kristina Volkova, *Fishy Behavior: Persistent effects of early-life exposure to 17α-ethinylestradiol*, 2015

111. Björn Sjöstrand, *Att tänka det tekniska: en studie i Derridas teknikfilosofi*, 2015

112. Håkan Forsberg, *Kampen om eleverna: gymnasiefältet och skolmarknadens framväxt i Stockholm, 1987–2011*, 2015

113. Johan Stake, *Essays on quality evaluation and bidding behavior in public procurement auctions*, 2015

114. Martin Gunnarson, *Please Be Patient: A Cultural Phenomenological Study of Haemodialysis and Kidney Transplantation Care*, 2016

115. Nasim Reyhanian Caspillo, *Studies of alterations in behavior and fertility in ethinyl estradiol-exposed zebrafish and search for related biomarkers*, 2016

116. Pernilla Andersson, *The Responsible Business Person: Studies of Business Education for Sustainability*, 2016

117. Kim Silow Kallenberg, *Gränsland: svensk ungdomsvård mellan vård och straff*, 2016

118. Sari Vuorenpää, *Literacitet genom interaction*, 2016

119. Francesco Zavatti, *Writing History in a Propaganda Institute: Political Power and Network Dynamics in Communist Romania*, 2016

120. Cecilia Annell, *Begärets politiska potential: Feministiska motståndsstrategier i Elin Wägners 'Pennskaftet', Gabriele Reuters 'Aus guter Familie', Hilma Angered-Strandbergs 'Lydia Vik' och Grete Meisel-Hess 'Die Intellektuellen'*, 2016

121. Marco Nase, *Academics and Politics: Northern European Area Studies at Greifswald University, 1917–1992*, 2016

122. Jenni Rinne, *Searching for Authentic Living Through Native Faith–The Maausk movement in Estonia*, 2016

123. Petra Werner, *Ett medialt museum: lärandets estetik i svensk television 1956–1969*, 2016

124. Ramona Rat, *Un-common Sociality: Thinking sociality with Levinas*, 2016

125. Petter Thureborn, *Microbial ecosystem functions along the steep oxygen gradient of the Landsort Deep, Baltic Sea*, 2016

126. Kajsa-Stina Benulic, *A Beef with Meat Media and audience framings of environmentally unsustainable production and consumption*, 2016

127. Naveed Asghar, *Ticks and Tick-borne Encephalitis Virus–From nature to infection*, 2016

128. Linn Rabe, *Participation and legitimacy: Actor involvement for nature conservation*, 2017

129. Maryam Adjam, *Minnesspår: hågkomstens rum och rörelse i skuggan av en flykt*, 2017

130. Kim West, *The Exhibitionary Complex: Exhibition, Apparatus and Media from Kulturhuset to the Centre Pompidou, 1963–1977*, 2017

131. Ekaterina Tarasova, *Anti-nuclear Movements in Discursive and Political Contexts: Between expert voices and local protests*, 2017

132. Sanja Obrenović Johansson, *Från kombifeminism till rörelse: Kvinnlig serbisk organisering i förändring*, 2017

133. Michał Salamonik, *In Their Majesties' Service: The Career of Francesco De Gratta (1613–1676) as a Royal Servant and Trader in Gdańsk*, 2017

134. Jenny Ingridsdotter, *The Promises of the Free World: Postsocialist Experience in Argentina and the Making of Migrants, Race, and Coloniality*, 2017

135. Julia Malitska, *Negotiating Imperial Rule: Colonists and Marriage in the Nineteenth century Black Sea Steppe*, 2017

136. Natalya Yakusheva, *Parks, Policies and People: Nature Conservation Governance in Post-Socialist EU Countries*, 2017

137. Martin Kellner, *Selective Serotonin Re-uptake Inhibitors in the Environment: Effects of Citalopram on Fish Behaviour*, 2017

138. Krystof Kasprzak, *Vara–Framträdande–Värld: Fenomenets negativitet hos Martin Heidegger, Jan Patočka och Eugen Fink*, 2017

139. Alberto Frigo, *Life-stowing from a Digital Media Perspective: Past, Present and Future*, 2017

140. Maarja Saar, *The Answers You Seek Will Never Be Found At Home: Reflexivity, biographical narratives and lifestyle migration among highly-skilled Estonians*, 2017

141. Anh Mai, *Organizing for Efficiency: Essay on merger policies, independence of authorities, and technology diffusion*, 2017

142. Gustav Strandberg, *Politikens omskakning: Negativitet, samexistens och frihet i Jan Patočkas tänkande*, 2017

143. Lovisa Andén, *Litteratur och erfarenhet i Merleau-Pontys läsning av Proust, Valéry och Stendhal*, 2017

144. Fredrik Bertilsson, *Frihetstida policyskapande: uppfostringskommissionen och de akademiska konstitutionerna 1738–1766*, 2017

145. Börjeson, Natasja, *Toxic Textiles–towards responsibility in complex supply chains*, 2017

146. Julia Velkova, *Media Technologies in the Making–User-Driven Software and Infrastructures for computer Graphics Production*, 2017

147. Karin Jonsson, *Fångna i begreppen? Revolution, tid och politik i svensk socialistisk press 1917–1924*, 2017

148. Josefine Larsson, *Genetic Aspects of Environmental Disturbances in Marine Ecosystems–Studies of the Blue Mussel in the Baltic Sea*, 2017

149. Roman Horbyk, *Mediated Europes–Discourse and Power in Ukraine, Russia and Poland during Euromaidan*, 2017

150. Nadezda Petrusenko, *Creating the Revolutionary Heroines: The Case of Female Terrorists of the PSR (Russia, Beginning of the 20th Century)*, 2017

151. Rahel Kuflu, *Bröder emellan: Identitetsformering i det koloniserade Eritrea*, 2018

152. Karin Edberg, *Energilandskap i förändring: Inramningar av kontroversiella lokaliseringar på norra Gotland*, 2018

153. Rebecka Thor, *Beyond the Witness: Holocaust Representation and the Testimony of Images–Three films by Yael Hersonski, Harun Farocki, and Eyal Sivan*, 2018

154. Maria Lönn, *Bruten vithet: Om den ryska femininitetens sinnliga och temporala villkor*, 2018

155. Tove Porseryd, *Endocrine Disruption in Fish: Effects of 17α-ethinylestradiol exposure on non-reproductive behavior, fertility and brain and testis transcriptome*, 2018

156. Marcel Mangold, *Securing the working democracy: Inventive arrangements to guarantee circulation and the emergence of democracy policy*, 2018

157. Matilda Tudor, *Desire Lines: Towards a Queer Digital Media Phenomenology*, 2018

158. Martin Andersson, *Migration i 1600-talets Sverige: Älvsborgs lösen 1613–1618*, 2018

159. Johanna Pettersson, *What's in a Line? Making Sovereignty through Border Policy*, 2018

160. Irina Seits, *Architectures of Life-Building in the Twentieth Century: Russia, Germany, Sweden*, 2018

161. Alexander Stagnell, *The Ambassador's Letter: On the Less Than Nothing of Diplomacy*, 2019

162. Mari Zetterqvist Blokhuis, *Interaction Between Rider, Horse and Equestrian Trainer– A Challenging Puzzle*, 2019

163. Robin Samuelsson, *Play, Culture and Learning: Studies of Second-Language and Conceptual Development in Swedish Preschools*, 2019

164. Ralph Tafon, *Analyzing the "Dark Side" of Marine Spatial Planning–A study of domination, empowerment and freedom (or power in, of and on planning) through theories of discourse and power*, 2019

165. Ingela Visuri, *Varieties of Supernatural Experience: The case of high-functioning autism*, 2019

166. Mathilde Rehnlund, *Getting the transport right–for what? What transport policy can tell us about the construction of sustainability*, 2019

167. Oscar Törnqvist, *Röster från ingenmansland: En identitetsarkeologi i ett maritimt mellanrum*, 2019

168. Elise Remling, *Adaptation, now? Exploring the Politics of Climate Adaptation through Post-structuralist Discourse Theory*, 2019

169. Eva Karlberg, *Organizing the Voice of Women: A study of the Polish and Swedish women's movements' adaptation to international structures*, 2019

170. Maria Pröckl, *Tyngd, sväng och empatisk timing–förskollärares kroppsliga kunskaper*, 2020

171. Adrià Alcoverro, *The University and the Demand for Knowledge-based Growth The hegemonic struggle for the future of Higher Education Institutions in Finland and Estonia*, 2020

172. Ingrid Forsler, *Enabling Media: Infrastructures, imaginaries and cultural techniques in Swedish and Estonian visual arts education*, 2020

173. Johan Sehlberg, *Of Affliction: The Experience of Thought in Gilles Deleuze by way of Marcel Proust*, 2020

174. Renat Bekkin, *People of reliable loyalty…: Muftiates and the State in Modern Russia*, 2020

175. Olena Podolian, *The Challenge of 'Stateness' in Estonia and Ukraine: The international dimension a quarter of a century into independence*, 2020

176. Patrick Seniuk, *Encountering Depression In-Depth: An existential-phenomenological approach to selfhood, depression, and psychiatric practice*, 2020

177. Vasileios Petrogiannis, *European Mobility and Spatial Belongings: Greek and Latvian migrants in Sweden*, 2020

178. Lena Norbäck Ivarsson, *Tracing environmental change and human impact as recorded in sediments from coastal areas of the northwestern Baltic Proper*, 2020

179. Sara Persson, *Corporate Hegemony through Sustainability–A study of sustainability standards and CSR practices as tools to demobilise community resistance in the Albanian oil industry*, 2020

180. Juliana Porsani, *Livelihood Implications of Large-Scale Land Concessions in Mozambique: A case of family farmers' endurance*, 2020

181. Anders Backlund, *Isolating the Radical Right–Coalition Formation and Policy Adaptation in Sweden*, 2020

182. Nina Carlsson, *One Nation, One Language? National minority and Indigenous recognition in the politics of immigrant integration*, 2021

183. Erik Gråd, Nudges, *Prosocial Preferences & Behavior: Essays in Behavioral Economics*, 2021

184. Anna Enström, *Sinnesstämning, skratt och hypokondri: Om estetisk erfarenhet i Kants tredje Kritik*, 2021

185. Michelle Rydback, *Healthcare Service Marketing in Medical Tourism–An Emerging Market Study*, 2021

186. Fredrik Jahnke, *Toleransens altare och undvikandets hänsynsfullhet–Religion och meningsskapande bland svenska grundskoleelever*, 2021

187. Benny Berggren Newton, *Business Basics–A Grounded Theory for Managing Ethical Behavior in Sales Organizations*, 2021

188. Gabriel Itkes-Sznap, *Nollpunkten. Precisionens betydelse hos Witold Gombrowicz, Inger Christensen och Herta Müller*, 2021

189. Oscar Svanelid Medina, *Att forma tillvaron: konstruktivism som konstnärligt yrkesarbete hos Geraldo de Barros, Lygia Pape och Lygia Clark*, 2021

190. Anna-Karin Selberg, *Politics and Truth: Heidegger, Arendt and The Modern Political Lie*, 2021

191. Camilla Larsson, *Framträdanden: Performativitetsteoretiska tolkningar av Tadeusz Kantors konstnärskap*, 2021

192. Raili Uibo, *"And I don't know who we really are to each other": Queers doing close relationships in Estonia*, 2021

193. Ignė Stalmokaitė, *New Tides in Shipping: Studying incumbent firms in maritime energy transitions*, 2021

194. Mani Shutzberg, *Tricks of the Medical Trade: Cunning in the Age of Bureaucratic Austerity*, 2021

195. Patrik Höglund, *Skeppssamhället: Rang, roller och status på örlogsskepp under 1600-talet*, 2021

196. Philipp Seuferling, *Media and the refugee camp: The historical making of space, time, and politics in the modern refugee regime*, 2021

197. Johan Sandén, *Närbyråkrater och digitaliseringar: Hur lärares arbete formas av tidsstrukturer*, 2021

198. Ulrika Nemeth, *Det kritiska uppdraget: Diskurser och praktiker i gymnasieskolans svenskundervisning*, 2021

199. Helena Löfgren, *Det legitima ägandet: Politiska konstruktioner av allmännyttans privatisering i Stockholms stad 1990–2015*, 2021

200. Vasileios Kitsos, *Urban policies for a contemporary periphery: Insights from eastern Russia*, 2022

201. Jenny Gustafsson, *Drömmen om en gränslös fred: Världsmedborgarrörelsens reaktopi, 1949–1968*, 2022

202. Oscar von Seth, *Outsiders and Others: Queer Friendships in Novels by Hermann Hesse*, 2022

203. Kristin Halverson, *Tools of the Trade: Medical Devices and Practice in Sweden and Denmark, 1855–1897*, 2022

204. Henrik Ohlsson, *Facing Nature–Cultivating Experience in the Nature Connection Movement*, 2022